The Human Use of Animals

THE HUMAN USE
OF ANIMALS

Case Studies in Ethical Choice

F. BARBARA ORLANS, PhD
Senior Research Fellow
Kennedy Institute of Ethics
Georgetown University

TOM L. BEAUCHAMP, PhD
Professor, Department of Philosophy,
and Senior Research Scholar
Kennedy Institute of Ethics
Georgetown University

REBECCA DRESSER, J.D.
The John Deaver Drinko-Baker and Hostetler Professor of Law,
and Professor, Center for Biomedical Ethics, School of Medicine
Case Western Reserve University

DAVID B. MORTON, BVSc, PhD, MRCVS
Professor, Department of Biomedical Science and Ethics
The Medical School, University of Birmingham, England

JOHN P. GLUCK, PhD
Professor, Department of Psychology
University of New Mexico

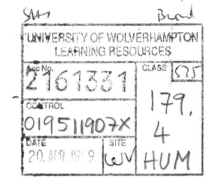
New York   Oxford
OXFORD UNIVERSITY PRESS
1998

Oxford University Press

Oxford   New York
Athens   Auckland   Bangkok   Bogota   Bombay
Buenos Aires   Calcutta   Cape Town   Dar es Salaam
Delhi   Florence   Hong Kong   Istanbul   Karachi
Kuala Lumpur   Madras   Madrid   Melbourne
Mexico City   Nairobi   Paris   Singapore
Taipei   Tokyo   Toronto   Warsaw

and associated companies in
Berlin   Ibadan

Library of Congress Cataloging-in-Publication Data
The human use of animals : case studies in ethical choice /
F. Barbara Orlans . . . [et al.].
p.   cm.   Includes bibliographical references and index.
ISBN 0-19-511907-X — ISBN 0-19-511908-8 (pbk.)
1. Animal experimentation—Moral and ethical aspects—Case studies.
2. Animal welfare—Moral and ethical aspects—Case studies.
I. Orlans, F. Barbara.
HV4915.H85   1997   179'.4—dc21   97-8594

9 8 7 6 5 4 3 2 1

Printed in the United States of America
on acid-free paper

Preface

This book is the first volume of case studies devoted to the ethical issues of human interactions with animals. The sixteen cases that follow the introduction cover biomedical research, cosmetic safety testing, behavioral research, wildlife research, educational teaching, food and farming, companion animals, and religious rites. Each case develops the facts of the narrative together with an analysis of the ethical issues. The number of cases dealing with the use of animals in various types of research reflects what the authors believe to be the high level of public interest in this area.

The introduction provides an overview of the central moral issues present in many of the later cases. It discusses differing views about ethics and professional ethics, the moral standing of animals, animal minds, the relevance of evolutionary biology, committee review of research protocols, the justification of animal research and possible alternatives, types of moral philosophy, and case study analysis as a method of study in ethics. Cross-references between the introduction and the individual case studies are provided for the guidance of readers.

Each of the five authors to this book comes from a different disciplinary background: physiology, philosophy, law, veterinary medicine, and psychology. The authors are also almost evenly split in national origins: three from the United States and two from the United Kingdom. Each author has read, commented on, and redrafted the work of the other authors in order to ensure a coherent work that reflects the appropriate disciplinary points of view.

Some of these cases have benefited from spirited discussions of early drafts at four intensive courses sponsored by the Kennedy Institute of Ethics at Georgetown University and one at the Poynter Center, Indiana University, Bloomington. The courses are part of an ongoing summer program for college faculty and students. They are intended to stimulate interest in teaching about animal ethics and to help develop new instructional materials.

Preparation of this manuscript was funded through a grant (SBE 91–21191) from The National Science Foundation, Ethics and Values Studies Program, to Barbara Orlans and Tom Beauchamp. Other financial support has been generously provided by The Kinnoull Foundation. We wish to thank Ralph B. Dell, Michael DeVita, and Peter Flanagan for some helpful comments, and Julia Fentem for supplying us with some valuable information. For comments that helped us frame some of the theoretical parts of chapter 1, we wish to thank Carl Cohen, David DeGrazia, Raymond Frey, Hugh LaFollette, and Tom Regan. In preparing this edition we have been ably assisted in bibliographical research and editorial matters by Emily Wilson and Moheba Hanif.

Washington, D.C.   F. B. O.
June 1997   T. L. B.
                                                      R. D.
                                                 D. B. M.
                                                 J. P. G.

Contents

V WILDLIFE RESEARCH

VI EDUCATION

VII   FOOD AND FARMING

VIII   COMPANION ANIMALS

IX RELIGIOUS RITES

I

INTRODUCTION

1

MORAL ISSUES ABOUT ANIMALS

In a famous public dispute between Juan Ginés de Sepúlveda and Bartolomé de Las Casas in 1550 and 1551, questions about the lawfulness of the Spanish conquest of American Indians were formally debated. Sepúlveda argued that the Indians were idolatrous, sinful, and less than fully human. Las Casas regarded the conquests as violations of natural justice, viewed the Indians as fully human, and saw love and kindness as the only legitimate forces for dealing with them. As the debate wore on, it became ever clearer that it was centrally about whether the Indians were human or subhuman and about whether Europeans could throw off all ordinary restraints of justice and humanity in their interactions with the Indians.[1]

Many believe that today's debates about human-animal interactions are fundamentally similar: The issues are about whether the nonhuman nature of other animals is morally relevant, and if it is relevant, what humanity and justice permit us to do with animals. But even this way of framing the questions is subject to the most spirited controversy. Many people think that questions of humanity and justice have nothing to do with deciding the permissibility of our treatment of animals. The cases in this book are intended as a source of reflection on these and many other questions about human-nonhuman interactions. The cases, all recent, have emerged from areas of public policy and professional practice in the use and treatment of animals.

The goal of this introduction is to provide a framework for moral thinking about human-nonhuman relations. In the first section, a few problems about the nature of morality, professional morality, and the moral community are discussed. In the second and third sections some psychological and biological questions about animal minds and Darwinian theory receive attention. In the fourth section, issues about the moral standing of animals are examined. Then, in the next section, some relevant types of systematic moral philosophy are considered, followed by two sections that treat issues in the justification of our treatment of animals and our evaluation of research involving animals. Finally, there is a section, that discusses methods of using case studies.

MORALITY AND THE MORAL COMMUNITY

The term *morality* refers to a body of learnable standards of right and wrong conduct so widely shared in society that they form a secure (although incomplete) communal consensus. Morality comprehends many standards of conduct that we refer to as "moral rules" and "human rights." Like natural languages and political constitutions, core parts of morality exist before we become instructed in its relevant rules and regulations. As we develop and mature, we learn moral responsibilities together with other social obligations, such as legal obligations. Eventually we learn to distinguish general social rules of law and morals from rules binding only members of special groups, such as the members of a profession. That is, we learn to distinguish general *social morality* from *professional morality*.

Social Morality

The morality shared by all morally serious persons in all societies is not *a morality*; it is simply morality, or what is sometimes called "the common morality." This morality is universal insofar as it contains fundamental ethical precepts found wherever morality is found. In recent years, the favored category has been universal human rights,[2] but parts of morality are also found in standards of obligation and virtue. This body of norms constituting our shared social morality will here be called "morality in the *narrow* sense." There are no distinctive moralities in this narrow sense, only morality.

However, there are distinctive moralities in a *broad* sense of the word. Morality in this broad sense recognizes divergent moral norms and positions that spring from particular cultural, philosophical, religious, and other sources. One reason ethical norms pertaining to animals vary from society to society, and even from person to person, is that permissible treatment of animals falls in the realm of morality in the broad sense. Morality in the narrow sense has nothing to say specifically about animals, although it does supply the core concepts and principles on the basis of which we can reflect on appropriate treatment of animals.

Many attempts have been made in the history of philosophy, political theory, and law to formulate the precepts of morality in the narrow sense in order to show that these precepts do not depend, as do customs and positive law, on local codifications. These controversies cannot be considered here, but some examples of universal morality deserve mention. The following are universal precepts (stated in the form of obligations) that all morally serious persons in all moral traditions accept:

1. Tell the truth.
2. Respect the privacy of others.
3. Protect confidential information.
4. Obtain consent before invading another person's body.
5. Do not kill.
6. Do not cause pain.
7. Do not incapacitate.
8. Do not deprive of goods.
9. Protect and defend the rights of others.
10. Prevent harm from occurring to others.

All rules on this list can in some circumstances be validly overridden by rules with which they contingently conflict. For example, in order to protect the rights of one person, a person might have to disclose confidential information about another person. Still to be decided, of course, is how morality helps us understand the ethics of human interactions with animals, especially our moral obligations to animals and any correlative rights that animals might have.

Professional Morality

But first we need to examine professional obligations—including the obligations of professionals such as veterinarians whose lives are often devoted to animal welfare. Just as there is a general common morality across society, with shared principles and rules, so most professions contain, at least implicitly, a professional morality with widely shared standards of behavior. In professional contexts some measure of morality is transmitted informally, but formal instruction and attempts at the codification of professional morality have increased in recent years. These efforts have addressed many problems of ethics in those professions engaged in research involving animal subjects and in regulations that establish professional responsibility—most prominently in codes of professional ethics, codes of research ethics, and government-sponsored reports and rules.

Particular codes written for groups such as veterinarians, biologists, physicians, and psychologists are sometimes defended by appeal to general norms in the common morality. Usually, however, professional codes are attempts to discover and develop an inchoate morality that is accepted in the profession itself and to expand the commitments of that morality. A professional code emphasizes these role obligations, which may be obligations either to animals or to other humans. (For examples, see the cases in chapter 13, on veal crates, and chapter 15, on practices of tail docking.)

Sometimes these codes *develop* an inchoate professional morality, as has occurred in fields that use animals as research subjects. Research is not our only use of animals, but it is a major use, and it occurs in fields that have recognized a need for codes of conduct and conformity to federal regulations. The following types of responsibility are often cited in the fields on which we will concentrate in this book:

Responsibilities to Animals
Avoidance of Unnecessary Pain, Deprivation, and Suffering
Welfare Protection by Improving the Environment
Searching for Alternatives to the Use of Animals
Setting Policies and Performing Professional Review

Responsibilities to Society
Avoidance of Unnecessary Harm-Causing Activities
Disclosure of Risks to Health and the Environment
Disclosure of Procedures Involving Animals
Maintaining Public Trust

Responsibilities to Employers and Funding Sources
Codifying Responsibilities in Formal Codes of Ethics
Protecting Privileged Information
Reassessing Policies, Goals, and Commitments
Adhering to Contracts, Laws, and Professional Standards

Responsibilities to Professional Colleagues
Reporting Data, Methods, Studies, and Results
Reporting Unacceptable Behavior and Conditions
Teaching Responsibilities
Promoting Standards in Codes of Practice

This outline of topics in the professional morality of those responsible for the use, protection, or care of animals should be understood as a representative rather than exhaustive list. No responsibility on this list is absolute, and none takes a ranked precedence over any other.

Morality in the Animal World

We earlier defined *morality* in terms of learnable standards of right and wrong conduct so widely shared in society that they form a secure communal consensus. Many have thought that we can find morality in analogous ways in some parts of the animal world. However, whether good evidence exists of an internal morality displayed by animals is controversial. Some observers believe it is little more than human fantasy to suppose that animals act morally; other observers find close similarities between the behavior of humans and nonhuman animals.[3]

The most difficult question is whether animals have a capacity to make moral *judgments* about members of their social group—for example, when those members are violating fixed expectations of conduct and deserve punishment or some form of rebuke. That animals intentionally reprimand and punish members of their group seems clear, but whether they use moral standards and make judgments is far less certain—and possibly even a deep mystery.

A more frequently heard suggestion is that animals have dispositions to behave morally that are created by evolutionary pressures. For example, the hypothesis of "reciprocal altruism" holds that two or more animals who reciprocally assist one another by acts such as grooming, aiding in distress, and protecting mates gain an evolutionary advantage.[4] Animals who refuse to cooperate in these ways, when it is expected, will cease to be aided and suffer as a result. An extension of this hypothesis is that some animals in cooperative societies help other animals even when they know it is highly unlikely that those helped will ever be in a position to return the favor—a purer altruism that is more distanced from reciprocity.

Charles Darwin, who was conversant with eighteenth-century moral philosophy, seemed to deny that animals make moral judgments, while affirming that they have moral dispositions. For example, he thought that animals do not really make judgments of blame when they are punishing their peers for misbehavior, but do have dispositions of love, affection, and generosity. (See below on "moral sense".) There are still today many controversies about whether animals show sympathy for or compassion toward other animals, exhibit mercy, express gratitude, engage in selfless acts of rescue, and the like.

If one understands morality in terms such as the ten substantive rules listed previously, together with the adoption of an impartial attitude, then it seems unlikely that animals have a morality, or act morally by applying rules. To act lovingly, protectively, and generously is not necessarily (even for humans) to act on general moral principles and is certainly not to act impartially in regard to all affected by the action. Perhaps animals "act morally" in some respects but lack critical dimensions of acting morally in other respects. Or perhaps animals have nothing at all to do with morality? These questions will occupy us at several points in this introduction.

Membership in the Moral Community

Two further and profoundly important questions about morality and animals need to be addressed: Which creatures belong to the moral community? and To which creatures does one owe moral obligations?

It has long been a matter of pervasive belief in the human community that one or two properties account for a creature's membership in the moral community—that is, for being properly an object of moral concern so that a creature's interests have weight in decisions made in regard to the creature. The first property is that of being *human* (or, perhaps, having *personhood*); the second property is that of being *rational*. Does either property, or both together, rightly determine who belongs to the moral community?

This question is particularly important for the cases in this volume, because if animals have no place in the moral community—no moral standing— then it appears that humans owe nothing to animals and can do with animals as they wish. On one account, we owe obligations to the humans who own animals, but not to the animals owned. On this account, if you poison your neighbor's barking dog, you violate a moral obligation that you have not to destroy your neighbor's property, but you do not violate any obligation to the animal. The neighbor is injured by your action; the dog who is killed is not injured. Animals are no different than plants in the neighbor's garden; if you poison them, you have wronged the neighbor only, not the plants.

Many people find this conclusion deeply counterintuitive, and some judge it flatly false and offensive. Others think these questions are difficult to judge because they are at the outer boundaries of proper moral concern (like questions about moral obligations to future generations of humans and obligations to the environment). To sort through these issues requires that we examine several underlying issues about the nature of animals and about their moral standing, if any.

ANIMAL MINDS

A general consensus exists today that many nonhuman species of animals have minds. Little agreement exists, however, about the levels and types of mental activity in these animals or about the ethical significance of their mental activity.

Historical Background

For several figures in the history of philosophy, including Aristotle and Immanuel Kant (see below), animals do not lack minds, but they do lack reason, which is sufficient to exclude them from the moral community. Other philosophers believe that animals do reason. Still other major philosophers have viewed animals as lacking all mental capacity—all feeling and even consciousness. Their views are directly relevant to our present inquiry: If animals are devoid of mind, they are like plants. They are little more than matter in motion, lacking not only moral sensitivity, but mental sensitivity. This view has important representatives in the history of philosophy and science.

Descartes

The most important representative was the French philosopher, physical scientist, and mathematician René Descartes (1596–1650). Descartes was the major figure whose views Darwin later had to confront—and presumably refute. Unlike Darwin, Descartes primarily found dissimilarities between human and nonhuman creatures. He argued that nonhuman creatures lack the capacity to feel pain and do not even have minds in the normal sense. Animals are automata who:

> act naturally and mechanically, like a clock which tells the time better than our judgment does. Doubtless when the swallows come in spring, they operate like clocks. The actions of honeybees are of the same nature, and the discipline of cranes in flight, and of apes in fighting. . . . All [animal motions] originate from the corporeal and mechanical principle.[5]

Descartes also held that the lack of language and abstract reasoning in animals demonstrates a lack of mind.[6] As a consequence, he maintained, humans are absolved of any crime or guilt in killing, eating, and experimenting on animals. These views were accepted by many scientists and philosophers of the seventeenth and eighteenth centuries, but other investigators who used animals at the time took a different approach. They recognized that animals felt pain, but they did not see such pain as a matter of moral concern or as a form of cruelty. After all, if humans had dominion over animals, how could a respectable use such as experimentation violate standards of good stewardship? Descartes and these other thinkers also influenced theologians in need of a theodicy (a theory to vindicate the goodness of God in the face of evil). They had to account for alleged animal suffering; and now they could argue that either there was no suffering or the suffering was a proper exercise of dominion—possibly even a moral obligation. These views were as powerful in England as in France—the two major countries at the time for developments in both science and philosophy.[7]

Hume

A powerful alternative to Descartes was offered a century later by the Scottish philosopher and historian David Hume (1711–1776), who regarded Descartes's views as an example of the excesses of adherence to a dogmatic philosophical theory. Without suggesting the theory of evolution, Hume anticipated some features of later Darwinian thinking about animal minds. He believed that when the terms *understand* and *reason* are used properly, they refer to recognizing on the basis of experience (understanding) and making causal inferences (reasoning). Hume believed that animals can both understand and reason:

> Animals, as well as men, learn many things from experience, and infer, that the same events will always follow from the same causes. By this principle they become acquainted with the more obvious properties of external objects, and gradually, from their birth, treasure up a knowledge of the nature of fire, water, earth, stones, heights, depths, &c. and of the effects, which result from their operation. The ignorance and inexperience of the young are here plainly distinguishable from the cunning and sagacity of the old, who have learned, by long observation, to avoid what hurt them, and to pursue what gave ease or pleasure. . . .
>
> In all these cases, . . . the animal infers some fact beyond what immediately strikes his senses; and this inference [of reason] is altogether founded on past experience.[8]

Hume attributed rationality, or at least the capacity to reason, to some animals, on grounds that these animals are significantly *like humans* in the principles of their nature, their patterns of learning, and their powers of inference. Hume cited, as evidence of thought, the adaptivity of many animals in obtaining food, their ingenious strategies, and their use of tools.

But he attributed more to animals as well. In *A Treatise of Human Nature,* he included whole sections on not only *reason* in animals but also *love* in animals and *pride* in animals.[9] He discussed sympathy and cooperative schemes in the animal world. In each case, he found the capacities of nonhuman animals analogous to human capacities. He argued that a philosophy with a proper breadth to grasp understanding and other mental powers would have to explain animal cognitive skills as well as parallel human skills. Likewise, we would have to explain the "evident" continuities between the human and the animal, as well as the discontinuities, such as the nonhuman animals' apparent lack of a sense of virtue and vice.

Contemporary Issues

Close observers of animal behavior today generally agree with Hume that many animals have capacities to understand and have developed complicated, sometimes elaborate forms of social interaction and communication (whether these qualify as "linguistic" or not). Intelligence and adaptation in animal behavior, as explored by ethologists and psychologists, is often inexplicable without acknowledging that animals exhibit understanding, intention, thought, imaginativeness, and various forms of communication. Certain facts of *mental* life in other creatures do not seem any more in doubt than facts about *physical* processes in these creatures. That a dog feels sick or that a bear is angry is often not more doubtful than that a child is sick or a spouse angry. We may not know the nuanced character of these mental states in others, but we often know when we have correctly attributed mental states such as pain to animals.

Donald Griffin has argued in his two influential books, *Animal Thinking* and *Animal Minds*,[10] that many complex actions, often novel in the circumstances, suggest adaptive and creative forms of judgment. Typical examples are innovative forms of defense, use of tools, adaptation to sudden and threatening changes in an environment, intentional movements and sounds to communicate or convey feelings, creative forms of play, constructing shelters and prey-catching devices, and the like. Different scientists give different explanations for these behaviors—for example, in terms of contingencies of reinforcement or in terms of cognitive abilities—but any type of explanation offered to account for an animal's behavior can also be invoked to explain parallel forms of human behavior.

If one attributes capacities such as intention, understanding, emotion, choice, belief, and thought to animals, then they are credited with properties relevantly similar to human capacities, and therefore, some argue, they merit whatever moral protections humans enjoy by virtue of having the same properties.[11] Unfortunately, we understand very little about the inner lives of animals, or even about how to connect many forms of observable behavior with other forms of behavior. We have difficulty understanding a concept like *intention* in animals because of the gaps involved in the inference from human to mental thought. Forms of communication are similarly difficult to grasp. We understand little in many cases about how animal noises (for example, those of killer whales) relate to animal behavior, or about why these noises occur under one set of conditions, but not under others. It is difficult to peer into the mental life of another species, even one as close to us in the evolutionary scheme as other primates.[12]

Neither evolutionary descent nor the physical and functional organization of an animal system (the conditions responsible for its having a mental life) gives us the depth of insight we would like to have in understanding the animal's mental states. Nor does observation of behavior yield adequate understanding. Even when we have as full an explanation as can be obtained under current scientific standards, we still have to decide about an animal, as about a brain-damaged human, whether the individual really has certain attributed mental states, really acts intentionally, and the like—or is just acting *as if* he or she had such states.

The behavioral and life sciences together with the philosophy of mind shed only limited light on animal mental states—such as alleged depression or happiness—and on questions of whether animals act intentionally by planning to trap their prey, build nests, protect their young, and the like. (Several cases below deal with this issue. See especially chapter 9, "Monkeys Without Mothers.") There remain many questions about what we are entitled to infer based on our limited knowledge about physiology and behavior, as well as how this knowledge would affect our thinking about ethics.[13]

DARWIN AND EVOLUTIONARY THEORY

In the circumstance of radical disagreement among great philosophers such as Descartes and Hume, Darwin stepped forth with a theory that was as philosophical as scientific, and as revolutionary as any ever presented in the history of science. In *The Descent of Man,* he catalogued many similarities in mental ability between humans and apes.[14] He observed, "It is a significant fact, that the more the habits of any particular animal are studied by a naturalist, the more he ascribes to *reason* and the less to *unlearnt instincts.*"[15]

We already have seen that prior to Darwin many biologists and philosophers argued that despite the anatomical similarities between humans and apes, humans are distinguished by the possession of *reason, speech,* and *moral sensibility.* Darwin thought, by contrast, that there is ample empirical evidence that animals have various powers of deliberation and decision making, excellent memories, imagination, and the like.

Darwin criticized the hypothesis that major cognitive differences separate apes and humans in the respects proposed by previous thinkers such as Descartes.[16] The ultimate import of his theory is that it is not only complex biological structures and functions that are shared in the evolutionary struggle, but psychological abilities and traits as well. From enzymes and proteins to memory and inference, remarkable continuities are present across the species. Any animal able to use mental abilities to choose between alternative forms of behavior is likely to be advantaged in the evolutionary process. It would be odd, Darwin suggested, if only humans had achieved any measure of this massive evolutionary advantage. Darwin's approach was to reject an account that hypothesized large gaps between the species and to adopt instead a continuity model.

Degrees of Mental Power

Darwin argued that despite "enormous differences" in *degree* of "mental power" between humans and apes, no fundamental difference exists in *kind* between humans and many forms of animal life. He believes that the apes are highly intelligent, similar to humans in emotional responses such as terror, rage, shame, and maternal affection; similar in character traits such as courage and timidity; and even similar in the use of systems of communication that approximate human language and human conceptual abstraction. Moreover, Darwin argues, a greater gap exists in the intelligence level of, for example, apes and marine life than between apes and humans. What we find in nature are "numberless gradations" in mental power, with apes and humans on the high end. In a revealing sentence Darwin maintained, "It is a pure assumption to assert that the mental act is not essentially of the same nature in the animal as in the man." (See the analysis of geese in the work of Konrad Lorenz mentioned in the case of force-feeding geese.)

Darwin challenged, modestly anyway, the above-mentioned views about self-consciousness and higher-level abilities. He wrote in an 1872 work on the emotions in animals:

> It may be freely admitted that no animal is self-conscious, if by this term it is implied, that he reflects on such points, as whence he comes or whither he will go, or what is life and death, and so forth. But how can we feel sure that an old dog with an excellent memory and some power of imagination, as shewn by his dreams, never reflects on his past pleasures or pains in the chase? And this would be *a form* of self-consciousness.[17]

Language

Darwin has some particularly interesting, though underdeveloped views about language. He takes it as proven empirically that animals communicate through sounds and gestures. He says "the habitual use of articulate language [verbal speech] is peculiar to man, but he uses, in common with the lower animals, inarticulate cries to express his meaning, aided by gestures and the movements of the muscles of the face." Darwin goes on to note that "our cries of pain, fear, surprise, anger, together with their appropriate actions, and the murmur of a mother to her beloved child are more expressive than any words"—and these are forms of expression shared by humans and many species of animals. Darwin also maintains that animals such as parrots and dogs can respond to and make associations with articulate sounds, much as humans do. (See the case of the African gray parrot named Alex in chapter 14.)

The direction of Darwin's argument is to deny that human language is different in kind from that of other creatures, though it is different by degree. Obviously his conclusions depend on the richness of the concept of a "language." In a minimalist view, a language is a system of conventions that allow communications to occur by members of a community. Clearly animals have this measure of language. But if an enriched notion of language is used, requiring syntactical rules, sentences, true and false statements, creative use of conventional symbols, and the like (as Descartes may have assumed), then perhaps no animals other than the human animal will qualify.

Use of this enriched notion suggests that if nonhuman animals have nothing corresponding to syntax in a language, then there is a sharp break in the evolutionary scheme. Darwin had no direct response, but in general he was leery of sharp-break theses. He tried to account for all major differences in terms of the development of the brain, which he thought more advanced in humans than in animals. He tried to account for differences in rationality similarly. Just as some educators today speak of several different forms of intelligence or IQ in children, Darwin thought several forms and degrees of rationality could be found in animals: means-to-end reasoning, spatial perception, capacity to improvise and cope successfully and to manipulate the environment, desires and beliefs joined together in action, capacity to sense and avoid harmful conditions, and so on. (For an exploration of these themes, see the case of "Apes and Language: Washoe and Her Successors" in chapter 7.)

The Moral Sense (Conscience)

In chapter 3 of *The Descent of Man,* Darwin argued that the human moral sense, or conscience, is itself the product of evolution. "Social instincts," meaning dispositions to act in certain ways, have become built into human nature; and "the moral sense is fundamentally identical with the social instincts." The latter instincts allow us to set aside self-interest to act in the interests of others. The moral sense or conscience thereby becomes an advanced sense of obligation and a form of sympathy extended to a larger social group. Darwin thought that some humans display a high level and other humans a low level of moral responsiveness; the highest level of morality is reached when persons extend their sympathies beyond their own group and indeed beyond their own species to all sentient creatures.

Darwin described conscience as "the most noble of all the attributes" found in the human animal: "I fully subscribe to the judgment of those writers who maintain that of all the differences between man and the lower animals, the moral sense or conscience is by far the most important." Though only humans possess conscience in the proper sense, this mental and moral capacity is not without analogues in the nonhuman animal world. Darwin argued that nonhuman animals have emotions such as love and sympathy, for both their kin and their larger social group. They have social instincts, enjoy companions, are sympathetic with the plight of those to whom they are close, help their fellows, knowingly risk their lives, grieve in the loss of life, are gratified by others' approval of their behavior. Darwin thus thought of animals as having altruistic dispositions, even if lacking in the higher level of conscience.

Although Darwin did not develop a detailed theory of the motivational structure of animals, he did maintain that animals act beneficently—that is, for the benefit of others. He argued that just as we can correctly attribute beneficence in humans based on their behavior, we can do the same for animals. His examples come from community organization, affection in companionship, play, mutual or reciprocal provision of services, mothers caring for offspring, the adoption of helpless orphans, caring for the wounded or invalids, attending to elderly parents, feeding the blind, and intentional exposure to danger in order to protect others.

So convinced was Darwin of the validity of his inferences that he attributed extraordinary, apparently selfless acts of bravery to animals, calling it moral heroism. He believed that some animals can act altruistically, even if they have no conception of altruistic behavior and no rules of obligation requiring such behavior. Although Darwin lacked sophisticated ethological and psychological studies on which to base this claim, it seems certain that he would take many studies conducted in the twentieth century as confirmations of his own highly anecdotal manner of proceeding. Recent work in the evolution of altruism seems to confirm the importance of his hypotheses.

In summary, Darwin looked less for differences across species than for similarities across the species. His view was that whatever moral, physical, and mental qualities humans possess evolved through gradual series of processes that also occur elsewhere in nature. The faculties of reason and speech are no different in their origin than are the tooth of the snake, the fin of the fish, and the beak of the buzzard:

> [T]he difference in mind between man and the higher animals, great as it is, certainly is one of degree and not of kind. . . . If it could be proved that certain high mental powers, such as the formation of general concepts, self-consciousness, etc. were absolutely peculiar to man, which seems extremely doubtful, it is not improbable that these qualities are merely the incidental results of other highly advanced intellectual faculties; . . . The half-art, half-instinct of language still bears the stamp of its gradual evolution.

Darwin also thought that animals possess "mental concepts," including abstract or general concepts. When you say "squirrel" and your dog begins looking in trees and circling, Darwin thought the dog has an abstract idea of a squirrel ("a general idea or concept") and an idea that "some animal is to be discovered and hunted." Part of Darwin's motivation in this argument is to show that rational abilities in humans are the products of natural selection, as they are for other animals. Therefore, we do not need a special accounting (such as God's infusion of a rational soul) in order to explain the human species.

Moral Implications

Darwin's psychology of animals has many moral implications. His theory debunks the traditional idea that we have magical capacities that distance us from the rest of the animal kingdom. We are not "the rational creature," as Aristotelians, Cartesians, Kantians, and other philosophers had suggested; we are one among all the other rational creatures. To give up the thesis about distinctive rationality is obviously a consequential moral matter, because it undermines the common view that human beings are fundamentally different and deserve unique or sole moral consideration. The implications of Darwinism are therefore deep and profound.

Pre-Darwinian philosophers such as Descartes and Kant can easily be excused for their inadequate understanding of the common evolution of species of animals and the closeness of the human animal to some of those species. Their ignorance was nonculpable. Today's moralists, scientists, and industrialists have a far better understanding. Nonetheless, appreciating the implications of Darwinian thought for the ways in which we presently conceive and use animals is a very difficult task. Perhaps the most difficult assignment is to figure out whether animals have moral standing.

MORAL STANDING

Problems about whether animals act morally, whether they are part of the moral community, and whether they have higher-level mental capacities are connected to other attitudes and assumptions that have been at work for centuries.[18] In Western history, animals have typically been treated as not being able to act morally and as not having any moral (or legal) *standing*. In the first chapter of the first book of the Bible, God is reported to have granted humans dominion over animals.[19] For centuries, down to the present day, the presumption of human supremacy has been influential in discussions of moral standing.

What Is Standing?

The term *standing* has been transported into ethics from law, where *standing* is "[o]ne's place in the community in the estimation of others; one's relative position in social, commercial, or moral relations; one's repute, grade, or rank" *(Black's Law Dictionary)*. Animals have been given almost no legal standing in British and American systems of law.[20] However, recent discussions about fetuses, infants, the brain-damaged, the mentally retarded, and animals have appropriated the term *standing,* while stripping away its distinctly legal meanings. In a *weak* sense, standing refers to a status, grade, or rank of moral importance. In a *strong* sense, standing means to have rights, or the functional equivalent of rights. (For an example of such an attribution of rights, see the case of oncology research with mice in chapter 4.)

The mainstream approach in some areas of recent moral philosophy has been to ask whether an entity is the *kind* of entity to which moral principles or other moral categories can be applied. It is now generally agreed that one attributes a more significant standing to an animal by granting that it is relevantly like an intact adult human being. Its standing would be still further enhanced by attributing something like personhood or autonomy to it. A category such as "person" or "autonomous agent" elevates the animal to a position approximating that occupied by those who have rights.

An example is found in *The Great Ape Project* by Paola Cavalieri and Peter Singer.[21] They argue that the great apes are *persons,* just as humans are *apes.* (This issue is present in the case of Washoe in chapter 7, on apes and language, and also in chapter 2, on baboon-human liver transplants.) It is no accident that the central theme of their project is the personhood of the apes. The more status one can give an animal on the model of personhood, the higher the standing of the animal. A widely shared view today is that if animals have capacities for understanding, intending, and suffering (or having desires, preferences, and other major psychological capacities), these morally significant properties themselves confer *some* moral standing. But do animals have standing by virtue of these properties; and, if so, how much standing do they have? (For a case that raises these issues in terms of the intelligence of birds, see chapter 14, "Fowl Deeds.")

The Model of Human Properties

Distinctively human properties have always played a pivotal role in these controversies, because these properties supposedly distinguish humans in the relevant ways from animals and justify the ways in which we traditionally allow human interests to rank higher, have more value, and count for more whenever they are in conflict with the interests of animals. Much of the recent discussion about standing has centered on the criteria for being a person, under the assumption that all and only persons have the relevant distinctive properties for which we are looking. Several philosophers have produced arguments along the following lines:[22] One is a person if and only if one possesses certain cognitive properties that give an entity moral standing. As a corollary, anything lacking these properties lacks moral standing, and therefore does not possess rights.

These philosophers try to distinguish persons from nonpersons on the basis of cognitive capacities—in particular those possessed by intact adult humans but lacking in others. A list of the conditions for being a person similar to the following has been put forward by several writers:

1. Self-consciousness (of oneself as existing over time)
2. Capacity to engage in purposive sequences of actions
3. Capacity to appreciate reasons for acting

4. Capacity to communicate with other persons using a language
5. Capacity to make moral judgments
6. Rationality

Many believe that more than one of the above conditions is required to be a person. It allegedly follows that fetuses, newborns, profoundly brain-damaged humans, and most if not all animals fail the cognitive criteria, and so do not have the moral standing conferred by the category of person.

As long as one requires high-level cognitive criteria, animals may not be able to qualify for significant moral standing. But if one appeals to less demanding cognitive capacities, such as intention, understanding, desire, preferences, suffering, and having beliefs, animals will likely acquire a significant range of moral protections. For example, if a high-level qualifying condition such as the capacity to make moral judgments is eliminated and conditions like intention and understanding are substituted, then it becomes plausible to find the cognitive capacities needed for moral standing in (at least some) animals.

The main issue in the cases in this book is whether there is something very special about humans or human relationships—for example, properties humans or human communities possess that give humans alone a unique and perhaps uniquely high moral standing. The belief persists in contemporary philosophy, religion, science, and popular culture that we can pinpoint what makes us special, that is, the special-making property or properties found in a species that confer moral standing or status.

Suppose that dogs and ducks are not persons, because they lack some critical property. Which property do they lack? A property often cited is the first on the above list of six properties—namely, self-consciousness, or a conception of oneself persisting through time. Animals, many believe, lack this capacity, and so lack both the capacity to plan for the future and to understand the past. The hypothesis is that although animals exhibit goal-directed behaviors such as building a nest, they do so without any sense of self, which is thought to be essential to personhood or to any condition that confers moral standing.[23]

Critics of the demand for high levels of cognitive criteria deny that there are *morally* significant cognitive differences between healthy adult humans and animals in the way presented in cognitivist theories, even if they agree that there are at least some *psychologically* significant cognitive differences. This strategy is used by Cavalieri and Singer, for example.

How Much Do Cognitive Criteria Count?

Will cognitive criteria take us very far in our examination of the moral standing of animals? Perhaps some creatures deserve moral standing if they do not possess even a single cognitive capacity. Perhaps a *noncognitive* property may be sufficient to confer some measure of moral standing.[24] At least two kinds of properties need to be considered: (1) properties of sensation (or perception), and (2) properties of emotion.

First, consider sensation. As Jeremy Bentham long ago pointed out (see below), the capacity to feel pain might by itself be sufficient for conferring a significant moral standing, and pain is not on the aforementioned list of cognitive criteria. Lack of personhood therefore did not for Bentham imply a lack of moral status or standing. In an extension of such ideas, Donald Griffin has recently argued that there is no good reason to place much weight on the distinction between perceptual awareness in animals and a reflective consciousness, though traditionally we have made sharp distinctions in many species between the two that affect animals' moral standing. Griffin proposes multiple levels of mentation that are shared across species, from basic pain receptors to intentionality.[25]

Second, consider emotion. The emotional lives of animals have long been avoided in scientific literature, where attributions of emotion, intention, and the like have been criticized as an unscientific abandonment of critical standards and precise measurements, as well as an importing of an unsupported anthropomorphism. The emotions have also been little discussed in moral writings about animals. Yet many good reasons exist for attributing a range of emotions to animals, and the basis is as good as we have for the attribution of pain and suffering. (See the cases of apes and language in chapter 7 and of pound animals in chapter 16 for examples of such attribution.) In Griffin's early work *The Question of Animal Awareness*[26] and in the popular best seller *When Elephants Weep: The Emotional Lives of Animals,*[27] we find recent returns to the Darwinian theme that animals experience love, joy, anger, fear, shame, compassion, and loneliness—the full range of emotions often omitted in literature on animals.

Even if these noncognitive properties of sensation and emotion are not sufficient by themselves to confer moral standing, they may be important factors in determining which creatures deserve moral standing.

Speciesism

One of the most widely discussed topics about moral standing is so-called speciesism. A speciesist is one who believes that the interests of members of the species *Homo sapiens* are to be favored over the interests of members of any other species.[28] Species membership therefore determines whether a creature has moral standing or moral rights. The speciesist believes that different forms of treatment are justified entirely on the basis of biological and psychological differences in the species.

The term *speciesism* is often used pejoratively by analogy to racism and sexism; in this usage, speciesism is understood as an *improper* failure to respect the lives and rights of animals merely because they are other than human. Just as gender, race, IQ, accent, national origin, and social status, for example, are not relevant properties in morals, neither is species. "To each according to species" seems as morally irrelevant and unfair as "To each according to one's skin color."

However, speciesism need not be understood in this pejorative manner. Some speciesists willingly and even enthusiastically accept the label if it is used descriptively rather than pejoratively. How the term should be used cannot be debated here; it deserves note only that *speciesism* has become a central term in the debates about animals and that it is used in different ways. It also should be noted that one who rejects speciesism need not be committed to the view that all animals are equal in their properties or in their moral standing. The antispeciesist usually claims only that one cannot determine anything about standing based on species membership alone.

One speciesist response is that humans have a natural feeling of kinship and closeness with members of their own species, just as some human family members are closer to other family members.[29] In both cases, natural feelings create stronger obligations to members of the relevant group—the family, on the one hand, and the species on the other. These premises seem correct, but it is difficult to assess what they prove. Does the argument justify all forms of action based on close-knit relationships? For example, can military persons favor military persons, members of the upper class members of the upper class, members of one race the members of their race, members of one gender the members of their gender? If one can detect an unjustifiable bias at any point in schemes of natural closeness, is speciesism invalidated?

Another defense of speciesism is that certain properties associated with the human species—in particular, the cognitive properties discussed previously—give humans a special moral standing; it is not species membership alone that justifies special treatment for humans. From this perspective, it just so happens that those who possess these properties are of one species. This argument runs the risk, however, of permitting (or even demanding) the same treatment for members of the human species who lack these same properties (such as the mentally handicapped and brain-damaged persons) as the treatment of nonhuman animals. This problem, which is presented in the case of "Apes and Language" in chapter 7, as well as in chapter 11 on dissection, will now be further considered through an examination of moral philosophies.

MORAL PHILOSOPHIES

Many figures in the history of philosophy have attempted to develop a systematically organized set of moral principles together with a justification of the system—a moral philosophy that allegedly organizes and integrates the moral life. Such a system would integrate virtually all the topics that we have thus far considered: the nature of morality, moral standing, and the like. The present section describes a few general theories that have played and continue to play a particularly significant role in the discussion of animals and ethics—in particular, utilitarian theories, Kantian (and deontological) theories, and rights theories.

Some knowledge of these types of moral philosophy is indispensable for reflective study in animal ethics, because the field's literature frequently draws on the terminology, arguments, methods, and conclusions of these accounts. In almost every case in this volume, one or more of these theories could be employed in assessing the morality of what was done or should be done, what is permissible, and the like.

Utilitarianism

Utilitarian theories have been the most widely discussed type of theory in the development of ethical issues about animals. Utilitarianism is rooted in the thesis that an action or practice is right (when compared to any alternative action or practice) if it leads to the greatest possible balance of good consequences or to the least possible balance of bad consequences in the world as a whole for all affected parties. Utilitarians hold that there is one and only one basic principle of ethics: the *principle of utility,* which asserts that we ought always to produce the maximal balance of positive value over disvalue—or the least possible disvalue, if only undesirable results can be achieved.

Four conditions must be satisfied for a theory to qualify as utilitarian:

1. *The Principle of Utility.* First, utilitarians require actors to maximize the good. We ought in every circumstance to produce the greatest possible balance of value over disvalue (or the least possible balance of disvalue) for all affected parties—whatever that balance is *and* however it is distributed. For example, we ought to maximize the *public benefits* of scientific research, the availability of healthy food, the pleasures of zoos, and such. But what is the good or the valuable as the utilitarian conceives it?

2. *A Standard of Goodness.* Utilitarians say that the goodness or badness of consequences is to be measured by items that count as primary goods or utilities. Many utilitarians agree that ultimately we ought to look to the production of what is always valuable and does not vary from one subject to the next, but other utilitarians interpret the good as that which is subjectively desired or preferred. In the ethics of animal treatment, this question about the nature of values is usually less significant than issues about *whose* values will be considered, and whether they will be considered equally (see below).

3. *Consequentialism.* All utilitarian theories are consequentialist. That is, actions are morally right or wrong according to their consequences, rather than by virtue of any intrinsic moral features they may have, such as fidelity, friendship, or trust. In many cases in this book we will see that certain consequences for human health, survival, and pleasure seem to matter over everything else in the way some people make moral decisions.

4. *Impartiality.* Finally, all parties affected by an action must receive impartial consideration. Any partiality that is allowed toward particular individuals must itself have a strict utilitarian justification.

Whose goods are to be counted and who is to be treated impartially are systematically ambiguous questions in many (though not all) utilitarian theories. Given this ambiguity, we might obtain different recommendations from two committed utilitarians in a particular case: Action *A* would be recommended if *only human* goods and interests are considered, whereas action *B* would be recommended if the goods and interests of *all affected animals* are to be considered. It is easy to imagine how different our environmental policies might be if we had to consider both the interests of animals and those of humans—especially if we had to give them *equal* consideration. There is therefore a general problem in utilitarianism about what constitutes "the general welfare" and "all those affected by an action." Whose welfare is at stake in the utilitarian formula? The members of the human species? All sentient animals?

The simplest and apparently the most consistent alternative is to maintain that species properties and differences are irrelevant and therefore that the welfare of all sentient animals is to be considered. The morally relevant consideration, in this interpretation of utilitarianism, is who or what has the relevant experiences, feelings, pleasures, and the like—not what kind of being it is.

Bentham's theory

Among the earliest and most significant utilitarian writings were those of Jeremy Bentham (1748–1832). He never quite resolved this problem, but he did offer some historically influential thoughts that suggest an answer and that have been widely quoted in the animal ethics literature. Bentham argued that animals, like humans, have the capacity to feel pain and therefore deserve moral protections. He reasoned that even though there are important differences between humans and animals, there are also important and relevant similarities, the chief being the capacity of sentience—that is, the capacity to experience pleasure, pain, and suffering.

Lack of the traits making for human personhood did not for Bentham imply a lack of moral status or standing, because the capacity for experiencing pain was itself sufficient for conferring at least some significant moral standing. This reasoning underlies a famous statement made by Bentham: "The question is not, Can they [nonhuman animals] *reason?* nor, Can they *talk?* but, Can they *suffer?*"[30] Bentham used this approach as a way of grounding obligations to animals themselves, rather than to human owners of the animals. We have duties to animals not to cause them pain and suffering, and these duties are independent of any duties we may have to the owners of the animals.

Bentham's thesis enjoys plausibility. Moral claims on behalf of animals do not in any obvious way have anything to do with obligations to owners or with the animals' intelligence, self-consciousness, personality, or any other such fact about them. It is pain, suffering, and overall welfare—not rationality or self-awareness—that provide the reason many critics of our uses of animals resist the way primates are used in biomedical experimentation, rabbits used in cosmetics research, and chickens raised for the market.[31] (See the cases below in chapters 3, 6, 9, 14, and 16.)

Contemporary theories

Influential contemporary utilitarians such as Peter Singer maintain that many animals have desires and preferences about their futures and that they experience pain and suffering.[32] Singer maintains that we need to justify our involvement of animals on a basis that takes account of their interests—utility from the animal's perspective. He argues that this utilitarian perspective "makes it more difficult to claim that a genuinely utilitarian approach favors animal experimentation in general or as an institution," although "some individual experiments— those that do not involve any or very much suffering for the animal, and promise major benefits for humans or animals—may be defensible on utilitarian grounds."[33]

Another influential utilitarian thinker in the debates about animal ethics is Raymond G. Frey, who sees practical implications of utilitarianism that are starkly different from Singer's conception, although their underlying utilitarian ethical theories are rather similar. Frey argues that the value of any life, human or nonhuman, is contingent on its quality and its quality is contingent on the goods (utilitarian properties) in that life. Although animal life is typically not as rich and therefore not as well endowed with goods as human life, some animals have lives that are more valuable than other animals, including human animals. The lives of dogs, cats, and chimps, for example, are more valuable than the lives of mice, rats, and worms, and if the life of a human infant is less rich than the life of an adult chimpanzee, infants have less moral standing than adult chimpanzees.[34]

This comparative-value and quality-of-life analysis allows Frey to maintain that (1) we should maximize utility for all affected parties, not merely the human species, and that (2) for humans and animals alike, life is valuable only under certain conditions. Life loses value when its riches or valued components are stripped away. As a life becomes progressively less valuable, it has a progressively reduced moral standing that makes it increasingly more vulnerable to use in the riskier sides of biomedical and behavioral research. Frey's utilitarian theory opens up the possibility that humans with a sufficiently impoverished or substandard existence may justifiably be treated exactly as we treat animals at the same level of existence. They can be used for research, mined for organs, and so on.

On both utilitarian accounts—Singer's and Frey's—species membership is not a factor in making moral judgments. It is not one's species, but the quality of one's life (its utility) that counts in offering moral protections and in dropping moral protections. There is no consistent way to draw nonarbitrary *moral* lines based solely on species differences between human and animal life that will exclude one and include the other in the scope of justified activities.

However, these two utilitarians differ over numerous issues. Frey allows for more extensive use of animals than does Singer. Frey also must, as a result of his utilitarian commitments, countenance the use of defective humans in biomedical research.[35] Singer believes it is an extremely unattractive feature of all accounts like Frey's that they allow some human persons to be drafted without consent as research subjects and then harmed or killed, just as we treat animals. Singer has pointed out that this line of argument leaves not a *narrow* but a *broad* range of human subjects unprotected:

> [C]ertain categories of human beings—infants and mentally retarded humans—actually fall below some adult dogs, cats, pigs, or chimpanzees on any test of intelligence, awareness, self-consciousness, moral personality, capacity to communicate, or any other capacity that might be thought to mark humans as superior to other animals. Yet we do not think it legitimate to experiment on these less fortunate humans in the ways in which we experiment on animals.[36]

In the end, Singer is in favor of increasing protections for vulnerable animals and humans; Frey is in favor of increased access to both. In part their differences can be accounted for by the consequentialist character of utilitarianism. Singer and Frey have radically opposed conceptions of the consequences of adopting one set of principles and practices rather than another. If they could agree on the consequences of human experimentation, animal experimentation, vegetarianism, and the like., they likely would agree in both theory and practice.

Many contemporary moralists reject utilitarianism of all types. Two relevant reasons are that (1) utilitarianism requires too much unfounded speculation about consequences and lacks the backbone of any firm principle,[37] and (2) utilitarianism requires a balancing of goods and harms that seems, on occasion, to violate rights or leave minorities vulnerable to abuse. To use a criticism proffered by moral philosopher Tom Regan, utilitarians suggest that "there is nothing wrong with a matador's painfully draining the life from a bull, for example, provided only that enough people find the spectacle sufficiently pleasant. . . . When it comes to how humans treat other animals, utilitarian theory seems better suited to defending rather than reforming the *status quo.*"[38] This type of problem with utilitarianism has driven many, including Regan, to look for a more satisfactory general theory. (Practical examples of this problem are found in almost every case in this book; for a somewhat unusual twist, see the case in chapter 15 on docking the tails of dogs.)

Kantianism and Deontological Theories

A second type of theory departs significantly from utilitarianism. Often called *deontological* (that is, holding that some features other than or in addition to consequences make actions obligatory), this type is now increasingly called *Kantian,* because of its origins in the theory of Immanuel Kant (1724–1804).

Kant's legacy

For Kantians the rightness or wrongness of at least some actions can be determined *no matter what the consequences are.* For example, if killing animals for sport is morally wrong, then it is *categorically wrong* and would be wrong even if many persons would be deprived of great pleasure or economic benefits by forbidding the killing. A bulwark is thereby erected against utilitarian balancing of consequences. Kant regards all considerations of utility and self-interest as secondary, because the moral worth of an agent's action depends exclusively on the moral acceptability of the rule on the basis of which the person is acting. An action has moral worth only when performed by an agent who possesses a good will, and a person has a good will only if moral obligation based on a universally valid rule is the sole motive for the action.

Kant's supreme principle, also called "the moral law" and "the categorical imperative," is expressed in several ways in his writings. Most pertinent, for our purposes, is the requirement to never treat persons as means to one's own ends. Kant words it as follows: "One must act to treat every person as an end and never as a means only."[39] This form of the imperative demands that we treat other persons as "ends in themselves," as having their own autonomously established goals, and that we never treat others purely as the means to our own self-determined goals. To give a simple example, Kant's principle does not mean that we cannot use human research subjects in nontherapeutic research, but it does mean that we cannot use them without appropriate consent and that the consent cannot be obtained manipulatively.

Kant once stated his views on using persons as means to ends as follows: "*Unlike objects or animals,* humans are never to be used merely as a means to another's ends." "Animals," he says, "must be regarded as man's instruments, . . . as means to an end. That end is man."[40] From this perspective, animals have a reduced or instrumental value because of their status *as subhuman ani-*

mals, and this reduced value permits us to value them exclusively, or at least largely, in terms of their value to humans.[41]

Kant further argued that we have no direct obligations to animals, only indirect ones: "If a man shoots his dog because the animal is no longer capable of service, he does not fail in his duty to the dog, because the dog *cannot judge;* but his act is inhuman and damages in himself that humanity which it is his *duty to show towards mankind.*"[42] A person should not be cruel to animals because such cruelty will make the person cruel in dealings with other persons, not because it violates an obligation to the animal.

Kant and many later Kantians have maintained that *human dignity* places humans in a privileged position in the order of nature. The idea of human dignity is that humans have properties (rationality, souls, creation in the image of God) that place them in a fundamentally different category from animals. For example, only human beings intentionally perform actions that are motivated by *reason* and by *moral rules.* Animals are intelligent, but they do not act on moral reasons or exhibit a rational will. A person's dignity—indeed, "sublimity"—comes from being his or her own moral lawgiver, that is, from being morally autonomous.[43] However, this analysis is precarious for humans too, because it fails to confer any dignity on humans who lack the capacity for autonomy.[44] How can these humans be ends in themselves if they lack the critical properties for being such ends? If there are no obligations to weak, vulnerable, and morally incapacitated humans, they can legitimately be treated as means, just like nonhuman animals. But if there are obligations to these humans, then why are there no obligations to similarly situated animals? Kantians have had difficulty in responding to this line of inquiry while remaining faithful to the full range of commitments of Kant's moral theory.

Inherentism

A noticeably different attack and set of conclusions is found in a type of deontological theory called "inherentism," which has been developed by Tom Regan. Regan views animals, like humans, as having significant value meriting moral protection because they are "subjects of a life." Regan adopts Kant's idea that individuals are "ends in themselves" and defends "the postulate of inherent value."[45] Regan's conviction, unlike Kant's, is that both humans and animals are experiencing subjects with their own *inherent value.* Irrespective of any specific cognitive capacities, all experiencing subjects have a moral standing that protects against their being treated in certain ways that reduce their lives to the status of mere resources for others. (For discussions, see the ethical-issues sections in the cases in chapter 2 on human-baboon liver transplants, chapter 10 on the death of a bird, and chapter 15 on docking the tails of dogs.)

On the one hand, Regan rejects claims like those of Frey that humans who have abundant intellectual, artistic, and moral skills have more inherent value and can justly compel animals to serve human needs and interests.[46] The levels of these traits have nothing to do with inherent value, from his perspective. On the other hand, Regan's theory requires what he calls a fairly rich psychology for animals that includes beliefs, desires, intentional acts, and the like. There is no inherent value for Regan without such properties, leaving the inherentist open to the problem that the lower the level of the traits the less the inherent value would seem to be—a view noticeably similar to Frey's. Yet Regan's theory presumably moves sharply away from a utilitarian account in which values can be weighed, balanced, and traded off and in which the value of a life is related to the quality of life of the subject that possesses it.

Regan accepts the postulate of inherent value for animals for two reasons. First, he views it as arbitrary to exclude animals from the realm of creatures with inherent value, once we recognize that the subject-of-a-life criterion gives us obligations directly to the animals. Second, he believes our considered reflective beliefs about morals support his contentions.[47] One need not stretch very far to see the explosively controversial character of each claim.

Inherentism is, as Regan says, an abolitionist philosophy. It is thoroughly opposed to recreational hunting, sports that exploit animals, scientific research involving animals, use of animals for food, and so on. That inherentism would radically reform contemporary human society is not questioned by anyone. The center of the dispute has been over whether inherentism has provided or can provide an adequate justification to sustain such reforms. Many believe it fails for one or more of three reasons: (1) it cannot adequately defend a set of criteria for attributing inherent value to animals; (2) it rules out all balancing of costs and benefits (so characteristic of utilitarian theories); and (3) it confers upon animals too many rights, at the same time stripping humans of some of their rights.

Rights Theories

Much of the modern ethical discussion about animal ethics and about public policy governing the use of animals has turned on the language of rights. Western political tradition itself has developed from a conception of rights. Historically, the notion of rights emerged from a need to check the sovereign power of states—to protect citizens against oppression, unequal treatment, intolerance, arbitrary invasion of privacy, and the like. Given this history, it is not surprising that many framers of declarations about protections for animals chose rights language as the basic terminology for expressing their views about animals. Eventually the movement to protect the interests of animals became known as the "animal rights movement." (See the the case in chapter 17 of religious sacrifice for an example of the importance of rights language for both humans and nonhuman animals.)

The vital role of civil, political, and legal rights in protecting the individual from societal intrusions is now beyond serious dispute, but the ideas that (1) animals have such rights and (2) that rights provide the basis of ethical and political theory have both been strongly resisted—for example, by many utilitarians, who see the idea of rights as undercutting the risk-benefit calculus at the heart of utilitarian reasoning. Animals have traditionally served the utilitarian interests of society, rather than enjoying the protections of rights. The idea of animal rights has therefore been regarded by some as an innovative doctrine, and some even view it as a radical doctrine. Nonetheless, the idea that animals have rights has come to be one of the most important ideas found throughout the literature of animals and ethics.

Rights are important in this volume not only because of themes of animal rights, but also because of the rights of groups that seek to protect animals and groups opposed to animal-protectionism. Rights of the public also play a role. In one case below, in chapter 5, two of the central questions are, what does the public have a right to know about animal experimentation? and what rights do institutions have to keep that information private? In particular, the case turns on whether animal welfare organizations have a legal or a moral right to information about animal experiments conducted at state institutions as well as rights to attend meetings about the experimental work and approval of the protocols.

The nature and function of rights

Rights are justified claims that individuals, groups, and institutions can make upon others or upon society. To have a right is to be in a position to control what others are required to do.[48] Rights give parties a claim based on a system of rules that authorize those parties to affirm, demand, or insist upon what is due to them. If an individual or group possesses a right, others are validly constrained from interfering with the exercise of that right. A right, then, is a justified claim or entitlement, validated by moral principles and rules.[49]

Many writers in moral philosophy believe that rights are directly connected to obligations, so that whenever someone has a right someone else has an obligation, and whenever someone has an obligation someone else has a right. For example, if a state has an obligation to provide goods such as food or health care to needy citizens, then any citizen who meets the relevant criteria of need can claim an entitlement to food or health care. This analysis suggests a *correlativity* between obligations and rights.[50]

This thesis is extremely important, because if one acknowledges that humans have *obligations* to animals, then animals have all the *rights* that are correlative to these obligations (rights not to be interfered with or to be provided with something). If a research investigator has an obligation to animal subjects to feed them and abstain from extremely painful procedures during the conduct of research, then animal subjects have rights to be fed and not to have the pain inflicted. Anyone who recognizes obligations of this sort (see below) must recognize correlative rights for animals.[51]

Opposition to animal rights

Because many writers on the ethical treatment of animals take human obligations to animals to be either self-imposed obligations or obligations owed only to the owners of animals, they deny that animals themselves have moral rights. The so-called rights of animals are not truly rights; they are only ways of restating various provisions that have been or could be made by humans for the protection of animals. They believe that rights theory and rights language are misplaced in the discussion of animals. A more appropriate vocabulary, from this perspective, would be either *charity* or *moral ideals.* On this conception, obligations of beneficence toward animals are captured by conceptions of kindness, compassion, and generosity, but the language of rights is misplaced.

Carl Cohen has defended a robust and influential version of this position. He aims to show "why animals have no rights." He argues that activities of making claims occur only within a community of moral agents who can make claims against one another and are authorized to do so. Since claiming a right occurs only within a community of moral agents authorized to make such claims, rights "are necessarily human; their possessors are persons" with the ability for moral judgment and the ability to exercise moral claims, and animals cannot have rights because they lack these abilities. Cohen concludes, "In conducting research on animal subjects, therefore, we do not violate their rights, because they have none to violate."[52]

Defenses of animal rights

Despite the principled character of this position, many obligations owed to animals do not seem merely self-imposed, or indirect, and in that case animals would have whatever rights correspond to the obligations we owe to them. Joel Feinberg has argued that animals can have rights because they have, or at least can have, interests that we are obligated to protect.[53] For example, he believes animals have the right to be treated humanely, which follows from an obligation of justice. Feinberg and others have argued that we have a strong moral obligation not to cause unnecessary suffering in animals, and that correlative to this obligation for us are rights for animals—even if the fulfillment of that obligation has the consequence of losing benefits for humans.

Feinberg's views contrast sharply with Cohen's, and it is instructive to note where the two philosophers' views diverge, just as we noted differences in the case of utilitarian and deontological theories above. Cohen acknowledges that we have obligations to animals and maintains that "the grounds of our obligations to humans and to animals are manifold." However, Cohen goes on to maintain that, in qualifying for rights, being inside the moral community, as humans are, is a critical difference from being outside it, as animals are. Feinberg, by contrast, suggests that animals have rights that are correlative to the obligations we have to them. On this account, Cohen is mistaken in claiming that they have no rights. The view Cohen should have defended, from the perspective of a defender of animal rights, is that animals have all and only those rights that are correlative to human obligations in regard to them.

Rights exercised by surrogates

A related matter concerns whether some party, human or nonhuman, can have a right if the party is not *competent* to exercise the right. The usual answer to this question is that a rights holder need not be able to assert rights in order to have them. For example, when infants, the comatose, and mentally disabled individuals are not able to claim their rights, claims can be made for them by legitimate representatives, or surrogates.

At least one of the functions of members of review committees established to protect the interests of research animals could be (and sometimes is) to see that prevailing policies of protection are properly implemented and that pain and suffering are minimized. If members of these committees have obligations to ensure that agony to animals is minimized, then they could be viewed as established to protect the rights of animals.

Conclusion

To summarize this section, both rights theories and Kantian-deontological theories sharply contrast with utilitarian theories. For the latter, obligations are fixed entirely by relative consequences; the obligatory action is the one that produces the best consequences. Kantianism and rights theory take principled exception. Both place an emphasis on respect for the individual. As Alan Donagan has put it, the emphasis (particularly for Kantians) is on the principle that "[i]t is impermissible not to respect every human being, oneself or any other, as a rational creature."[54] Not consequences, but respectfulness is at the center of both Kantian theory and rights theory. Individuals cannot be treated as means to even very good ends, as is permissible in utilitarianism.

These theories are powerful tools for thinking about the issues in the cases and about one's moral commitments. Those who master this theoretical material should find that it helps significantly in the quality and precision of moral thinking. At the same time, it is important to appreciate the limits of the theories. They require thoughtful specification of their principles and cannot be mechanically applied to achieve resolutions in the cases. As we have seen, the values defended in these theories can be and have been turned in very different directions in the attempt to grasp the moral dimensions of the human-nonhuman relation.

THE JUSTIFICATION OF HUMAN USES OF ANIMALS

The centerpiece of moral philosophy has often been thought to be how to justify a moral position. Usually we do not need to deliberate very hard to justify our moral decisions, but occasionally the whole point of the enterprise is to justify or find a failure of justification in some proposed practice, policy, or course of action. Nowhere is this truer than in literature on animals, whether the topic is food production, hunting, sport and recreation, wildlife conservation, or religious sacrifice. Historical practices as well as innovative policies all stand in need of justification.

The analysis here will concentrate on research involving animals, both because of its centrality to the chapters below and because a more developed literature exists on the subject. However, the points made could be generalized to the many other human uses of animals found in the cases below.

The Concept of Justification

The term *justification* has several meanings in English, but in its customary sense, to justify is to show to be right, to vindicate, or to furnish adequate grounds for. The objective of justification is to establish one's case by presenting sufficient grounds for action. For example, one might attempt a justification by appealing to preexisting rules, such as those in codes of ethics, or to authoritative institutional agreements and practices, or to the moral convictions in which we have the highest confidence and believe to have the lowest level of bias. In each case, appeals are made to the most compelling moral reasons for the proposed course of action.

However, a reason can be a *good* reason without being *sufficient* for justification. There is always a need to distinguish a reason's relevance to a moral judgment from its final adequacy in support of that judgment.

General Justifications for the Use of Animals in Research

Many cases in this volume center on research of some type: biomedical, behavioral, museum collecting, and safety testing for cosmetics (including toxicity testing). At least since the scientific and philosophical writings of Claude Bernard (1813–1878), research involving animal subjects has been widely regarded as essential for scientific and medical advances.[55] Many believe today that further advances in diabetes, hypertension, cancer, and AIDS research will occur only if animals are involved. Likewise in veterinary schools, advances in the treatment of animals often require that the animals are used in research.

However, all research is morally troublesome when subjects are exposed to a significant level of risk. Normally when we present a risk or cause a harm, the burden of proof for the action is on the person who initiated it. This simple point about burden of proof leads to questions about justification. Under what conditions, if any, is such research, as well as other ways in which we treat animals, justified? Does it make a difference whether the subjects are human or nonhuman, and, if so, why?

Almost everyone agrees that the general justification for using both human and animal subjects in research is that benefits to be gained from research are substantial and that the disease, displeasure, and harm that could be expected to result from forgoing such investigations would be exceedingly grave. Medical and veterinary research has produced benefits of the highest importance for humans and animals alike, thereby lending credibility to claims that research is essential. These claims are especially attractive when there is historical evidence that a useful way to attack problems of illness and lack of information in the relevant scientific fields is the use of human or nonhuman animal subjects.[56]

Intact, live animals respond to research interventions in a manner that cannot always be simulated through research techniques that rely on nonanimal systems. For example, administering a drug to a rat may produce a complex reaction that affects multiple physiological systems. This response cannot always be understood through computer modeling or the manipulation of cells in tissue culture. Human subjects could be substituted for animal subjects in many cases, but the painful, invasive, and even lethal character of much animal research poses insuperable moral problems for proposals that human subjects be used.[57]

However, the absence of a justification for using human subjects does not by itself justify using animal subjects. If the goals of research cannot be carried out using humans because of the suffering that would be inflicted, the justification for inflicting the same or similar suffering on animals is far from established. A complicating problem is that at present we have no shared conception of what counts as a justifiable "harm" and a justifiable "risk" of harm for an animal. If a "harm" is defined as a thwarting, defeating, or setting back of a nontrivial interest, then many harms are suffered by animals in biomedical research and elsewhere.[58]

A related problem is that we lack a shared conception of what counts as a significant benefit. Research in the behavioral sciences that uses animals has had a long history of controversy about whether its results are significant contributions to knowledge. The more questionable the benefits, the more difficult is the justification of causing harm to animals. Although scientists rightly point out that we often do not see the utility in scientific experiments until some time after their completion, this fact is not sufficient to justify all forms of experimentation. The key question seems to be, when knowledge will be gained but there is no clear application or rationale for its use, should we declare the information trivial or should we allow experts in science to determine when a line of approach is promising? (See chapter 8, which examines research on animal aggression.)

It is also unclear whether research that exceeds a certain threshold or upper limit of pain, suffering, anxiety, fear, and distress can be justified. In research with human subjects, it is conventional to insist both on thresholds—for example, upper levels of risk, pain, and discomfort—and on a balancing of benefits and potential costs. If the threshold of harm is not exceeded, benefits of the research may justify the risks and costs involved in using humans or animals; but if the threshold is exceeded, the research cannot be justifiably conducted, irrespective of its value and potential. For such a threshold to be meaningful, careful guidelines would have to be prepared for investigators and review committees in planning and evaluating research, including a grading of research procedures as to their noxious, aversive, and painful properties. (For examples of possible needs to set thresholds in research, see chapter 4, on oncology research with mice.)

The argument against a firm threshold in our use of animals is that any criterion proposed will be too restrictive. It will impede or block some valuable research or some use of animals in educational training, food production, and the like (see, for example, the case of force-feeding geese in chapter 12). In particular, setting a threshold might prevent the balancing of risks and benefits in critical areas of clinical research, and therefore would cause us to forgo forms of knowledge with vital benefits for humans.

In the end, the main problem may be less *whether* we should require a threshold in research with animals than *how and where* to draw the threshold line. The threshold also may need to be drawn in different places for different species. For example, we now set the threshold of suffering, anxiety, fear, and distress differently for primates than we set it for species "below" primates. A justification for this differential treatment is itself needed, but the point is that we already employ the principle that it is justified to vary the threshold in accordance with species differences.

The Justification of Particular Research Protocols

The *general* justification of research in terms of overall benefit needs to be revisited for each *particular* research protocol to see if that protocol is justified. From the fact that research is valuable in general, it never follows that any particular research protocol is warranted. We need a carefully reasoned demonstration that any particular research investigation will significantly contribute to the health, safety, and welfare of future persons (or, in some cases, animals) and that the information obtained will be of sufficient significance that it offsets associated animal pain and suffering.[59]

Pain and suffering

A careful assessment of types and levels of pain, suffering, and deprivation will need to be included in any such justification. There are imposing empirical problems of measuring how much pain is felt, whether analgesic drugs are adequate for intended analgesia, whether the animal conceives the experience as agony or torment, and the like. For example, researchers need to determine the precise impact of small-diameter holes drilled through the skull, just to the surface of the dura (outermost covering of the brain) of an experimental animal, if the protocol calls for this surgery. They will also need to determine what pain and suffering will later be experienced, even if proper anesthesia is used during the surgery.

Such questions are at the heart of the ethics and review of animal research. If anything deserves the most careful and detailed scrutiny, it is the effect of such interventions on the animals involved. Surprisingly, little is often reported on this subject in research protocols, at least in any detail, although reassurances are often given as to the benign character of the intervention, the adequacy of anesthesia and analgesics, and the overall comfort of the animal. The critical matter is that carefully reasoned conclusions be drawn, preferably by an independent assessment that is free of investigator or institutional conflict of interest. The absence of detailed and unbiased evaluations has led in the past to many criticisms about the way research is reviewed that could have been avoided if appropriate review had occurred. (See the cases of review in chapter 5, on the public's right to know, and chapter 8, on animal aggression studies.)

Mental and emotional reactions

Of equal importance with pain and suffering, and directly connected to them, is the impact of the intervention on the *mental* and *emotional* lives of animals. It is often said that during the course of animal research "indices of psychological well-being" will be monitored. Such indices are required in USDA regulations and by the American Psychological Association in its "Guidelines for Ethical Conduct in the Care and Use of Animals."[60] Persons examining justifications offered in defense of research protocols should always ask what role did information about psychological well-being play in the prior peer review of the research. Were mental states a part of the review process?

These matters are of the highest importance when evaluating invasive research that places animals in restraints and in unfamiliar surroundings. Many documents report only the *physiological* effects (on fibers, enzymes, and the like) of interventions, but the mental and emotional effects of the restraints are more pertinent to ethical review. To assume that the *psychological* lives of animals are, were, and will be unaffected would be more than precarious; it would be false.

In some countries, legal requirements compel investigators to categorize the invasiveness of their proposed work, as to the harm—pain, suffering, social deprivation, confinement, and such—that will befall the animals during the experiment. Even if no comparable *legal* requirements exist in a country, such evaluation is essential for moral justification.

Conclusion

Scientists commonly obtain new and valuable information from their investigations with animals. Science feeds on incremental new knowledge, and it is an important part of the justification of the research. But every scientific investigation that uses live subjects, human or nonhuman, requires a comprehensive assessment of benefits versus risks and costs. In the simplest terms the question is, how much new knowledge beyond that gained in previous investigations will be gained, and does the merit of the new knowledge *justify* the harms or costs to the animals (as well as the costs in dollars, an issue of another sort)?" No checks on a list of rules of humane care and treatment amounts to this judgment, and it is a confusion to suppose that research is justified merely by conformity to such rules.

Benefits for Humans and Costs for Animals

A related problem concerns the fairness of the way in which risks and benefits are balanced. Attempts to resolve problems of either the general justification of research or the justification of particular research protocols through broad risk-benefit and cost-benefit analyses is a strategy that demands particularly close scrutiny. Costs to animals can easily be ignored in institutional and public policies when the use of those animals benefits the larger human community. Humans receive the benefits, animals the costs. Animals are subjects or objects of sacrifice; humans are not. (Several cases in this book present this problem, but the case of religious sacrifice in chapter 17 presents it in a somewhat novel way.)

Animal welfarist proposals about research involving animals have often suggested that the main way to combat this problem is to appoint review committees that are truly impartial. Even under obligatory systems of review, as long as researchers themselves heavily populate the committees, with few animal advocates present, costs to animals are not as likely to be taken seriously as they would be if a more impartial committee were formed. The practical implication is that a committee of broad representation, with a mandate to weigh the cost of the research to the animals involved, might approve only a small segment of the research that is presently approved.[61]

This problem extends beyond *research* with animals. For example, there has been an active discussion of the problem in factory farming, which is designed to maximize economic efficiency and the yield of food. Some of the morally most troublesome cases of factory farming (see the cases of broiler chicken, veal, and goose-liver products, in chapters 12–14) have been defended by claiming that such farming produces the greatest good for the greatest number of people. But does this form of balancing, even if true, adequately consider the interests of animals? Can unnecessary suffering be justified by these considerations of economic efficiency?

Cost-benefit analysis is an essential tool of public policy, but deciding issues of animal welfare through cost-benefit tradeoffs may be morally less satisfactory than looking directly and sympathetically at the suffering involved by animals and placing a limit on that suffering through the thresholds previously mentioned.

ALTERNATIVES AND COMMITTEE REVIEW

Critics and proponents of animal research and testing alike have often urged that alternatives to the direct use of animals should be vigorously pursued.[62] The requirement to seek alternatives entails a search for ways to accomplish scientific goals while reducing the amount of pain and distress to animals. From the beginning, the movement to alternatives has been an attempt to promote the humane treatment of animals without compromising legitimate scientific and clinical aims. However, whether both aims can be coherently sustained has never been entirely resolved.

The Three Rs: Replacement, Reduction, and Refinement

Virtually all analytical treatments of problems of alternatives begin with three components originally presented in an influential treatise by William M. S. Russell and Rex L. Burch:[63] *replacement* of animals with nonanimal research methods (such as cell lines and computer models), *reduction* in the numbers of animals used in experiments, and *refinement* of experimental techniques to reduce the pain and suffering experienced by experimental animals.

Positive response to Russell and Burch's proposal of replacement, reduction, and refinement has gained momentum in recent years,[64] and many now argue that scientists are both morally and legally required to comply with the three-Rs conception. However, some scientists oppose the pursuit of alternatives on grounds that scientific study will inevitably be retarded or eliminated. The scientific community is divided over these issues. Some groups, such as the Society of Toxicologists, have actively promoted the three Rs as a matter of good ethics in scientific practice; other scientific groups believe that they have no such obligations. A similar split appears in various government agencies.[65] (See, further, the discussions in chapter 2 on liver transplants, chapter 3 on head injury studies, chapter 6 on cosmetic testing, chapter 8 on animal aggression studies, and chapter 11 on dissection of frogs.)

Replacement

Even strong defenders of animal research have frequently acknowledged that the *unnecessary* use of animals constitutes inhumane treatment and creates an obligation that we desist from animal experimentation, as long as alternative methods can be used to accomplish the same result.[66] Thus, there is widespread agreement that requirements of humane treatment take precedence over mere preferences that the researcher may have about the need for and use of animals in research. Although proponents of animal research are quick to point out that the day of complete animal replacement is difficult to envision, many support replacement insofar as it is consistent with scientific progress. (For a clinical applicaton, see the case in chapter 2 of human-baboon transplantation; for an unusual example of using "human volunteers," see the case of cosmetic testing in chapter 6; and for an example of alternatives to killing in wildlife studies, see chapter 10, "The Death of a Vagrant Bird.")

Reduction

Reduction refers to the incorporation of techniques and approaches that decrease the number of animals used in research. For example, reduced numbers could be achieved by carefully guided research, as opposed to freewheeling trial and error, by the elimination of an unnecessary repetition of experiments, by the incorporation of statistically well-planned experimental designs, and the utilization of the minimum number of animals required to provide statistically significant results. The admonition to reduce sometimes encourages researchers to question standard laboratory procedures and to make animal use decisions on different bases. (Again, see the case of cosmetic testing in chapter 6 for a different approach to reduction, and see chapter 8, on animal aggression studies.)

Refinement

The objective of refinement is the reduction of pain or distress by shifting, insofar as maintenance of the scientific integrity of the experiment allows, to a lower category of pain and distress.[67] For example, a design that caused significant distress or discomfort could be refined to produce a lower level of distress and discomfort. Many defenders of animal research acknowledge that investigators have an obligation to subject animals only to necessary pain.

Any convergence of opinion toward acceptance of the three Rs among both defenders and critics of animal research begins to weaken as the precise obligations of researchers and institutions are formulated. It is one thing to say that alternatives are desirable, another to say that we overuse or use too many animals in research. Some defend the three Rs as an ideal, while maintaining that instead of reducing the total number of animals at the present time "we should increase it" and that "enlargement in the use of animals is our obligation," as Carl Cohen puts it.[68]

Cohen and others believe that the use of animals has already been dangerously reduced in our pursuit of highly desirable goals and that if we do not use animals, then humans will have to be subjected to risks that animals could have borne in their place. This view is especially attractive if one believes that too much clinical experimentation with humans occurs prior to scientific animal studies.[69] However, it has proved difficult to document the empirical assumptions in this thesis about the number of animals and the use of humans.[70]

In assessing the role of alternatives in the evaluation of scientific protocols, it should be remembered that there are *three* Rs, not just the first R of replacement. It is easier to cast doubt on the value of replacement if one ignores the options (and the imperatives) of refinement and reduction. Refinements are generally the most feasible option, given the current state of knowledge.

Animal Welfare Regulations and Committee Review

In 1966 *Life* magazine ran a story entitled "Concentration Camps for Dogs" that portrayed various abuses of animals.[71] The ensuing outcry, together with efforts of animal welfarists, led in the United States to the 1966 Laboratory Animal Welfare Act. Provisions about adequate housing, food, cage size, and the like were staples of the bill, and these provisions have been expanded over the years by amendments and additional federal regulations. Also covered were provisions for transportation carriers, the handling of animals, oversight responsibilities, and the like.

Public Health Service (PHS) policy separately requires that each institution receiving federal support provide a written assurance that it will comply with federal regulations. This assurance establishes a minimum basis for animal welfare provisions at each institution, and requires use of its policies as the cornerstone of care at the institution.[72] PHS policy requires the creation of an Institutional Animal Care and Use Committee (IACUC), which is a mandated oversight committee that includes at least one veterinarian, one animal investigator, and one nonaffiliated public member. This committee has oversight responsibility for semiannual review of animal care and use, inspection, review of research protocols involving animals, recommending personnel training, and the suspension of improper activities.

Committee review

Review committees, in the United States and in many other countries, are established to examine protocols to see if they can be improved in various ways, including (as is implicit in current public policy) by reducing, replacing, or refining animal use. These committees serve as gatekeepers who determine whether the use of animals proposed is warranted. Since its modest beginnings,[73] a robust and increasingly international system for prior review of research with living subjects has evolved. Although each committee is likely to use both local and national standards, there is a broad consensus internationally on the types of moral rules that should govern human research, and a gradual evolution has occurred toward international guidelines on research with animals.

However, these rules are seldom specific, and whether these committees function adequately in their understanding of the available rules is a matter of controversy.[74] Inconsistencies in their deliberations have been noted, as has the lack of information about animal pain and suffering provided in the protocols of investigators and on the basis of which review occurs. The investigator's description of the project may only briefly describe the procedure, and committee approval is sometimes pro forma. Often missing is a serious assessment of the degree of animal pain or suffering, forms of analgesia, and the effect on animals of the experimental methods used. A search for alternatives is also often not adequately addressed. (See the case in chapter 8, on animal aggression studies.) The full protocol is not necessarily disclosed to the full committee. Based on the limited empirical evidence about these committees, little evidence exists of thorough review that is impartial and free of conflict of interest.

Institutions often point out that they have followed proper procedures of review and that all rules have been followed by duly constituted committees. This observation seems generally to be true both in the United States and in most countries with such requirements. But the real issue is not a *procedural* one about whether legal requirements have been followed; it is a *substantive* question about the actual work of these committees in discharging their moral responsibilities. (See, for example, the case of "What Does the Public Have a Right to Know?" chapter 6 below.)

These committees are often given extensive data about proposed scientific investigations. This data shows intricate planning, probing scientific hypotheses, and familiarity with the relevant literature. Rarely are the committees given anything comparable in detail by way of ethics materials or ethical defenses of the research. For an adequate ethics review, the ethical reasoning must be spelled out, just as the science has been specified. Such is rarely the case in these committees, leading to widespread suspicion about the quality and worth of the committees.

Many members of these committees would say that framing the issues in this way holds researchers to an unrealistically high ethical standard. They claim that if the review has been done "by the book," then one's moral responsibilities have been met. "The book" in the United States is, roughly speaking, the US Animal Welfare Act and its implementing regulations;[75] *International Guiding Principles for Biomedical Research Involving Animals,* by the World

Health Organization's Council for International Organizations of Medical Sciences (CIOMS);[76] and the *Public Health Service Policy on Humane Care and Use of Laboratory Animals* and *Guide for the Care and Use of Laboratory Animals.*[77]

How are we to evaluate the thesis that whenever review takes place under these guidelines the review is morally sufficient? There are three potential problems with such a claim: (1) One can follow the procedures and rules in "the book," but do so in a cursory and perfunctory manner. This often happens in the review of both human and animal research. (2) Those doing the review may be poorly trained for the work or have serious conflicts of interest. (3) Even if the experiments under review conform to "the book," that fact alone does not make them ethically acceptable, because the experiments may not be consistent with the most appropriate standards articulated in various parts of the profession, the public, and the scholarly literature on the subject. "The book" is not always up-to-date, comprehensive, or relevant.

For example, neither the CIOMS *International Guiding Principles,* which was never intended as a regulatory set of guidelines, nor the PHS policy is as rigorous and demanding as the highly respected Canadian *Guide to the Care and Use of Experimental Animals*[78] or the compact little *Australian Code of Practice.*[79] The point is that there are more and less comprehensive guides to review. Some use higher standards than others. No one has yet agreed on the middle ground or the minimal level of requirements, but for those who want to take the "moral high ground" in the review of research (as many institutions now say that they wish to), it is well to remember that there are many possibilities for basic standards.

Pain and suffering

Suggestions about replacement and reduction have been minor activities for many committees, but refinement has been a primary activitity for virtually all committees. Researchers with inadequate plans must modify their research design to improve analgesics and anesthetics used, as well as methods of euthanasia. Careful committee review considers whether immobilization for the animals is necessary, whether tumor burden in cancer research can be reduced, and the like.

However, the nature and role of animal pain and suffering has proved difficult for members of these committees to assess.[80] Suffering is even more difficult than pain, partially because of the breadth of the concept of suffering. The term *suffering* is generally used to include both discomfort and disease, as when animals are kept in unsanitary and crowded conditions that deprive them of freedom of movement. *Discomfort* is itself a broad notion and is often used to refer, for example, to tension, anxiety, stress, exhaustion, and fear.

Different empirical assumptions are at work in current literature about the degree to which animals suffer, including whether they suffer *more* or *less* than humans do. In the scientific literature, there is a tendency to assume that animals have different forms of pain reception and cannot anticipate or remember pain—and therefore suffer less than humans. A contrasting view is that animals suffer more, not less, because they have less understanding of the origin, nature, and meaning of pain. That is, an animal may be a captive of the momentary experience of pain, and without the capacity to deal with danger, injury, and the like. What can be processed and put in context by a human may be experienced as terror by a captive animal.[81]

The definition of "animal" and the differential treatment of species

The animal welfare community has attempted to protect all animals by appropriate laws. One of the most controversial aspects of animal welfare regulations in the United States is that birds, mice, and rats are not animals according to the definition of the word in the USDA regulations for the Animal Welfare Act. These species are therefore unprotected by the legislation. Approximately 85% of research and testing animals belong to these excluded species. The exclusion was introduced to reduce costs of USDA inspections, but it has had the effect of leaving many forms of research and even whole facilities totally uninspected and unregulated.

The moral issues reach beyond the obvious ones of unprotected animals and the potential unfairness involved in including some species under legal protections while excluding others for no morally relevant reason; there is also a problem of moral coherence in public policy. The PHS policy definition of "animal" (unlike that of USDA regulations) includes all vertebrates. Birds, mice, and rats are therefore included in its protections. The effect is that in institutions not included in PHS coverage (including industry and colleges not receiving PHS funding), research, testing, and education involving birds, mice, and rats is unregulated—a striking incoherence, and one confined to the United States.[82]

REASONING ABOUT CASES

Every subsequent part of this book contains cases involving human-animal relationships. The "case method," as it is often called, has long been used in several fields of inquiry as a basic method of instruction and decision making. However, only recently has philosophically oriented ethics drawn attention to the importance of case studies and the case method. The use of these methods is still controversial and unsettled.

Methods of Case Analysis

In the field of law the case method has come to be understood as a way of learning to assemble facts and judge the weight of evidence—enabling the transfer of that weight to new cases. This task is accomplished by generalizing and mastering the principles that control the transfer, usually principles at work in the reasoning of judges. Beyond the law, however, it is not clear that case analysis can or should proceed with such assumptions. In many fields, cases are developed to recreate a situation in which dilemmas are confronted so that persons can learn about moral reasoning by thinking their way through the dilemmas.

Daniel Callahan and Sissela Bok have suggested that in contemporary ethics "case studies are employed most effectively when they can readily be used to draw out broader ethical principles and moral rules . . . [drawing] the attention of students to the common elements in a variety of cases, and to the implicit problems of ethical theory to which they may point."[83] Yet it has proved difficult to apply theory, draw out principles, or find common elements in these discussions. Cases have not been used merely to illustrate principles or rules, because the latter are often too general to give us final resolutions in difficult situations.

The objective of using cases has more often been to develop a capacity to grasp problems and to find novel solutions that work in the context. This use of the case method springs from an ideal of education that puts the discussants in the decision-making role after an initial immersion into the facts of a complex situation. Theories and generalizations are reduced in importance, and the skills of thinking and acting in complex and uncertain environments are upgraded. The essence of the case method, so understood, is to present a situation replete with the facts, opinions, and prejudices that a person might encounter and to foster good decision making in such an environment.

This approach to case analysis makes no assumption that there is a *right* answer to any problem. Understanding argument and analysis is as important as understanding substantive principles and theories. These forms of understanding need not be seen as antagonistic or competitive, but the case method in many contexts has placed the premium on problem resolution rather than on analysis by appeal to theories in moral philosophy. It also avoids the authority-based method relied on in law schools and courts, where judges and the body of law are overriding authorities.

However, dangers are present in this approach to cases. Not much is drearier than a tedious exposure to the moral opinions of those ignorant of the philosophical materials outlined in the earlier sections of this introduction. Accordingly, case analysis is often enhanced by familiarity with the relevant parts of moral philosophy and the fields from which the case derives. Cases often play the roles of providing data and supplying the testing ground for theory. Revealing cases lead to modification and refinements of theoretical commitments, just as theory helps frame thinking about the case. Traditional moral philosophy, from this perspective, has as much to learn from the practical decision-making contexts presented in cases as decision makers stand to learn from theory.

Casuistry

Proponents of an ancient approach called "casuistry" have criticized the abstractness of the approaches found in the "Moral Philosophies" section above, in order to focus on the importance of the case in moral reasoning and practical decision making—especially nuanced cases in which judgments made cannot be brought under *general* norms such as principles and rules. Casuists are skeptical of principles, rules, rights, and theory divorced from history, circumstance, and experience. One can make successful moral judgments of agents and actions, casuists say, only when one has an intimate understanding of particular situations and an appreciation of the record of similar situations.

Casuists maintain that the forms of moral reasoning used in analyzing cases often make no appeal to principles, rules, rights, or virtues. They note that our actual moral reasoning about cases turns on the clever use of paradigm cases, analogies, models, classification schemes, and even immediate intuition and discerning insight. The paradigm case (or precedent-setting case) is especially important because we *reason* by appeal to such cases; we do not merely reason by applying general rules to cases. Using appeals to these sources, the casuist views practical ethics as a field that arises out of experience and professional practice.

The casuistic method is to start with cases whose moral features and conclusions have already been decided, and then to compare the salient features in the paradigm case (that is, the case with morally settled dimensions) with the features of cases in need of a decision. Analogical reasoning links one case to the next and serves as the primary model of moral reasoning.[84] Casuists do not dismiss principles altogether, but they do downgrade them in importance because they think moral reasoning starts at a different point.

Although casuistry is often presented as antitheoretical, it need not be so understood. A casuist emphasizes the importance of cases, but need not deemphasize the proper role for the theories presented in the previous section.

Reasoning Through Moral Problems

Many cases in this book present moral problems that are controversial and require careful moral reasoning. Facing and reasoning through problems to conclusions and choices is a familiar feature of the human condition. Often problems appear because some evidence or reason indicates that an act is morally right, and some evidence indicates that the act is morally wrong, but the evidence on both sides is inconclusive. Experimentation on animals, for example, is sometimes said to be a terrible dilemma for those who see the evidence in this way.

Nonetheless, there are practical ways of reasoning about what should be done in cases of dilemmas and other moral problems. First, in managing new, complex, or problematic cases, the first line of attack should be to specify further one's general moral commitments to see if ambiguities and problems can be eliminated. Direct application of principles and rules rarely works in hard cases, but progressive specification of the commitments of one's moral position may reduce the problems.

As a simple example of specification, consider the rule "Meetings of ethics committees considering animal research should be open to the general public." (See the case of the public's right to know in chapter 5.) Openness of discussion and adequate disclosure are worthy moral goals. However, sometimes these committees consider research strategies that involve private information or privileged information that cannot reasonably be made public. It does not follow from rules of public discussion that a research investigator's work should be destroyed or imperiled by public disclosure. Our rules against nondisclosure and acting in the public interest are not categorical demands, and we therefore need to specify our precise commitments to public disclosure and to the privacy of information. Unless abstract values are specified in concrete form, it is hard to see how deep moral conflicts are to be avoided.

Specification holds out the possibility of a continually expanding normative viewpoint that is faithful to initial beliefs (which are not renounced) and that tightens rather than weakens coherence among the full range of accepted norms. When we refashion our general moral commitments to make them suitable for particular cases and contexts, inventiveness and imaginativeness in their use is essential for moral reasoning. Here inventiveness that is faithful to general moral values is to be encouraged, not discouraged. Moral progress can be made in this way. Through progressive specification, practical ethics becomes increasingly more practical, while maintaining fidelity to basic principles and rules.

Another approach to hard cases is to *balance* values, not merely to *specify* them. Whereas specification entails a substantive development of the scope of norms, balancing consists of deliberation and judgment about the relative weights of different moral commitments. Specification and balancing can best be conceived as mutually facilitative approaches, methods, or strategies. Balancing is especially useful in individual cases, whereas specification is especially useful for developing policies that can govern a range of similar cases.

The metaphor of weights moving a scale up and down graphically depicts the balancing process, but it may also obscure what happens in the actual process of reasoning. Justified acts of balancing entail that *good reasons* be provided for a judgment. Conversely, poor reasoning is discounted. Thus, in weighing the various ethical positions that are presented in the analyses of the cases considered in this book, decisions are made in favor of arguments that further one's general moral commitment and rest on good reasons.

As an example of the metaphor of weights, suppose a veterinarian encounters an emergency case of a wounded animal that would require her to extend an already long day so that she would be unable to keep a promise to take her son on a school trip. She will then engage in a process of deliberation that leads her to consider how urgently her son needs to go on the trip, whether they could go later and catch up with the group, whether another veterinarian could handle the case, and so forth. If she determines to stay deep into the night with the injured animal, this obligation will have become overriding because she has a good and sufficient reason for her action. A life hangs in the balance, she has professional obligations, and she alone has the knowledge to deal adequately with the full array of the circumstances. Her action of canceling her evening with her son, painful and distressing as it is, can be justified by these reasons. Balancing is a good method for addressing problems in cases, but it always requires that good reasons be present.

Just the Facts

In using methods of case analysis and attempting to reason through cases, one temptation should be avoided. Those who study the facts of cases invariably desire more facts. They see a solution as dependent on knowing more than is given about what transpired. If additional data can be discovered, they think, it will become clear that the problems can be handled and the dilemmas disentangled. A related temptation is to doctor the known facts, thereby presenting a hypothetical case, rather than an actual case. Such hypothetical cases can at times be instructive, but the temptation to change the facts or look for others should usually be avoided. In all interesting cases only limited information is known, and one must treat the problem under these real-life conditions of information scarcity.

Professionals in many fields who work with animals work under such conditions day in and day out, and for them a case must be addressed as it is, and not as it might be in some possible world.

CONCLUSION

One of the best-known journals in practical ethics is the *Hastings Center Report*. This journal ran a special supplement on ethics and animals[85] and soon received a letter of response and complaint from Robert J. White, professor of surgery at the Case Western Reserve University in Cleveland: "I am extremely disappointed in this particular series of articles, which, quite frankly, has no right to be published as part of the *Report*," wrote White. "Animal usage is not a moral or ethical issue and elevating the problem of animal rights to such a plane is a disservice to medical research and the farm and dairy industry."[86]

White believes that including nonhuman animals in our ethical system is a "philosophically meaningless" ambition.[87] He represents a minor, and rather extreme, segment of the scientific community that has long been troubled by complaints about animal usage in science. For example, when the first Cruelty to Animals Act was passed in Great Britain in 1876, it brought a system of regulation and inspection detested by many British scientists, who viewed the act as an unjustified interference with their work. Antivivisectionists did not relish the act any more than scientists. They saw it as a meager attempt to appease public outcries, and the act spurred them on to even more vigorous protests.

In some respects the public controversy, over a century later, is no different.

No strong partisan in the debate today esteems government regulations in any nation in the world. Each partisan side is hostile to the other side. We should not mask how difficult these issues are and how strongly people feel about them. At the same time, we should not forget that moral thinking by reasonable persons has often taken us further than we might at the outset have thought we could go.

Discussions about the proper treatment of animals have been carried on in journals of ethics for many years without bitter partisanship and ill feeling. Indeed, many of the participants in opposite camps are close friends. The authors of the present book can only hope that the following cases will contribute to this more civil level of discourse, especially in the now extensive and sometimes angry debates occurring in politics and popular culture.

NOTES

1. See Lewis Hanke, *Aristotle and the American Indians* (London: Hollis & Carter, 1959), pp. 30–43; Henry R. Wagner, *The Life and Writings of Bartolomé de Las Casas* (Albuquerque: University of New Mexico Press, 1967), pp. 170–82.

2. See, for example, Ronald Dworkin, *Taking Rights Seriously* (Cambridge, MA: Harvard University Press, 1977); Judith Jarvis Thomson, *The Realm of Rights* (Cambridge, MA: Harvard University Press, 1990); Ruth Macklin, "Universality of the Nuremberg Code," in *The Nazi Doctors and the Nuremberg Code*, ed. George J. Annas and Michael Grodin (New York: Oxford University Press, 1992), pp. 240–57.

3. Various aspects of these questions are discussed in Jeffrey M. Masson and Susan McCarthy, *When Elephants Weep: The Emotional Lives of Animals* (New York: Delacorte Press, 1995), esp. chap. 8; Richard Dawkins, *The Selfish Gene* (Oxford: Oxford University Press, 1976); and James Rachels, *Created from Animals: The Moral Implications of Darwinism* (New York: Oxford University Press, 1990).

4. Cf. Robert M. Seyfarth and Dorothy L. Cheney, "Grooming, Alliances, and Reciprocal Altruism in Vervet Monkeys," *Nature* 308 (1984): 541–42; Richard Connor and

Kenneth Norris, "Are Dolphins Reciprocal Altruists?" *American Naturalist* 119 (March 1982): 358–74.

5. René Descartes, "Animals Are Machines," in Tom Regan and Peter Singer, eds., *Animal Rights and Human Obligations*, 2nd ed. (Englewood Cliffs, NJ: Prentice-Hall, 1989), pp. 17f. Hereafter, "Regan-Singer."

6. Descartes thought that animals have no capacity for the sophisticated abstractness of human thought. As a consequence, they fail to move beyond the particularities of sensual experience and reactions based on instinct and conditioning—the mechanical principles of their nature.

7. Anita Guerrini, "The Ethics of Animal Experimentation in Seventeenth-Century England," *Journal of the History of Ideas* 50 (1989): 391–407; Lloyd Stevenson, "Religious Elements in the Background of the British Anti-Vivisection Movement," *Yale Journal of Biology and Medicine* 29: 125–57.

8. "An Enquiry Concerning Human Understanding," in *Hume's Enquiries*, ed. L. A. Selby-Bigge and P. Nidditch (Oxford: Oxford University Press, 1975), sec. 9, par. 2.

9. Hume, *A Treatise of Human Nature*, ed. L. A. Selby Bigge and P. Nidditch (Oxford: Oxford University Press, 1978), 1.3.16; 2.1.12; etc.

10. Donald R. Griffin, *Animal Thinking* (Cambridge, MA: Harvard University Press, 1984); idem, *Animal Minds* (Chicago: University of Chicago Press, 1992), pp. 15–16 and chaps. 6–10.

11. Some of these problems not explored below are examined in Bernard Rollin, *The Unheeded Cry: Animal Consciousness, Animal Pain, and Science* (Oxford: Oxford University Press, 1989); Daisie Radner and Michael Radner, *Animal Consciousness* (Buffalo: Prometheus Books, 1989); Marian Stamp Dawkins, *Animal Suffering: The Science of Animal Welfare* (New York: Chapman and Hall, 1980).

12. See, for example, Dorothy L. Cheney and Robert M. Seyfarth, *How Monkeys See the World: Inside the Mind of Another Species* (Chicago: Chicago University Press 1990); "Monkey Responses to Three Different Alarm Calls," *Science* 210 (1980): 801–3; and "Vervet Monkey Alarm Calls: Semantic Communication in a Free-Ranging Primate," *Animal Behavior* 28 (1980): 1070–94.

13. Cf. Griffin's assessment in *Animal Minds*, pp. 245–52.

14. Charles Darwin, *The Descent of Man* (1871); all material cited from Darwin, unless otherwise noted, is from the selection of this work in Tom L. Beauchamp, Joel Feinberg, and James M. Smith, eds., *Philosophy and the Human Condition*, 2nd ed. (Englewood Cliffs, NJ: Prentice-Hall, 1989), pp. 107–10.

15. In *Origin of the Species* (1859), Darwin does not attempt to pinpoint a single ancestral origin of humans and apes, although he does try to trace a general line of descent from a primitive ape "low in the mammalian series."

16. For an engaging explication of Darwin's views, see Rachels, *Created from Animals*.

17. Charles Darwin, *The Expression of the Emotions in Man and Animals* (1872; Chicago: University of Chicago Press, 1965) (italics added).

18. See, for example, James C. Whorton, "Animal Research, Historical Aspects," *Encyclopedia of Bioethics*, ed. Warren Reich (New York: Free Press, 1995), pp. 143–47; Andrew N. Rowan, *Of Mice, Models, and Men: A Critical Evaluation of Animal Research* (Albany: State University of New York Press, 1984), chaps. 3–4.

19. *Genesis* 1:26.

20. Gary L. Francione, *Animals, Property, and the Law* (Philadelphia: Temple University Press, 1995), chap. 4. He argues that the law of standing has been coupled to the law of property and that the law understands animals as property.

21. Paola Cavalieri and Peter Singer, *The Great Ape Project* (New York: St. Martin's Press, 1993); *Etica Animali* 8(1996), special issue devoted to the Great Ape Project.

22. See Michael Tooley, "Abortion and Infanticide," *Philosophy and Public Affairs* 2 (Fall 1972): 37–65; "In Defense of Abortion and Infanticide," in *The Problem of Abortion,* ed. Joel Feinberg, 2nd ed. (Belmont, CA: Wadsworth Publishing Company, 1984), pp. 120–34; Mary Anne Warren, "On the Moral and Legal Status of Abortion," *Monist* 57 (January 1973); Wayne Sumner, *Abortion and Moral Theory* (Princeton, NJ: Princeton University Press, 1981).

23. See, as examples, Allen Buchanan and Dan Brock, *Deciding for Others: The Ethics of Surrogate Decision Making* (Cambridge: Cambridge University Press, 1989), pp. 197–99, 261–62; Gerald Dworkin, *The Theory and Practice of Autonomy* (New York: Cambridge University Press, 1988), esp. pp. 15–20; David DeGrazia, "The Moral Status of Animals," *Kennedy Institute of Ethics Journal* 1 (1991): 58.

24. See the outstanding work on this topic in David DeGrazia, *Taking Animals Seriously: Mental Life and Moral Status* (New York: Cambridge University Press, 1996.) Another and more technically correct way to put the point is to say that even if some cognitive criteria do turn out to form a sufficient condition of moral standing (and so to confer moral protection), these criteria may only be sufficient conditions of moral standing, not necessary conditions.

25. Griffin, *Animal Minds,* esp. p. 248. See also Rosemary Rodd, *Biology, Ethics, and Animals* (Oxford: Clarendon Press, 1990).

26. Donald R. Griffin, *The Question of Animal Awareness: Evolutionary Continuity of Mental Experience* (New York: Rockefeller University Press, 1976), 2nd ed., 1981.

27. Masson and McCarthy, *When Elephants Weep.*

28. See Peter Singer, *Animal Liberation,* 2nd ed. (New York: New York Review of Books/Random House, 1990), p. 6. This book has been the most widely influential work in the animal liberation movement.

29. Mary Midgley, *Animals and Why They Matter* (Athens: University of Georgia Press, 1984); Jeffrey Gray, "On the Morality of Speciesism" and "Reply" *Psychologist* 4 (1991): 196–98, 202–3.

30. Jeremy Bentham, *Introduction to the Principles of Morals and Legislation* (1789; New York: Hafner, 1948), chap. 17, sec. 1. See the Bentham selection in Regan-Singer, p. 26. Bentham reasons as follows: "If the being eaten were all, there is very good reason why we should be suffered to eat such of them as we like to eat: we are the better for it, and they are never the worse. They have none of those long-protracted anticipations of future miserys which we have. The death they suffer in our hands commonly is, and always may be, a speedier, and by that means a less painful one, than that which would await them in the inevitable course of nature. . . . But is there any reason why we should be suffered to torment them? Not any that I can see. Are there any why we should *not* be suffered to torment them? Yes, several. . . ."

31. See, for example, Dawkins, *Animal Suffering;* A. H. Flemming, "Animal Suffering: How It Matters," *Laboratory Animal Science* 37 (January 1987, Special No.): 140–44; Andrew N. Rowan, "Animal Anxiety and Animal Suffering," *Applied Animal Behaviour Science* 20 (1988): 135–42; Richard Ryder, *Victims of Science: The Use of Animals in Research* (London: Davis-Poynter, 1975).

32. Singer, "Comment," *Between the Species* 4, no. 3 (Summer 1988): 203, and "The Significance of Animal Suffering," *Behavioral and Brain Sciences* 13 (1989): 9–12; on underlying claims about preferences, pain, and suffering, see Dawkins, *Animal Suffering.*

33. Peter Singer, "Animal Research, Philosophical Issues," in *Encyclopedia of Bioethics,* vol. 1, p. 150.

34. Raymond G. Frey, "Moral Standing, the Value of Lives, and Speciesism," *Between the Species* 4, no. 3 (Summer 1988): 191–201, esp. p. 196. See also his "Medicine and the Ethics of Animal Experimentation," *The World & I,* April 1995, pp. 358–67, and his early and influential book *Interests and Rights: The Case Against Animals* (Oxford: Clarendon Press, 1980).

35. Raymond G. Frey, "Medicine, Animal Experimentation and the Moral Problem of Unfortunate Humans," *Social Philosophy and Policy* 13 (1996): 181–211; "Autonomy and the Value of Animal Life," *Monist* 70 (January 1987): 50–63; "Animals, Science and Morality," *Behavioral and Brain Sciences* 13 (1990): 22; "Animal Parts, Human Wholes: On the Use of Animals as a Source of Organs for Human Transplants," in *Biomedical Ethics Reviews 1987,* ed. James M. Humber and Robert F. Almeder (Clifton, NJ: Humana Press, 1987).

36. Peter Singer, "Animal Experimentation: Philosophical Perspectives," in *The Encyclopedia of Bioethics,* ed. Warren Reich (New York: Free Press, 1978), vol. 1, p. 81. See further the discussion of this problem in chapter 12 below on force-feeding of geese.

37. See Evelyn B. Pluhar, *Beyond Prejudice: The Moral Significance of Human and Nonhuman Animals* (Durham, NC: Duke University Press, 1995); and Stephen R. L. Clark, *The Moral Status of Animals* (Oxford: Clarendon Press, 1977).

38. Tom Regan, "Animals, Treatment of," *Encyclopedia of Ethics,* ed. L. C. Becker and C. B. Becker (New York: Garland Publishing, 1992), vol. 1, p. 43.

39. Immanuel Kant, *Foundations of the Metaphysics of Morals* (1785), Lewis White Beck, trans. (Indianapolis: Bobbs-Merrill Company, 1959), p. 47.

40. Kant, *Foundations,* p. 47 (italics added).

41. For problems with Kant's vision of animals as instruments to our ends, see Mary Midgley, "Persons and Non-Persons," in *In Defense of Animals,* ed. Peter Singer (Oxford: Basil Blackwell, 1985), esp. pp. 56–57; Alexander Broadie and E. Pybus, "Kant's Treatment of Animals," *Philosophy* 49 (1974): 375–76.

42. Kant, "Duties in Regard to Animals," in Regan-Singer, pp. 23–24 (italics added).

43. Kant, *Foundations,* p. 58. Kant added that the dignity deriving from this capacity is of a priceless worth that animals do not have: "[Each person] possesses a dignity (an absolute inner worth) whereby he exacts the respect of all other rational beings. . . . The humanity in one's person is the object of the respect which he can require of every other human being." Kant, "The Metaphysical Principles of Virtue," pt. 1, James W. Ellington trans., in Kant, *Ethical Philosophy* (Indianapolis: Hackett Publishing Co., 1983), pp. 97–98.

44. See Tom Regan, *The Case for Animal Rights* (Berkeley: University of California Press, 1983), pp. 178, 182–84.

45. Regan, *Case for Animal Rights,* pp. 236–37; idem, "Animals, Treatment of," p. 44; and selection in Regan-Singer, p. 111.

46. Regan, *Case for Animal Rights,* pp. 236–37.

47. Ibid., pp. 240, 243, 258–61.

48. Cf. H. L. A. Hart, "Bentham on Legal Rights," in *Oxford Essays in Jurisprudence,* 2nd ser., ed. A. W. B. Simpson (Oxford: Oxford University Press, 1973), pp. 171–98.

49. See Joel Feinberg, *Social Philosophy* (Englewood Cliffs, NJ: Prentice-Hall, 1973), p. 67.

50. See David Braybrooke, "The Firm but Untidy Correlativity of Rights and Obligations," *Canadian Journal of Philosophy* 1 (1972): 351–63.

51. In evaluating such claims, it should be recognized that not all uses of the word *obligation* entail correlative rights. For example, we sometimes refer to obligations of charity, and no person can claim another person's charity as a matter of right. In this instance, obligation takes the form of a self-imposed obligation and is *not literally a moral (or a legal) obligation.* The correlativity relation holds only for moral obligations that everyone similarly situated would have—namely, those required by a system of law or social morality.

52. Carl Cohen, "The Case for the Use of Animals in Research," *New England Journal of Medicine* 315 (1986): 865–70, esp. pp. 865–66.

53. Joel Feinberg, "The Rights of Animals and Future Generations," in Regan-Singer, pp. 190–96.

54. Alan Donagan, *The Theory of Morality* (Chicago: University of Chicago Press, 1977), pp. 63–66.

55. Claude Bernard, *An Introduction to the Study of Experimental Medicine,* trans. Henry C. Greene (New York: Dover, 1957), pp. 59ff; see also Nicolaas A. Rupke, ed., *Vivisection in Historical Perspective* (London: Croom Helm, 1987).

56. In the discussion that follows, it is generally assumed that the term *animals* refers exclusively to nonhuman vertebrates—although it is not assumed that the question of research involving invertebrates does not deserve ethical analysis.

57. For several aspects of this problem, see J. A. Smith and K. M. Boyd, eds., *Lives in the Balance: The Ethics of Using Animals in Biomedical Research,* the Report of a Working Party of the Institute of Medical Ethics (Oxford: Oxford University Press, 1991).

58. See a debate on this issue involving Andrew Rowan, Neal D. Barnard, Stephen R. Kaufman, Jack Botting, Adrian R. Morrison, and Madhusree Mukerjee in *Scientific American* (February 1997): 79–93.

59. See US Congress, Office of Technology Assessment, *Alternatives to Animal Use in Research, Testing, and Education* (Washington: GPO, 1986); William Paton, *Man and Mouse: Animals in Medical Research* (Oxford: Oxford University Press, 1984).

60. APA, Committee on Animal Research and Ethics (Washington: APA, 1985, as revised 1993).

61. See Rebecca Dresser, "Standards for Animal Research: Looking at the Middle," *Journal of Medicine and Philosophy* 13 (1988): 123–43; Lawrence Finsen, "Institutional Animal Care and Use Committees: A New Set of Clothes for the Emperor?" *Journal of Medicine and Philosophy* 13 (1988): 145–58.

62. See F. Barbara Orlans, *In the Name of Science* (New York: Oxford University Press, 1993), chap. 5 and appendix B.

63. W. M. S. Russell and R. L. Burch, *The Principles of Humane Experimental Technique* (London: Methuen and Company, 1959; reprint, Dover Publications and Potters Bar, UK: Universities Federation for Animal Welfare, 1992).

64. For example four prestigious academic institutions in the United States have created centers for the study and development of animal alternatives. These include the In Vitro Toxicology Laboratory at the Rockefeller University, the Center for Alternatives to Animal Testing at the Johns Hopkins University, the Center for Alternatives at the University of California, Davis, and the Center for Animals and Public Policy at the Tufts University School of Veterinary Medicine. In addition, the partners of the European Union have founded an alternatives research center in Italy.

65. See A. N. Rowan and K. A. Andrutis, "Alternatives: A Socio-Political Commentary from the USA," *ATLA* 18 (1990): 3–10; H. Lansdell, "The Three Rs: A Restrictive

and Refutable Rigmarole," *Ethics and Behaviour* 3 (1993), esp. p. 183; NIH, *Plan for the Use of Animals in Research* (Washington: NIH, 1993); Gary Francione, "Access to Animal Care Committees," *Rutgers Law Review* 43 (1990): 1–14.

66. Cohen, "Case for the Use of Animals in Research," pp. 866, 868.

67. See F. Barbara Orlans, "Research Protocol for Animal Welfare," *Investigative Radiology* 22 (1987): 253–58.

68. Cohen, "Case for the Use of Animals in Research," pp. 868–69.

69. Ibid., p. 869; and also Cohen's "Animal Experimentation Defended," in S. Garattini and D. W. van Bekkum, eds., *The Importance of Animal Experimentation for Safety and Biomedical Research* (Boston: Kluwer Academic, 1990): 7–16, esp. p. 15.

70. The authors of the present book have searched every available database for a study that would confirm or refute such claims and have not found significant studies on the point.

71. *Life,* 4 February 1966, pp. 22–29.

72. The US Public Health Service policy is published in two parts: Institute of Laboratory Animal Resources, National Research Council, *Guide for the Care and Use of Laboratory Animals* (Washington: National Academy Press, 1996); and Office of the Director, NIH, *Public Health Service Policy on Humane Care and Use of Laboratory Animals* (Washington: NIH, revised 1986; reprint, March 1996).

73. R. A. Whitney Jr. "Animal Care and Use Committees: History and Current National Policies in the United States," *Laboratory Animal Science* 37 (January 1987), Special Supplement, pp. 18–21.

74. Orlans, *In the Name of Science,* chaps. 6–7; Rebecca Dresser, "Review Standards for Animal Research: A Closer Look," *ILAR News* 32, 1990 no. 4: 2–7.

75. 7 USC 2131–59 (1993). Regulations implementing this act are in 9 CFR, subchapter A, pts. 1–3.

76. Council for International Organizations of Medical Sciences (CIOMS), World Health Organization, *International Guiding Principles for Biomedical Research Involving Animals* (1984) (Geneva: CIOMS)..

77. *Public Health Service Policy on Humane Care and Use of Laboratory Animals* (Bethesda, MD: NIH, Revised 1986).

78. Canadian Council on Animal Care, *Guide to the Care and Use of Experimental Animals,* vols. 1–2 (Ottawa: Canadian Council on Animal Care, 1980, 1984). See also its "Ethics of Animal Investigation" (revised 1989), a set of principles.

79. National Health and Medical Research Council, *Australian Code of Practice for the Care and Use of Animals for Scientific Purposes,* as revised 1989 (Canberra: Australian Government Publishing Service, 1990).

80. On the background and nature of the problem, see Rollin, *The Unheeded Cry: Animal Consciousness, Animal Pain, and Science,* chap. 5, esp. pp. 118ff.

81. See Bernard Rollin, "Animal Pain," in Regan-Singer, pp. 60ff.

82. See Orlans, *In the Name of Science,* pp. 58–60.

83. Daniel Callahan and Sissela Bok, *The Teaching of Ethics in Higher Education* (Hastings-on-Hudson, NY: Hastings Center, 1980), p. 69.

84. John Arras, "Principles and Particularity: The Role of Cases in Bioethics," *Indiana Law Journal* 69 (1994): 983–1014; Albert Jonsen and Stephen Toulmin, *The Abuse of Casuistry* (Berkeley: University of California Press, 1988), pp. 11–19, 66–67, 251–54, 296–99; Albert Jonsen, "Practice versus Theory," *Hastings Center Report* 20 (1990): 32–34; idem, "Casuistry as Methodology in Clinical Ethics," *Theoretical Medicine* 12 (1991): 299–302.

85. "Animals, Science, and Ethics," *Hastings Center Report* 20 (May/June 1990), Special Supplement, pp. 1–32.

86. *Hastings Center Report* 20 (November/December 1990), Letters, p. 43. See also R. J. White, "Animal Rights versus Human Rights", *Surgical Neurology* 30, no. 5 (November 1988): 410–11.

87. Robert J. White, "Anti-Vivisection: The Reluctant Hydra," *American Scholar* 40 (1971): 503–12, esp. p. 507.

II

BIOMEDICAL RESEARCH

2

BABOON-HUMAN LIVER TRANSPLANTS: THE PITTSBURGH CASE

In the summer of 1992, physicians at the University of Pittsburgh performed a lengthy operation to replace the failing liver of a 35-year-old man with the liver of a 15-year-old male baboon. The man's own liver had been destroyed by the hepatitis-B virus. He also had been infected with human immunodeficiency virus (HIV, the virus that causes AIDS) for at least five years. The patient was deemed ineligible for a human liver transplant because it was feared that the new organ would also be destroyed by the hepatitis. Baboon livers are believed to be resistant to this disease.[1]

Although more than 25 doctors observed the surgery, the patient's identity was kept confidential.[2] By the time the transplant was performed, he required continuous hospital care and had lapsed into a coma. The physicians felt that he was near death and in urgent need of a replacement liver.[3]

Five days after the operation, the patient was able to eat and walk, and after one month, he was transferred out of the intensive care unit. However, he suffered from several infections, renal failure, and other health problems that required treatment. About two months after the procedure, the patient was readmitted because he had become jaundiced. Two weeks later, he had a massive stroke and died.[4]

Physicians attributed the patient's death to an infection that had entered his brain. The HIV infection did not appear to contribute to the death. Surgeon

Thomas Starzl speculated that the transplant team's extreme concern that the patient's body would reject the liver led them to oversuppress the patient's immune system.[5] On autopsy the liver appeared healthy, but physicians could not rule out rejection as a partial cause of the patient's death.[6] Autopsy results also engendered speculation that the baboon liver is metabolically unable to function in a human being.[7]

Despite the patient's death after a relatively short period, his doctors were optimistic. According to Starzl, "The state of the liver after more than 70 days was really remarkably good."[8] Starzl was particularly pleased by the baboon liver's ability to regenerate to the larger adult human's size, as well as by the presence of baboon DNA in the patient's blood, heart, and other parts of his body.[9] On the basis of the results in their first attempt, the Pittsburgh group planned to undertake future baboon-human liver transplants.[10] At a meeting in the spring of 1993, Starzl predicted, "It would not be surprising if successful xenotransplantation [in humans] were achieved within the next 6 to 12 months."[11]

Public reaction to the transplant was varied. The event sparked protests by animal advocates outside the hospital. Animal welfare and animal rights groups criticized the treatment of animals as "spare parts." They argued that xenografts should be a last resort when all alternative methods to increase the supply of transplant organs are proven inadequate.[12] Some scientists and other commenta-

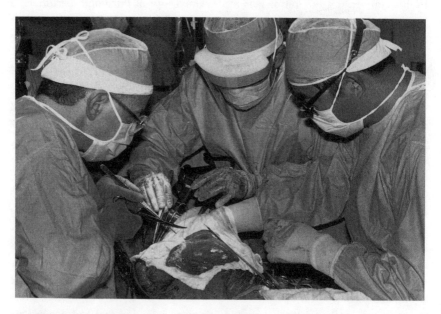

Surgeons at the University of Pittsburgh Medical Center preparing the baboon liver for the first such transplantation into a human being in the summer of 1992. Credit: University of Pittsburgh Medical Center.

tors also viewed the transplant as premature and unsupported by adequate data indicating that it could successfully prolong the patient's life.[13] A speaker at the spring meeting where Starzl expressed his optimism about xenografts said Starzl "vastly overstates the potential for xenotransplantation."[14] Concern was also expressed about the risk that baboon organs could infect human recipients with contagious viral infections, which could lead to a serious epidemic.[15]

The baboon whose liver was taken came from a large colony of baboons operated by the Southwest Foundation for Research and Education, in San Antonio, Texas. This procedure required killing the baboon. Although he was screened for the presence of disease, the Pittsburgh researchers reportedly did not inform the foundation that they planned to use him as a xenograft source. An associate at the foundation said that if they had known the intended use, "[g]reat effort would have been made to find a 'cleaner' baboon."[16] In fact, the baboon was infected with several viruses, as is common among baboons. According to many scientists, diagnostic tests are not available for many viruses infecting nonhuman primates.[17]

HISTORICAL CONTEXT

Cross-species transplantation, also called xenografting, was first attempted in the early twentieth century. Since then there have been numerous cases in which physicians sought to extend human life by substituting a nonhuman animal's kidney, heart, or liver for that of a human patient. In the most successful case, a patient in the early 1960s survived for nine months after receiving a chimpanzee kidney. Because of the poor outcomes, few nonhuman-to-human transplants were performed after the 1960s.[18]

Organ rejection is a major barrier to cross-species transplantation. The human immune system is designed to attack foreign tissue. Even human-to-human transplants (allografts) are vulnerable to failure due to the recipient's hostile immunologic response to the new organ. The greater the immunologic difference between the organ source and recipient, the greater the chance of organ rejection. Transplants between members of the same species are most likely to succeed, and transplants between members of species with similar genetic background have a better chance of working than those between members of distantly related species. Scientists refer to genetically similar species as "concordant," and distantly related species as "discordant."[19]

Beginning in the 1980s, a variety of new developments enabled transplant teams to improve their success rates in performing human-to-human transplants. Much of their increased success was due to the advent of more powerful immunosuppressive drugs, which reduce the possibility of rejection without destroying the body's ability to stave off infection. The availability of these drugs, together with other research advances, has made some scientists hopeful that future xenografts will fare better than they have in the past.[20]

A new phase of xenografting began in 1984, when Dr. Leonard Bailey and his colleagues at Loma Linda University Medical Center replaced a human infant's heart with that of a baboon. The "Baby Fae" case attracted public and scientific interest, even though this patient met the same fate as her predecessors, dying twenty days after the surgery.[21] After this case, scientists pursued further research on xenografts between a variety of nonhuman species. The Pittsburgh baboon liver xenograft was based on this work, as well as on the belief that liver xenografts were less susceptible to rejection than other vital organs.[22]

Besides the recent Loma Linda and Pittsburgh attempts to implant nonhuman organs as permanent replacements for human ones, physicians have begun to use nonhuman organs as "bridges" to sustain patients temporarily until human organs can be procured. In a few cases, physicians have maintained the lives of patients by using pig livers and cells to cleanse the patients' blood for a short period before human livers were located.[23] In addition, scientists have performed transplants of baboon bone marrow in hopes of repairing the immune systems of people with AIDS.[24]

ETHICAL ISSUES IN THE USE OF ANIMALS

Xenografts raise a number of issues about the ethics of research on animals, including several of the basic issues explored in the introduction to this volume.

Utilitarian Issues of Harm and Benefit

To perform the Pittsburgh transplant, investigators killed a healthy male baboon in his early adult years. The xenograft proposal was reviewed by the University of Pittsburgh's Institutional Animal Care and Use Committee and approved on grounds that harm to the animal was justified by the procedure's potential contribution to human health and the advancement of knowledge.

To evaluate this utilitarian justification of animal use requires assessment of the relevant harms and the benefits. (See chapter 1.) On one utilitarian calculus, the benefits of the research, especially for humans, outweigh both the harms to experimental animals and the risks to human subjects. On a competing utilitarian calculus, the harms and risks outweigh the benefits. Harms to the donor-baboon and potential harms to human beings—the recipient as well as other humans who might become infected with a virus should an epidemic ensue—are all factors in the utilitarian calculus.

Harms involved in xenografts

First, what harms, if any, were experienced by the animal? The procedure itself probably did not impose significant experiential burdens on the baboon. We can assume that death occurred when he was fully anesthetized and was not painful or distressing to the animal. He probably experienced some fear, distress, and the like at being removed from his customary habitat and companions, transported to Pittsburgh, and subjected to various tests and procedures preliminary to the terminal surgery he underwent. The more significant harms to the animal probably occurred during his life in captivity.

In her book *Almost Human,* primatologist Shirley Strum describes the rich and complex lives of baboons living in troops on the African savannah.[25] Individual baboons have a variety of intricate and demanding social relationships with other members of their troops. They engage in a multitude of activities, including communication, reciprocal grooming, play, and infant care, which is performed by both sexes. Although life in captivity offers protection from certain natural and human threats encountered by freely ranging baboons, it also provides baboons with many fewer opportunities to exercise their normal mental, social, and physical capacities. It is possible that captive baboons experience frustration and other forms of subjective deprivation from their relatively sterile environments. The extent of these experiential deprivations probably varies according to the degree to which the animals are confined, isolated from their conspecifics and other animals, and so forth.

Potential benefits involved in xenografts

Successful organ transplantation (whether from a human or a nonhuman) supplies the benefit of extending the lives and reducing the suffering of human beings, whose cognitive lives and social relationships in most cases make preservation of life especially valuable. Physicians and researchers have turned to xenografts because there is a serious shortage of human organs available for transplantation. Although polls report that a high percentage of Americans respond that they would be willing to donate their organs, they often do not follow through with these intentions. Because the most suitable organs come from patients who have died as a result of sudden trauma, family members may be too preoccupied with their grief to respond positively to a request for donation. As a result of the shortage, many people have died because no organs were available. Others who would benefit from kidney transplants can survive only by undergoing dialysis, which is more costly and less effective than a transplant would be. In 1992 it was estimated that nearly 15,000 people on the transplant waiting list would not receive the organs they needed.[26]

Many efforts have been and are being made to increase the number of people who donate their own or their deceased relatives' organs. For example, several laws now require hospital personnel to ask the families of all patients who have died about organ and tissue donation. Programs to educate the public and hospital personnel about the need for organs have also been implemented. Physicians have made efforts to improve organ preservation in persons who have died so as to increase the number of organs medically suitable for transplantation.[27]

Proposals to alter existing human organ procurement practices and policies also have emerged. Examples of such strategies include: (1) providing monetary compensation to persons who promise to donate their organs upon death and to families who agree to donate the organs of their deceased relatives; (2) adopting "presumed consent" laws that permit tissue and organ procurement from persons who will undergo an autopsy and have failed during their lives to record their opposition to organ removal; (3) more extensive use of living human volunteers as sources of kidneys, livers, lungs, bone marrow, and pancreases, although these procedures present some degree of risk to the donor; and (4) developing mechanical devices as replacement organs.

A variety of ethical, social, and technical impediments make it unlikely that any of these strategies will meet the demand for organs in the foreseeable future. Moreover, even if they were able to meet the existing need, it is probable that the waiting list for organs would then expand to include others who would benefit from transplants but are not now on the list due to their age, medical condition, financial status, or residence in underdeveloped countries.[28] Given that none of these alternatives is satisfactory, xenografting remains an important experimental procedure in the attempt to benefit humans by extending their lives. The hope is that xenografts will eventually alleviate at least some of the current scarcity of transplantable organs, saving the lives of many humans who would otherwise die.

Loss of a Life

What did the baboon liver "donor" lose by being denied the opportunity to live out his natural life? Here a mere utilitarian assessment in terms of harms and benefits may not be the most appropriate way to frame the issues about what the animal has lost. Perhaps this baboon has been wronged without being harmed, in the standard sense of *harm*. To take the animal's life caused a loss, but perhaps did not cause a harm. What is this loss, and what ethical issues are at stake? (On some of the underlying issues about the value of animal life, see chapter 1.)

The losses involved in a premature death are difficult to assess for human beings, but even more difficult for animals because we understand so little about their mental life. One reason we view even a completely painless premature death as a moral issue for humans is that it cuts short the individual's desires and hopes about the future. Another reason is such a death often has negative effects on family, friends, and others whose lives were touched by the now absent individual.[29] As we discussed in chapter 1 of this volume, these human losses may have parallels in the animal world. It seems reasonable to say that the loss sustained in the baboon's death was a function of his cognitive abilities and relationships with others. Whether or not baboons have a sense of the future and an ability to plan for the future is unclear, although Strum's work indicates that baboons in the wild possess an extensive capacity for short- and long-term memory. She also observed that most male baboons had adult female and infant "friends," and that it was possible, though uncertain, that some baboons who died were missed by their families and friends.

Some might argue that the moral costs of ending a captive baboon's life are reduced because the captive animal has a less rich cognitive and social existence than a wild baboon. We do not know the exact nature of the Pittsburgh baboon's prior opportunities for cognitive activity, nor do we know the extent and nature of his relationships with baboon companions or companions of other species. In light of what we do know, however, we should acknowledge the possibility that this baboon's death constituted a loss that requires justification beyond the utilitarian benefits that flow from use of the animal.

Alternatives to the Baboon Xenograft

It has long been held that researchers have obligations to perform their work without animals, if possible, and with the minimum number of animals, if not. Were there any realistic alternatives to killing a baboon in this effort to save a human life? If so, how important is this moral issue? Is this issue again reducible to a utilitarian calculation of harms and benefits, or are there reasons to favor alternatives that are independent of the harm-benefit calculus?

As we have seen, attempts to increase the rates of human organ donation have been inadequate to meet the demand. In the Pittsburgh case, it was believed that a human liver would not provide the patient with long-term survival, since the hepatitis virus would probably attack the human organ.

Other nonhuman species are possible candidates for organ sources. Chimpanzees have an estimated 99% genetic similarity with humans; thus, chimpanzee-human transplants have a higher chance of success than those between the more distantly related humans and baboons. Chimpanzees, however, are believed to possess even more complex cognitive and social abilities than baboons, so that a chimpanzee's death would arguably amount to an even greater ethical cost than that of a baboon. Moreover, chimpanzees are an endangered species, and may not be imported from their native habitats for research purposes. The captive US population available for lethal research is extremely limited and is unlikely to grow substantially in the foreseeable future, because chimpanzees reproduce at a relatively slow rate.[30]

Baboons are viewed as more attractive organ sources than other nonhuman primates because they are "common and easy to grow in captivity."[31] Yet there are reportedly no more than three thousand captive baboons available for research in the United States at present.[32] Moreover, baboons also require relatively lengthy periods between the births of their offspring. Although baboons are plentiful in Africa, it would be costly and impractical to capture them for transplantation programs. For these reasons, it is believed that baboon organ transplantation could not in itself produce an adequate supply of vital organs.[33]

Wild and domestic baboons also harbor viruses that make them less than ideal organ sources for humans.[34] Although scientists are able to screen animal donors for some pathogens, screening tests are not available for all baboon viruses. Moreover, a human organ recipient could be vulnerable to an as yet undiscovered animal disease. In the worst-case scenario, a contagious disease could spread to other persons exposed to the xenograft recipient. Would it be ethically defensible to expose others to this small but serious threat, in order to advance the xenograft recipient's interests?

The limited supply of potential primate organ sources, as well as concern about disease transmission and the ethical propriety of using a "distant family member"[35] in lethal research, have led researchers to target instead certain livestock species as the ultimate xenograft sources. Many scientists have selected pigs as the ideal source, in light of the pig's physiological similarities to humans and its easy availability. The major existing impediment to success is the extreme rejection reaction that accompanies transplantation between such discordant species. However, many scientists believe that genetic engineering techniques eventually will enable them to produce pigs and other donor animals that do not provoke the hostile immune response that occurs when a normal nonprimate organ is implanted into a human. In addition, though there is some risk of disease transmission, scientists believe that potentially harmful viruses might be more easily be avoided in pigs.[36]

Some animal advocates have responded that the loss of a pig's life is no less ethically troubling than the loss of a baboon's life, because pigs are sentient, cognitively complex mammals. Even pigs, they argue, are "subjects of a life" (see chapter 1) who have the right not to be killed merely for the benefit of others, human or nonhuman.[37] Animal advocates who do not subscribe to this theory still oppose current xenografting work on grounds that efforts to increase the rate of human organ donation should be pursued instead.[38] Before turning to an examination of whether xenografting holds promise for genuine benefit to humankind, one more proposed alternative to xenografting deserves consideration.

Is Xenografting Speciesist?

Speciesism is the view that members of a particular species (in this case *Homo sapiens*) are superior to other species, simply by virtue of the individual's membership in that species. Those who believe that xenografting is speciesist argue that some human beings are more appropriate donors than some nonhuman donors. Again, this argument is independent of questions of the harm-benefit calculus. It has often been argued that speciesism is an unwarranted form of discrimination against animals even if a favorable harm-benefit analysis exists. (On the nature of speciesism, see chapter 1.)

Human cadavers are now the primary source of livers for transplantation. Although physicians at a few facilities have achieved some good outcomes by transplanting segments of livers taken from live, competent, and consenting human donors into biologically related recipients, it is unclear whether this procedure will be successful in the long run.[39] Even if it is, many patients in need will not be fortunate enough to have immunologically compatible relatives willing to expose themselves to the risks of live donation. There also is concern that relatives will feel undue pressure to agree to donate to a very ill family member. In response to this situation, some commentators believe that we are morally obligated to look elsewhere for an expanded source of human vital organs.

Current law permits whole organs to be removed solely from humans who meet the legal criteria for death: irreversible cessation of either respiratory and circulatory function or total brain function. Some opponents of xenografting have argued that it would be ethically acceptable to obtain organs for transplant from severely brain-damaged humans now defined as alive.[40] Anencephalic infants, who are incapable of consciousness because they lack a functioning cortex and who inevitably die within a short time after birth, are one possible source. Permanently unconscious human children and adults are another.

Why not change the law, xenograft opponents ask, to permit these patients' families to donate their relatives' organs? These human organs would not only provide recipients with a much better chance of survival, given their greater genetic compatibility, they would also come from individuals who, unlike many animals, have no capacity for cognition, emotion, or social interaction. On this view, it would be more defensible to kill a permanently unconscious human being to obtain transplant organs than to kill a conscious living nonhuman mammal for this purpose.

Other critics of the status quo contend that it is difficult to defend using nonhuman primates and other mammals as transplant sources while excluding as sources mentally disabled humans with mental capacities equivalent to those of the animals.[41] The highly controversial opinion of one observer is, "If a primate's capability was higher than that of a human—say, a severely mentally handicapped child—I think it would be appropriate to support the opposite approach of Baby Fae, [which would be] a transplant from a child to save the life of a healthy baboon or chimpanzee."[42]

Those opposed to using mentally compromised humans as organ sources believe that the practice would pose too great a threat both to mentally disabled people and to the general ethical principle of respect for human life.[43] In their view, such a move would violate society's basic moral prohibition on using one human being solely for the benefit of another, a prohibition that became prominent after the horrors of Nazi experimentation on nonconsenting persons and related problems in medical and research ethics.

ETHICAL ISSUES IN HUMAN EXPERIMENTATION AND HEALTH POLICY

In reaching an overall moral assessment of xenografting, the ethical questions raised by the use of animals as organ sources for humans cannot easily be isolated from ethical questions raised by (1) the use of humans as research subjects in the xenograft experiments and (2) the use of both health care and animal resources in pursuing these projects. Few people doubt that xenografting is providing useful scientific information and could someday provide major scientific and health care benefits. But is that time near, and are we using resources appropriately in pursuing these goals?

Experimentation on Human Beings

Although prior human-animal transplants had been performed, the Pittsburgh case constituted the first attempt to implant a baboon liver into a human being. In contrast to purely therapeutic interventions, scientists and physicians undertake experimental procedures in humans for two major reasons: (1) to benefit the experimental subject and (2) to produce knowledge that could help other people in the future. At this stage in its development, xenografting remains an experimental procedure with an unproven potential for therapeutic benefit.

As part of the government's program to protect the rights and interests of human research subjects, experimentation on human beings is governed by special institutional and regulatory requirements. All proposals for such experimentation must be reviewed by an institutional review board (IRB), which must include community and nonscientist members. The IRB review process is designed to ensure that research proposals comply with applicable regulatory requirements.[44] Prior to conducting human studies, scientists must lay a solid foundation in animal and other types of research suggesting an intervention's potential value to human beings.

The IRB also considers the ethical justification for conducting research on particular groups of human beings. Certain population groups, such as children and mentally disabled persons, are regarded as needing special protection from the potential harm that research participation can inflict. It is generally agreed that members of these vulnerable groups should not be among the first humans to experience a novel procedure, medical device, or drug.[45] The Baby Fae xenograft was criticized on this basis, although Dr. Bailey contended that his choice of an infant was supported by the near-absence of human infant organs available for transplant and his belief that the infant immune system would be less likely than an adult's to reject a nonhuman organ (a belief which later was shown to be erroneous).[46]

The first baboon liver recipient was an adult man with no reported mental impairment that could compromise his capacity to understand and consent to the risks entailed in the procedure. Two significant questions remain, however. One is the extent of the information that was disclosed to him before he made his decision to go forward with the transplant. Without having more information on the consent form and the process by which consent was obtained, it is impossible to judge whether the Pittsburgh liver recipient was sufficiently forewarned about both the poor outcomes in prior human-nonhuman transplants and the potential experiential burdens that could accompany any prolonged life the baboon liver was able to provide him. We do not know, for example, whether he was told that even if the procedure prolonged his life, he might never be healthy enough to leave the hospital.

The second significant ethical question concerns the propriety of asking a terminally ill person to undergo such an unproven procedure. Although terminally ill persons are often viewed as having "nothing to lose" from participating in a research protocol, this attitude is unjustified. Experimental interventions can hasten a terminally ill person's death; they can also compromise the quality of the life that remains. Terminally ill research subjects whose deaths might otherwise have been relatively comfortable may instead suffer added pain, distress, and other experiential harms. At the same time, dying patients are especially vulnerable to the influence of any unrealistically positive expectations expressed by the research team.

Critics of the Pittsburgh xenograft contended that it was inappropriate to propose the surgery to "someone who may have felt he had little choice."[47] Apparently, members of the university's IRB did not believe that either concerns about the procedure's burdens, or the subject's vulnerable status as a terminally ill patient, were serious enough to merit a decision disapproving the xenograft. Indeed, the committee gave its approval for Starzl's team to conduct up to four baboon-human liver transplants.[48]

The apparent ease with which protocols are often approved for human subjects has its parallels in the approval of protocols for the use of animals. Many critics believe that both forms of review need considerable tightening.

Problems in Health Policy

Temporary xenografts are ineffective in decreasing the number of humans who die for want of a replacement organ. They do, however, provide an opportunity to collect data that could advance the goal of developing successful long-term xenografts; transplant surgeons anticipate that the work done to date will have precisely this effect. Moreover, it is possible that at some future time newly developed immunosuppressive drugs, innovations in transplantation techniques, or genetic manipulations of pigs or other species will produce xenografts capable of serving as long-term replacement organs in humans.

Is this goal one that society ought to pursue vigorously through experimental transplantation, or should it be pursued in alternative ways? This question must be considered in the context of a broader set of issues about organ transplantation as representative of the "high-tech" approach to health care. Millions of people in the US lack access to basic health care because they do not have the money to pay for it. Is it appropriate to devote scarce health care resources to developing a procedure such as xenografting, which is destined to remain expensive and can help only a relatively small number of the people in need of health care?[49] Similarly, is it appropriate to devote scarce resources in the form of research animals to developing a procedure such as xenografting?

Some commentators have raised similar questions about the entire transplantation enterprise. Renée Fox and Judith Swazey, two sociologists who have personally observed and written on organ transplantation for many years, recently announced that they are "leaving the field," partially because of their concerns about the inequities present in the existing health care system.[50]

Others challenge this perspective. They contend that organ transplantation is a wise investment of our health care dollars.[51] As for xenografts, these analysts say, it is too early to tell whether they will eventually confer substantial long-term survival benefits on recipients, but there is no reason to think they will not.[52] Moreover, some claim that successful xenografting could actually reduce the current costs of organ procurement.[53]

Fox and Swazey are not troubled solely by the disproportionate share of resources they believe is now devoted to organ transplantation. They also attack what they call the "death-denying" attitudes underlying the current state of affairs. In their view, the "overly zealous medical and social commitment to the endless perpetuation of life and to repairing and rebuilding people through organ replacement" produces extreme suffering in the many patients who, because their replacement organs fail to function properly, die after a period of prolonged discomfort or survive with a quality of life that is unacceptable to them.[54] Patients who have received organs from animals are a prime example, though their numbers are small.

CONCLUSION

It remains to be seen whether society is ready to engage in a reassessment of the current campaign to increase the supply of organs or organ substitutes for transplantation. Although there is evidence that some people are beginning to question the wisdom of the current emphasis on the high-tech rescue medicine that transplantation exemplifies, there are also solid indications that the goal of conquering organ failure has strong support among many health care practitioners and policy makers. Following the Pittsburgh baboon liver transplant, it was announced that teams at several other hospitals were "gearing up for similar operations in the near future."[55] One company developing genetically altered pigs has plans for immediate xenograft trials.[56] Support for xenografting seems unlikely to diminish in the next few years.

NOTES

1. Thomas E. Starzl et al., "Baboon-to-Human Liver Transplantation," *Lancet* 341 (9 January 1993): 65–71; Lawrence K. Altman, "Terminally Ill Man Gets Baboon's Liver in Untried Operation," *New York Times,* 29 June 1992, p. A1.
2. Altman, "Terminally Ill Man," p. A1.
3. Starzl et al., "Baboon-to-Human," p. 66.
4. Ibid., pp. 67–68.
5. Ibid., p. 70.
6. Ibid.
7. Andrew A. Skolnick, "Transplantation Pioneer Predicts Successful Xenotransplantation Soon," *Journal of the American Medical Association* 269 (16 June 1993): 2958.
8. Franklin Hoke, "Undaunted by Death of First Baboon Liver Recipient, Interdisciplinary Transplant Team Looks to the Future," *Scientist* 28 (September 1992): 1.
9. Starzl et al., "Baboon-to-Human," pp. 67, 70.
10. Starzl and his team performed a second baboon-to-human transplant on January 10, 1993. This patient died from an infection after 26 days, never having fully regained consciousness. "Baboon Liver Recipient Dies after Infection," *New York Times,* 6 February 1993, p. A7.
11. Skolnick, "Transplantation Pioneer," p. 2951. Starzl's group had not performed any more baboon liver transplants as of August 1997, however. At a meeting in June of 1995, he expressed doubt that xenotransplantation was close to clinical success. Mark J. Hanson, "The Seductive Sirens of Medical Progress," *Hastings Center Report* 25 (September/October 1995): 5.
12. Lantz Miller, "Baboon Liver Transplant Stirs Hope and Rage," *Lab Animal* 21 (October 1992): 8; Sally Squires, "Organs from Animals," *Washington Post,* 14 July 1992, p. Z9.
13. Hoke, "Undaunted by Death," p. 6.
14. Skolnick, "Transplantation Pioneer," p. 2951.
15. Rachel Nowak, "Hope or Horror? Primate-to-Human Organ Transplants," *Journal of NIH Research* 4 (September 1992): 37.
16. Nowak, "Hope or Horror?" p. 37. To address this concern, the US Public Health Service is preparing rules for clinical investigations of xenografts. US Department of Health and Human Services, "Draft Public Health Service Guideline on Infectious Diseases in Xenotransplantation," *Federal Register* 61 (23 September 1996): 49920–32.

17. Louisa E. Chapman et al., "Xenotransplantation and Xenogenic Infections," *New England Journal of Medicine* 333 (30 November 1995): 1498–1501.

18. Council on Scientific Affairs, American Medical Association, "Xenografts: Review of the Literature and Current Status," *Journal of the American Medical Association* 254 (20 December 1985): 3353–55; Arthur Caplan, "Ethical Issues Raised by Research Involving Xenografts," *Journal of the American Medical Association* 254 (20 December 1985): 3340.

19. John Najarian, "Overview of In Vivo Xenotransplantation Studies: Prospects for the Future," *Transplantation Proceedings* 24 (April 1992): 733–38.

20. Hoke, "Undaunted by Death," p. 6.

21. Alexander M. Capron, "When Well-Meaning Science Goes Too Far," *Hastings Center Report* 15 (February 1985): 8–9; George J. Annas, "Baby Fae: The 'Anything Goes' School of Human Experimentation," *Hastings Center Report* 15 (February 1985): 15–17.

22. Skolnick, "Transplantation Pioneer," p. 2951.

23. Ravi S. Chari, "Brief Report: Treatment of Hepatic Failure with In Vivo Pig-Liver Perfusion Followed by Liver Transplantation," *New England Journal of Medicine* 331 (1994): 234–37; Hilde L. Nelson, "Perfusion by Pig," *Hastings Center Report* 23 (March/April 1993): 4.

24. The results thus far are equivocal. Lawrence K. Altman, "Baboon Cells Fail to Thrive, but AIDS Patient Improves," *New York Times,* 9 February 1996, p. A8.

25. Shirley Strum, *Almost Human* (New York: W.W. Norton, 1987).

26. Brian McCormick, "Medicine, Law Urged to Focus More on Organ Donations," *American Medical News,* 7 September 1992, p. 6.

27. Arthur L. Caplan, "Is Xenografting Morally Wrong?" *Transplantation Proceedings* 24 (April 1992): 722–24; Robert Arnold and Stuart Youngner, "Back to the Future: Obtaining Organs from Non-Heart-Beating Cadavers," *Kennedy Institute of Ethics Journal* 3 (1993): 103–11.

28. Caplan, "Is Xenografting Morally Wrong?" pp. 722–24.

29. Peter Singer, *Practical Ethics* (Cambridge: Cambridge University Press, 1979), pp. 72–92.

30. Dennis O. Johnson, "The Need for Using Chimpanzees in Research," *Lab Animal* (July/August 1987): 19–23.

31. Miller, "Baboon Liver Transplant," p. 8.

32. Marjorie Shaffer, "Baboon Liver in Man," *Medical World News,* 28 August 1992.

33. Rachel Nowak, "Xenotransplants Set to Resume," *Science* 266 (1994): 1148–51.

34. This has become a major concern in the debate over xenografting. For detailed discussion of the threat, see S. S. Kalter and R. L. Heberling, "Xenotransplantation and Infectious Diseases," *ILAR Journal* 37 (Winter 1995): 31–37; Jonathan S. Allen, "Xenotransplantation at a Crossroads: Prevention versus Progress," *Nature Medicine* 2 (January 1996): 18.

35. David Brown, "Cross Transplantation a Lure, If Not a Cure," *Washington Post,* 14 September 1992, p. A3 (quoting transplant surgeon John Najarian).

36. David Concar, "The Organ Factory of the Future?" *New Scientist* (18 June 1994): 24–29; Allen, "Xenotransplantation at a Crossroads," p. 20.

37. Tom Regan, "The Other Victim," *Hastings Center Report* 15 (February 1985): 9–10; Gary L. Francione, "Xenografts and Animal Rights," *Transplantation Proceedings* 22 (June 1990): 1044–46.

38. Squires, "Organs from Animals," p. Z9 (quoting Martin Stephens, of the Humane Society of the United States).

39. Caplan, "Is Xenografting Morally Wrong?" p. 723.

40. Peter Singer, "Xenotransplantation and Speciesism," *Transplantation Proceedings* 24 (April 1992): 728–32.

41. James L. Nelson, "Moral Sensibilities and Moral Standing: Caplan on Xenograft 'Donors,'" *Bioethics* 7 (1993): 315–22.

42. David Larson, Co-director of the Center for Christian Bioethics at Loma Linda University, as quoted by Suzanne E. Roy, in "We Can't Turn Animals into Spare Parts Shops," letter to the editor in *The New York Times,* 16 July 1992, A24 (quoting an interview published in the *Sacramento Bee*).

43. James L. Nelson, "Transplantation Through a Glass Darkly," *Hastings Center Report* 22 (September/October 1992): 6.

44. DHHS Protection of Human Research Subjects, 45 CFR sec. 46.101–117 (1993); Caplan, "Ethical Issues," p. 3343.

45. Caplan, "Is Xenografting Morally Wrong?" p. 726; Annas, "Baby Fae," pp. 15–16.

46. Olga Jonasson and Mark A. Hardy, "The Case of Baby Fae," *Journal of the American Medical Association* 254 (1985): 3359.

47. "Transplant Trials," *Time,* 29 September 1992, p. 18.

48. Squires, "Organs from Animals," p. Z9.

49. Nelson, "Moral Sensibilities and Moral Standing," p. 313.

50. Renée C. Fox and Judith P. Swazey, "Leaving the Field," *Hastings Center Report* 22 (September/October 1992): 14.

51. Caplan, "Is Xenografting Morally Wrong?" p. 724.

52. Robert M. Veatch, *Death, Dying, and the Biological Revolution,* rev. ed. (New Haven, CT: Yale University Press, 1989), pp. 204–5.

53. Squires, "Organs from Animals," p. Z9 (quoting Dr. John Najarian).

54. Fox and Swazey, "Leaving the Field," p. 15.

55. Squires, "Organs from Animals," p. Z9.

56. Claire O'Brien, "Yellow Light for Pig-Human Transplants," *Science* 271 (8 March 1996): 1357.

3

HEAD INJURY EXPERIMENTS
ON PRIMATES AT THE UNIVERSITY
OF PENNSYLVANIA

During the early morning hours of the Memorial Day holiday weekend, 18 May 1984, five men and women crept across the deserted University of Pennsylvania campus in Philadelphia. They entered the University's Head Trauma Research Center, where head injury studies on baboons were conducted under the direction of Thomas A. Gennarelli, associate professor of neurosurgery. They stole approximately thirty videotapes that had been made by the researchers to record the day-to-day experiments. The videotapes showed baboons in states of paralysis and incapacity and researchers who seemed indifferent to the distress of the animals. Before they left, the intruders also vandalized equipment used in the experiments and wrote on the lab wall their initials, ALF—Animal Liberation Front.

The ALF is a radical organization of about a hundred persons who conduct laboratory raids. Because the ALF is a clandestine group, another national animal rights group, People for the Ethical Treatment of Animals (PETA), handled the ALF's publicity and negotiations in the wake of the Pennsylvania incident. PETA claimed that the videotapes, which they had received from the ALF, provided documentation of repeated, significant violations of federal policies governing the humane use of laboratory animals, including inadequate anesthesia and disregard of legally required surgical asepsis. The experiments were required to be in compliance with two federal policies, one administered by the

National Institutes of Health (NIH),[1] and the other, the Animal Welfare Act, administered by the US Department of Agriculture (USDA).[2]

PETA released excerpts from the videotapes to the media. Major televised networks showed shocking pictures of a baboon repeatedly writhing on a table as a hydraulic piston hit the animal's head. The experimental procedure was to cement the baboon's head securely in a helmet and subject it to a sudden jerking movement delivered by a specially designed device that inflicted "acceleration injury," as in whiplash. The device could generate the equivalent of up to two thousand times the force of gravity. There was no penetrating wound and the neurological damage was caused by the movement of the soft brain mass inside the bony skull. Paralysis and coma were the results. The animals were maintained in their helpless states for up to two months after injury. They were then killed and their brains analyzed.

The investigators claimed that anesthetics were adequate during the procedure and the animals felt no pain, but this was strongly contested. The anesthetic methods used in the baboon studies were approved by the oversight committee of the University of Pennsylvania, but, after the raid, the "facts" about anesthetic use were disputed and assessed differently by different parties (as is not uncommon in discussions of adequate anesthesia for animals). Critics, who were convinced that the animals suffered pain, questioned the choice of anesthetics, dosage used, and overall drug regimen. This critical view was born out

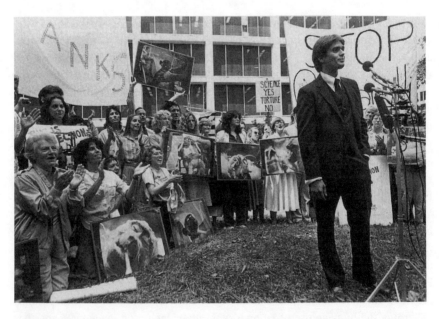

Animal rights demonstrators at the National Institutes of Health, Bethesda, Maryland, in July 1985, protesting against the NIH-funded head injury studies on baboons being conducted at the University of Pennsylvania. At the right is Alex Pacheco, chairperson of People for the Ethical Treatment of Animals. Credit: Montgomery County Journal.

by the subsequent NIH review, which found that violations of NIH's animal welfare policy occurred in anesthetic management.

The experimental sessions to produce the head injuries lasted several hours. In order to sedate the animal in their home cages, they were injected with the dissociative agent PCP, also known by the street-drug name of "angel dust." This drug was used for facilitating animal restraint; it is not a painkiller.

When the animals were brought to the operating room nitrous oxide was administered, the animals were instrumented surgically with blood and other monitors, and their heads were secured in metal helmets and fixed in place in the acceleration device. Nitrous oxide is an inhalant general anesthetic from which the animal can quickly recover consciousness and ability to experience pain. The nitrous oxide was withdrawn up to one hour before the head injury. According to the investigators, only if the experiment went "awry" was the nitrous oxide reinstituted. (Just how the experiments were thought to possibly go awry has not been discovered in any pertinent research document.)

A period of consciousness was needed before the injury for tests of motor reflexes. Under a general anesthetic the results would have been meaningless. Just before the injury, animals were seen in the videotape with their eyes open, twisting on the table in an attempt to turn their bodies over, and in one instance, a technician called out that the animal was "awake" immediately before the injury. Some animals received repeated head blows.

The investigators maintained that the purpose of the research was to develop an animal model to study the functional and anatomical effects of head injury, such as that which occurs in automobile accidents, football, and boxing. However, an investigation indicated that well-formulated scientific hypotheses may not have been tested. The lack of a testable hypothesis was considered poor science by some, but defenders of the work argued that the investigations provided basic information about pathological events.

The case stunned the biomedical community, brought public sympathy for PETA and others critical of animal experiments, and became a cause célèbre that sparked public debate. Media attention was worldwide, and within eighteen months of the raid, Congress enacted a new law that required more stringent oversight of laboratory animal care and use. As a direct result of this case, standards of treatment of laboratory animals have improved. Still today this case is considered one of the most significant cases in the history of the ethical issues involving animal subjects of research.

HISTORY OF THE HEAD TRAUMA STUDIES

There had been several warning signs even before the raids that all was not well regarding animal welfare in the baboon laboratory. The American Anti-Vivisection Society had made public protests about the experiments and, only five months before the raid, the University's Institutional Animal Care and Use Committee (the federally required oversight body) had unanimously found that they were "unable to approve the [baboon] project from the standpoint of the humane treatment of animals."[3] Some corrections were made, and three months later, in March 1983, the work was approved and resumed.

After the raid in 1994 PETA quickly put together a controversially edited, twenty-minute film from the sixty hours of footage of the stolen videotapes and provided several showings to the media. The edited version was entitled *Unnecessary Fuss,*[4] a title selected because Gennarelli stated that he was "not willing to go on record to discuss the laboratory studies because it had the potential to stir up all sorts of unnecessary fuss among those who are sensitive to those kinds of things."[5]

Within days of the raid a University of Pennsylvania spokesperson said that the ALF had leveled "false and misleading attacks on both the quality and integrity of the research . . . [A]fter careful review of procedures used in the laboratory, we are convinced that the actual treatment of the animals conforms to the guidelines for the humane care of experimental animals set forth by the National Institutes of Health."[6] Thomas W. Langfitt, chair of neurosurgery, claimed, "The experiments have provided extremely valuable information on the nature of severe, often irreversible brain damage."[7]

The most influential and oft-quoted defense came from the director of NIH, James B. Wyngaarden, who said that the University of Pennsylvania's head injury clinic is considered to be "one of the best labs in the world."[8] However, Wyngaarden's comments were denounced by the animal rights movement because of his conflict of interest; before he took the position of NIH director, he had been the chairman of the Department of Medicine at the University of Pennsylvania Medical School.

Two months after the first raid, the ALF made two other raids on the university within a few days of each other and thirteen animals were stolen from the veterinary school. An ALF spokesman said that these new raids were to protest the university's "failure to investigate allegations of animal abuse at the school."[9] (Indeed, it was not until 15 months after the first raid that the university issued its report of the formal investigation into the head injury studies.)[10]

The head injury studies were part of a larger program headed by Langfitt that covered both human and animal studies. In 1984 the total NIH grant award to Langfitt was approximately one million dollars: Gennarelli's animal studies received an award of approximately $330,000 per year.

Since federal money funded these experiments, the government was aroused. At congressional hearings on the raid, testimony was presented by representatives from NIH and USDA—two government agencies that had reviewed and approved the experiments. NIH teams of experts had repeatedly found the baboon experiments to be scientifically meritorious. None of the NIH external-review teams had raised issues about animal welfare. Only a few days before the raid, USDA inspectors uncovered only four violations of USDA regulations. However, spurred perhaps by the publicity surrounding the raid, the same veterinary inspector found 74 violations a few days later.[11]

PETA wanted to show *Unnecessary Fuss* at the congressional hearings, but NIH and USDA threatened not to attend if the showing were permitted. PETA then arranged public showings at a nearby church during the lunch break of the hearings. PETA's press release for this event stated: "The graphic footage shows violations of federal regulations and federal and state laws. Researchers perform painful surgery on animals without proper pain relief, reuse surgical instruments that have fallen on the floor, . . . and mock brain-damaged animals."[12] In one sequence in the film, a researcher can be heard to say, "The animal is off anesthesia" just before infliction of the brain injury. The film records the laboratory personnel ridiculing the injured animals for their inability to use their limbs.

The laboratory conditions depicted were such that it was hard going for many to watch the film. Students in some universities reported they felt nauseous and could not stay in the classroom for the duration of the film. Newspaper columnist Henry Mitchell reported that the film made him feel like vomiting, and he could not watch it all.[13] A reporter for *Science* described the tapes as ranging from "embarrassing to disastrous."[14]

The productivity of the baboon work was challenged in some quarters. Ten years were spent on developing the research model and no progress is known to have been made in devising therapeutic interventions or preventive equipment. Nedim Buyukmichi, a veterinarian and president of the Association of Veterinarians for Animal Rights, said that Gennarelli's experimental results were too inconsistent to give a reproducible model and "essentially nothing has come out of this research that hasn't already been known from studies of human head trauma."[15]

Criticisms about productivity of the work were discounted by defenders of Gennarelli's work, including an NIH review team who met subsequent to the raid and voted to renew the government grant for another five years. The funding agency wanted additional numbers of baboons to be used on the basis that the work was scientifically important. The research was also defended by the Society of Neuroscience, the professional association of which Gennarelli and Langfitt were members. The society's three-person investigative committee maintained that there is nothing morally wrong with causing severe head injury to baboons and found that Gennarelli had made "a convincing case that the procedures represent an ethical and humane way to produce an animal model of human head trauma."[16]

Gennarelli maintained to the university and in public that the information gained from the baboon model was a major contribution toward understanding the basic mechanisms responsible for brain damage in head-injured patients. Previously it had been thought that this type of injury could not be produced in experimental animals, thus rendering the research a major breakthrough. Gennarelli maintained that the baboons had been treated humanely.

DELAYS AND COMPROMISES

Institutional Responses

A year passed without progress toward a resolution of the controversy over this research. NIH, USDA, and the university were united in their opposition to PETA's allegations. NIH demanded that PETA unconditionally hand over the sixty-hour version of the tape, and refused to view the edited twenty-minute version on grounds of biased and unfair editing. PETA demanded that NIH include a person who was acceptable to both NIH and PETA to participate in the investigation "to assure that the investigation is verifiably fair and impartial."[17] NIH refused. About a year after the original raid, the tapes were handed over to the USDA and then to NIH.

After the raid, NIH's Office for Protection from Research Risks (OPRR) investigated PETA's allegations. On November 15, 1984, the compliance officer at OPRR wrote to PETA stating that OPRR had been unable to confirm the alleged misconduct because of PETA's failure to provide copies of the videotapes. Later, in May 1985, OPRR conducted a site visit to the head injury laboratory and in June 1985 NIH issued a public report that is described below.

Under some pressure from the University of Pennsylvania's law school, the university's vice provost for research, Barry Cooperman, formed a panel of faculty members to examine the controversial head injury experiments. (The university had originally planned to appoint an outside panel of investigators, but decided against it.) However, Cooperman refused to allow *Unnecessary Fuss* to be shown at the meeting. Thirteen law school professors, including Gary Francione, an animal activist, accused the university of stifling debate and suppressing evidence. Law professor Arnold Morris said, "It seems pretty peculiar that the tape that generated the discussion not be shown."[18] The meeting was angry and inconclusive.

Animal protection sympathizers were frustrated at the nature and slowness of the response from the scientific establishment. By comparison, after the first major raid on an animal facility by the ALF in 1981, known as the Silver Spring monkey case, NIH had acted within four weeks of the raid to halt government funding. However, officials at NIH had developed more cautious attitudes since the Silver Spring monkey case.

After a year in which no investigations were completed by NIH, USDA, or the university, it came as a shock to the animal activists and others to discover that NIH was set to renew Gennarelli's grant for another five years, starting August 1, 1985. Opposed to this funding, members of the animal rights movement urged members of Congress to take action. Some sixty members of Congress petitioned the Secretary of Health and Human Services Margaret M. Heckler to stop the funding of this laboratory. When no action was forthcoming, the activists undertook a major campaign of peaceful civil disobedience to press their case.

NIH Sit-In

Some fourteen months after the initial raid, several NIH offices were occupied by approximately one hundred animal activists from various parts of the US. According to an animal rights report, this sit-in was called "when it became obvious to PETA leaders that they were getting nowhere with letter writing, lobbying and the usual means of protest."[19] Media coverage of the protest was intense. After four days, Secretary Heckler instructed NIH to suspend the use of federal funds.[20]

Secretary Heckler's actions attracted criticism as well as praise. Among the critics, the Association of American Medical Colleges protested that this capitulation to the demands of an "irresponsible advocacy group" increases the vulnerability of academic institutions to further destruction of property and loss of research of incalculable value.[21]

Penalties Imposed

NIH completed a full investigation of compliance with NIH policy, and the investigating committee reported its findings on July 17, 1985. They found there was "material failure" of the university to comply with NIH animal welfare policy.[22] Among the areas of noncompliance cited were deficiencies in the management of anesthesia for the baboons, inadequacy of techniques to achieve sterile environment, inadequacy of the laboratory environment, and inadequate training of laboratory personnel. Experiments were not consistently conducted under the immediate supervision of qualified scientists, and adequate nursing care was not always provided. Use of pain-relieving drugs had not been adequate in either the pre- or post-injury period.

In September 1995, the president and provost of the university issued a public reprimand of Gennarelli and Langfitt for "less than satisfactory discharge of the responsibility expected of research faculty at the university."[23] In November 1985, USDA fined the University of Pennsylvania four thousand dollars for violations of the Animal Welfare Act in the baboon head injury lab.[24] The fine was small by comparison to the seventy million dollars the university had received that year from NIH. The fine was, however, symbolically important as a finding of wrongdoing and culpability.

Within nine months of the funding suspension and in response to the university having made some corrections, NIH removed its funding restrictions.[25] However, the baboon studies were not restarted because, by that time, the university had decided to suspend all research using primates at the head injury clinic.

ETHICAL ISSUES

The legal and policy questions in this case have sometimes overshadowed the heart of the case, which is the complex array of moral problems that it presents.

Thresholds and Balancing: Are There Unacceptable Procedures?

Some critics of the head injury studies argued that certain experiments should never be performed—irrespective of social benefits and the advancement of scientific knowledge—because the costs to the animals are too substantial. Candidates for unacceptable procedures are severe trauma including brain or spinal cord injury, severe burns, lethal doses of radiation, and primate studies of prolonged deprivation that produce severely abnormal mental states and behaviors in animals. Critics judge this class of experiments unacceptable even if it seems clear that human benefits may accrue from the experimental results.

The laws of several countries outlaw certain animal procedures.[26] The rationale is that the level of animal pain or suffering involved is too high, and exceeds what is morally acceptable. An analogy is sometimes made to human experimentation where there are certain procedures that can never be justified, irrespective of any useful scientific findings. (See the discussion of thresholds in the chapter 1 of this volume.) However, others argue that research procedures are never necessarily unacceptable when animal subjects are involved. From one perspective, since humans enjoy a sanctity of life not shared with other animals, it is permissible to use animals freely for human benefit. From this point of view, so long as certain conditions are satisfied—the scientific merit is high, the researchers are competent, and the potential for major human benefits in the form of vital knowledge or therapeutic treatment exists—then there should be no restrictions on upper limits of permissible animal pain or suffering.

How can this disagreement about acceptable procedures be resolved? What information should be required before deciding whether to allow a project? Who should decide what proposed projects should be approved? Should it be solely animal researchers, other academic scholars, the public, or representatives from the animal welfare community, or a mix of these?

From a utilitarian perspective, costs and benefits are weighed against each other in deciding whether a proposed experiment is justified (see chapter 1). Critics have noted problems with this rationale, however. Virtually all the costs fall on nonhuman animals and all the benefits on humans. The costs and benefits are, in this respect, incommensurable and cannot in any meaningful way be balanced. Is there justice in this distribution of costs and benefits? Whatever the answer, this approach enjoys wide acceptance and various schemes have been proposed to help make it practicable.[27] This takes us to the subject of harms and benefits.

Harms and Benefits

On any assessment of harms, the Pennsylvania baboon head injury experiments would be judged severe. Healthy baboons were subjected to irreversible brain damage, paralysis, and disability to the point of being unable to feed themselves. In addition to general harms suffered by all animals who are used in biomedical experiments (captivity, lack of control over their environment, and loss of life), they were deprived of their freedom. As experimental subjects, they were confined to life alone in a cage. As is often the case with animal experiments, these costs were certain for each and every animal used; they were not potential (as is generally the case with human benefits from research results).

In some countries (but not the United States), there is a legal requirement for investigators to categorize the invasiveness of their proposed work. The question is asked: What harm (pain, suffering, social deprivation, confinement, water deprivation, etc.) will befall the animals during the experiment? In Canada, the Netherlands, and the United Kingdom, national policy requires that the invasiveness of the procedure be categorized as minor, moderate, or severe. Minor procedures include simple blood sampling, and terminal experiments under anesthesia; the moderate-severity category includes frequent blood sampling, and insertion of indwelling catheters; and the severe category includes total bleeding without anesthesia, production of genetic defects, and severe trauma.

Categorizing experiments according to the degree of invasiveness seems essential to sound ethical decision making. The more invasive the experiment, the more stringent are the requirements for high social value of the results. The benefits of research are assessed according to criteria such as social value (improvement of human health), and scientific value (contributions to fund of scientific knowledge). The social value of some animal and human research to improving human health can be readily apparent, such as the development of a drug to correct high blood pressure. But for other research, often called "basic" research, there is no ready human application. The scientific value at the time lies exclusively in the contribution to new knowledge.

Opinions were divided on the level of benefits achieved with the baboon head injury study. The researchers themselves and the NIH funding committee judged there was social benefit, but their views were disputed. The researchers repeatedly avowed that this original work would lead to treatment that would help head-injured human beings, but details were not provided of specific applications of experimental results. If this work had presented a more direct contribution to applied therapies for human head injury, it might have been viewed by the public more sympathetically.

Scientists recognized that this basic research stood to make a contribution to original knowledge. Scientists are more likely than the general public to understand the value of basic research, and they rightly defend basic research on grounds that an understanding of pathological processes can and likely will lead, in the future, to ideas for prevention or treatment. The question is not whether this is a great benefit—it is—but whether the procedures essential to such research are warranted when they produce significant harms to animals.

Necessity Arguments and Alternatives

Arguments that research involving animals is "necessary" cover a number of important ethical questions. Among them are: Is it necessary to use an animal at all? Would the funds used for animal research be better spent elsewhere? Are severe procedures needed, or could they be modified? Is it necessary to use primates (the most highly developed and sentient species) or could a less sentient species be substituted? Could fewer animals be used and still maintain scientific validity?[28]

The public scrutiny of the baboon studies led some critics to believe that these experiments, as conducted, were not necessary. They argued, for example, that a diversion of funds from Gennarelli's research to greater efforts into *prevention* of head injury would bring greater benefits to human victims. Prevention would be enhanced, for instance, by requiring vehicular air bags, lowering speed limits, enacting motorcyclist helmet laws, and legislating against head blows in boxing. Thus, one should ask whether the resources spent on collecting data from animal studies might be put to more effective use elsewhere.

In the United States it is legally required that the principal investigators of research projects must "consider" alternatives to any procedure likely to produce pain or distress in an experimental animal.[29] Although the three Rs of replacement (with nonanimal methods), refinement (to eliminate or minimize animal pain), and reduction (of numbers of animal used) are not specifically described as such, the three Rs are inherent in several legal provisions (see chapter 1).

Replacement

Replacement is one of the three Rs (see chapter 1). Replacement alternatives include mathematical models, computer simulation, and in vitro biological systems. Could nonanimal model alternatives be substituted for the head-injury experiments? The rationale for seeking alternatives is that the animal studies involve a very high level of harm—so high that to many observers it is ethically unacceptable. But others argue that human head and spinal injury traumas are so terrible that even severely harming animals is justified. As the father of one head-injured boy said, he did not care how many baboons suffered if his son could be saved.

Using human survivors of naturally occurring trauma is a possibility, and indeed such work is conducted and is very productive. Also, some suggest that more use could be made of autopsy studies. There is no lack of human subjects since some four hundred thousand head-injured people are hospitalized each year in the United States.[30] But can the same research be performed on these subjects as on animals, and can progress be made quickly enough using only human subjects?

Problems are present in any attempt to rely only on human data for head injury studies. Ethical and legal restrictions apply to human subjects that do not apply to animal subjects and they impose constraints on the conduct and interpretation of data. Many scientists argue that both human and animal research is required to run side by side.

Problems are also present in using alternatives that involve neither human nor animal subjects. The University of Pennsylvania Head Trauma Research Center used exactly this argument. Gennarelli said he used some nonanimal replacement alternatives and found them useful. These included mathematical and computer models, gelatin simulations of brain material, and using the brains and nervous tissue of organisms lower on the phylogenetic scale with lesser cognitive abilities and pain perception, such as guinea pigs, rats, frog, squid, and crayfish.[31] Such studies can decrease the actual number of sentient animals used, but they may not be able to replace animal studies on all topics. The substitution of species lower on the phylogenetic scale was introduced by Gennarelli after the renewal of NIH funding for his research. The accelerator device previously used on the baboons was then transferred for use on minipigs, a breed of small pig specially developed for laboratory use. For the period 1991–96, NIH funded this head injury work on minipigs.

It can be argued that minipigs are a reasonable substitute for baboons on several grounds. First, work on pigs does not receive the same level of public criticism found in work on primates. Pigs are far less popular in the public eye. However, this objection seems more a matter of good public relations than good ethics. Second, physiologically and anatomically, pigs have been found to be good substitutes for humans. Third, pigs may suffer less than baboons because pigs may have less well developed nervous systems. Just how far apart pigs and baboons are in these mental capabilities is hard to judge, but they are not so far apart that pigs would not suffer at all.

Another reason for the substitution of other species, such as pigs, is that they are "purpose-bred," that is, raised specifically for research purposes. This carries a lesser ethical cost than capturing animals from the wild: Animals born and raised in captivity do not suffer the trauma of giving up a free life for permanent captivity. Today many baboons and monkeys used in research are also purpose-bred. But does this fact tip the balance in favor of justified use in studies such as those at the University of Pennsylvania?

Reduction

Reduction is also one of the three Rs (see chapter 1). Should the numbers of animals used have been reduced in this experiment? Gennarelli used two hundred baboons over the four years preceding the raid, approximately one animal per week. Whether fewer would have sufficed, given the design of the research, has never been determined.

The number of animals used is of particular significance when a procedure carries high ethical burdens. In these cases, the oversight committee can establish special restrictions such as requiring pilot studies to demonstrate that the welfare of the animals was satisfactory, permitting only a small number of animals to be used, allowing only highly competent laboratory personnel to do the work, and requiring significant oversight and re-review at frequent intervals. There is no indication that the university's oversight committee used these strategies. Apparently, the number of baboons used was determined by the convenience of the investigators to conduct the experiments.

Standards of Behavior of Laboratory Personnel

Are there certain standards of decorum, respect for animals, and concern for animal welfare that are requirements for all persons involved in animal research? The answer is yes. The American Association for Laboratory Animal Science (AALAS), a membership organization for laboratory veterinarians and technicians, has a *Code of Ethics*.[32] This code requires the "highest standards of personal conduct," the encouragement of the "highest levels of ethics within the profession of laboratory animal science," and the upholding of all laws and regulations relating to animal care, welfare, and experimentation. Unstated are any directives regarding what to do when faced with unethical behavior by other personnel.

In this case, the team of laboratory personnel seemed to have established its own way of dealing with the disabilities of injured animals, which included occasional mocking of the animals. Such lack of respect for injured animals is widely perceived as inappropriate, but some observers judged that in this case the researchers' behavior was excusable on grounds that it was little more than "gallows humor," such as is found, for instance, among some surgeons in the operating room and some neurologists who attend comatose patients. The only potentially interesting ethical issue at stake is whether "humor" of this sort fosters a general disrespect for vulnerable subjects, human and nonhuman, that deserves a rebuke wherever it is found.

A directly related issue is whether persons in these circumstances have a responsibility to speak up about observed infractions of standards by co-workers to see that they are corrected. During the several years of the Penn baboon studies, dozens of people were exposed to the laboratory environment. The great majority of codes of professional ethics require that observed infractions be reported to higher officials. These codes require that misrepresentation, fraud, unethical behavior, illegal behavior, or incompetence be reported. These codes generally recognize that a difference of opinion does not equate to unacceptable behavior; but they firmly insist that there is a moral obligation either to report or to correct observed infractions.

Institutional Responses to Raids and Underlying Problems

Institutional ethics

The University of Pennsylvania responded in contradictory ways to the allegations of mistreatment of animals: The day after the raid, university officials strongly defended the work; 16 months later, when it was obvious that the official government investigations had established infractions of the Animal Welfare Act, the university issued a reprimand of the two primary researchers. In between, the university had resisted inquiries, backed away from an outside investigative team, refused pressure from the university law school to open up the case with evidence for discussion, and conceded only minor infractions of the Animal Welfare Act. The university did not, for example, concede the inadequacy of the anesthetic regimen.

Institutions such as a university have a position of trust within a community. They serve the public and both develop and reflect community standards. There is, therefore, a standard of conduct of honesty, inquiry, and openness that can be expected—an academic ethics that is as professional as the conduct we expect of veterinarians and biomedical researchers.

The government also was deeply involved in this case since NIH funded the research. Important NIH officials rushed in to defend the head injury work before an inquiry had taken place. NIH significantly delayed any inquiry into the illegality of the research and, over a year after the raid, NIH review groups unconditionally approved the research for continued funding without requiring a report on the allegations.

What would have been appropriate institutional responses to the dramatic disclosures from the raid? What responsible institutional policies are needed to prevent a recurrence of similar events?

The ethics of raids

Both the initial laboratory raid—involving break-in, theft, and damage to property—and the NIH sit-in were illegal. The ALF continued its activities, raiding other facilities including the University of Oregon, Eugene; the University of California, Davis; the University of Arizona; the University of Pennsylvania again when sleep research of Adrian Morrison on cats was protested; and Michigan State University. According to data from the Association of American Medical Colleges, property damage from hostile activities against laboratories from 1985 to 1990 amounted to $3.5 million. No persons were ever identified to be charged of these illegal actions.

Are such illegal raids ever justified? A PETA spokesperson explained that raids and other illegal activities are last resorts used only when repeated and widespread legal methods had failed to yield results.[33] PETA judged such civil disobedience in a long tradition of justified responses to social injustices, but NIH director Wyngaarden said the raid on the head injury laboratory "carried civil disobedience to a level this society cannot tolerate."[34]

Is illegal entry always intolerable? Is property damage always intolerable? The justification depends, at least in part, on the wrong that is being protested and the level of injustice involved. For those who believed there was no wrong-doing on the part of the researchers, all illegal activities were wrong.

PETA supports destruction of property in cases of last resort, but never a harming of people. Yet occasionally animal rights protests have included arson and personal harassment of researchers. Researchers have suffered the loss of months or years of experimental results and have been publicly maligned in their neighborhoods. Although, in the United States, no person has suffered physical harm from animal rights activities, the anguish and mental suffering of some laboratory personnel is significant.

According to a government report, up until 1992 there were a total of 313 animal extremist incidents against "animal enterprises" (laboratories, factory farms, furriers, animal exhibits, and the like).[35] The peak year for "extremist incidents" was 1987 with 53 events. Since then, there was a decline to 11 incidents in 1992 by which time the raids were small-scale and haphazard.

Since 1992, the decline has continued. Although the raids have diminished, the ethical issues they raised are still debated.

Researchers Breaking the Law

After delay, the government inquiry substantiated the allegations made by the raiders, namely, that the researchers were violating several provisions of the animal protection laws. Historically, the USDA and NIH have not vigorously monitored research laboratories for compliance with the law. USDA and NIH have relied upon the animal rights movement to track potential violations, to collect evidence, and to notify the government regulators. The argument can be made that if the animal rights movement had not raided the head injury laboratories, researchers' violations of the law would have continued. So the raiders broke some laws in order to uncover legal infractions by others. How can these dual illegalities be measured against each other, and is it always morally wrong to break the law? What moral judgments can be made against researchers who break the animal protection laws, and what responsibilities does a university have to see that such laws are complied with?

NOTES

1. In effect at that time was the *NIH Guide for the Care and Use of Laboratory Animals,* 1979. Among the requirements were that each facility maintain an oversight committee and that pain-relieving agents be used where indicated.

2. In effect at that time was the *Animal Welfare Act* (7 USC 2131–2156), as amended 24 December 1970. Among other provision, the law requires use of pain-relieving agents and use of aseptic surgery for nonhuman primates.

3. Minutes of the University of Pennsylvania's Animal Care Committee of November 19, 1982, sent to all committee members from Moshe Shalev, recording secretary, December 1, 1982, pp. 1, 2. See "Evaluation of Experimental Procedures Conducted at the University of Pennsylvania Experimental Head Injury Laboratory 1981–1984," *National Institutes of Health,* 17 July 1985.

4. People for the Ethical Treatment of Animals, *Unnecessary Fuss* (videotape).

5. Paul Palango, "Brunt of Research Borne by Monkeys," *Toronto Globe and Mail,* 5 March 1983, p. 1.

6. Undated statement of Barry S. Cooperman, vice provost for research at the University of Pennsylvania.

7. *New York Times,* 20 May 1984, p. A17.

8. Jeffrey L. Fox, "Lab Break-In Stirs Animal Welfare Debate," *Science* 224 (22 June 1984): 1320.

9. Edward Colimore, "13 Lab Animals Are Stolen from Penn Vet School," *Philadelphia Inquirer,* 28 July 1984, pp. 1B, 4B.

10. University of Pennsylvania, *Report of the Committee to Review the Head Injury Clinical Research Laboratory of the School of Medicine,* 2 August 1985.

11. Jeffrey Goldberg, "Report Shows Violations in Animal Care: USDA Cites Lab with 74 Infractions," *Daily Pennsylvanian*, 8 April 1985, p. 1.

12. "Violations of Federal Law Shown in Footage to Be Released Wednesday, Capitol Hill," *News Release from PETA*, 17 September 1994.

13. Henry Mitchell, "Any Day," *Washington Post*, 21 September 1984, p. C4.

14. Fox, "Lab Break-In Stirs Animal Welfare Debate," p. 1319.

15. J. Dusheck, "Protesters Prompt Halt in Animal Research," *Science News* (27 July 1985): 53.

16. Robert E. Burke, "The Philadelphia Raid—the 'Next Taub Case'?" *Neuroscience Newsletter* (September/October 1984): 9.

17. Alex Pacheco, Chairperson, PETA, letter to Honorable Margaret Heckler, Secretary, US Department of Health and Human Services, Washington, DC, 13 November 1984, p. 1.

18. Jeffrey Goldberg, "Profs Blast Constraints on Animal Panel," *Daily Pennsylvanian*, 6 December 1984, pp. 1, 10.

19. Jim Mason, "Baboons Win Reprieve: Civil Disobedience, Protests Pay Off," *The Animals' Agenda*, September 1985, pp. 9–10.

20. "Statement by HHS Secretary Margaret M. Heckler on the University of Pennsylvania Head Injury Clinical Research Center Grant," *HHS News*, 18 July 1995, p. 1.

21. Quoted in "An Update on the Head Injury Laboratory," *Almanac Supplement* (University of Pennsylvania), 3 September 1985, p. 2.

22. "Evaluation of Experimental Procedures Conducted at the University of Pennsylvania Experimental Head Injury Laboratory 1981–1984." Report submitted to the Office of the Director, National Institutes of Health, 17 July 1985, p. 5.

23. Sheldon Hackney and Thomas Ehrlich, "On the Head Injury Laboratory: To the University Community," *Almanac* (University of Pennsylvania), 24 September 1985, p. 1.

24. "University of Pennsylvania Settles USDA Animal Welfare Act Charges," *News* (US Department of Agriculture Office of Information) 18 November 1985.

25. "Lab Animal Research Funding at University of Penn Re-instated," *NABR Update* (National Association for Biomedical Research), 24 March 1986, p. 1.

26. According to national law in the countries specified, outlawed procedures include: painful procedures on anesthetized animals paralysed with curariform drugs, and also killing an animal by use of strychnine, potassium chloride, nicotine, and certain other injectable agents (1985 law of the US); the use of animals for testing weapons, cosmetics, washing powders, and tobacco products (1986 law of Germany); experiments leading to intense suffering, anxiety, or severe pain (1993 law of Denmark); experiments involving severe pain and most use of animals to gain manual skills (1985 law of the UK); use of animals to produce monoclonal antibodies (1995 law in Switzerland).

27. Jane A. Smith and Kenneth M. Boyd, eds., *Lives in the Balance: The Ethics of Using Animals in Biomedical Research* (Oxford: Oxford University Press, 1991), pp. 138–44.

28. Smith and Boyd, *Lives in the Balance*, pp. 141–43.

29. Animal Welfare Act, as amended (7 USC §§ 2131 et seq.).

30. *NIH Report*, 17 July 1985, p. 1 of appended section entitled "A General Description of the Experimental Head Injury Laboratory."

31. F. Barbara Orlans, *In the Name of Science* (New York: Oxford University Press, 1993), pp. 128–52; Smith and Boyd, *Lives in the Balance*, chap. 4.

32. "AALAS Code of Ethics," *Contemporary Topics*, January 1995, p. 20. Adopted

by the Board of Trustees of the American Association for Laboratory Animal Science, 14 October 1994.

33. C. M. Jackson, "The Fiery Fight for Animal Rights," *Hastings Center Report* 19, no. 6 (1989): 37–39

34. John K. Ingelhart, "Health Policy Report: The Use of Animals in Research," *New England Journal of Medicine* 313 (8 August 1985): 398.

35. *Report to Congress on the Extent and Effects of Domestic and International Terrorism on Animal Enterprises* (Washington: US Department of Justice, 1993).

4

PATENTING ANIMALS:
THE HARVARD "ONCOMOUSE"

On April 12, 1988, Harvard University received the first patent ever issued for a multicellular living organism. Harvard applied for the patent after two researchers, Dr. Philip Leder and Dr. Timothy Stewart, developed the "oncomouse." The mouse was genetically engineered to make it unusually susceptible to cancer.[1] The United States Patent Office extended the patent beyond the genetically altered mice created by the Harvard scientists to cover any mammalian species in which the same genetic techniques were performed.[2]

To produce the oncomouse, Leder and Stewart first extracted a gene (the "oncogene") linked to cancer in many mammals, including humans. They then inserted the oncogene into a fertilized mouse egg, using a technique called microinjection. Next, they implanted the fertilized egg into an adult female mouse made receptive to pregnancy through hormonal treatment. The female mouse gave birth to offspring with the oncogene as part of their genetic makeup. Because they possess genes from sources other than their natural parents, the oncomice are called "transgenic" animals. The oncogene becomes part of the genetic material that the transgenic animals may pass on to their own offspring.[3]

The oncomice are widely viewed as offering an opportunity for scientists to gain a better understanding of how genes, environmental factors, and nutritional intake contribute to the development of cancer. Researchers anticipate that the mice will be especially sensitive animal models on which to evaluate the effectiveness of potential cancer treatments.[4] After receiving the oncomouse patent, Harvard granted an exclusive license for production and sale of the mice to the E. I. du Pont Co., which provided most of the financial support for the research.

The oncomice are provided to cancer researchers for about fifty dollars apiece, which is five to ten times the price of an ordinary laboratory mouse.[5] The mice are not actually sold; instead, the researcher is given a license to use them, with Du Pont retaining legal title to the animals. The researchers are authorized to reproduce up to one hundred of the mice without further cost. Commercial groups may be charged additional licensing fees, as well as royalties on oncomouse offspring. Du Pont also may reserve the right to claim a portion of any product developed from use of the oncomouse.[6]

To receive patent protection, inventors of organisms must demonstrate that the organisms are human creations that would not occur in the natural world. Creators of transgenic animals, such as the oncomouse, can meet this requirement because the research group manipulates the animals' genetic composition to include DNA both from the animals' biological parents and some other source, usually another species.

The first transgenic animal was made in 1982, when scientists produced a mouse twice as big as its siblings by giving it a rat growth-hormone gene. In just ten years, transgenic animals have become common in biomedical research laboratories, with a reported 62,000 produced in 1991 in Great Britain alone.[7] In

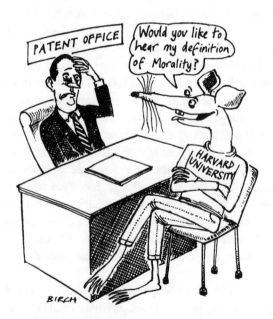

This cartoon appeared in Nature, *in 1993, when the patent for the Harvard "Oncomouse" was first announced. Credit: Nature.*

another sign of the rapid growth of transgenic animal research, a writer checking citations in the Medline database found 163 references to research on transgenic organisms in 1987; five years later, the number had increased to over 1,000.[8] Many transgenic animals contain human genes, particularly those animals designed to serve as models for human diseases.[9]

HISTORICAL CONTEXT

The Patent System

United States patent law has its roots in English patent law, which heavily influenced the US Constitution's provisions on the subject. The Constitution authorizes Congress to "promote the Progress of Science and useful Arts, by securing for limited Times to . . . Inventors the exclusive Right to their . . . Discoveries."[10] In response, Congress has enacted legislation setting forth the requirements for issuance of a patent. The currently applicable statute says, "Whoever invents or discovers any new and useful process, machine, manufacture, or composition of matter, or any new and useful improvement thereof, may obtain a patent."[11]

To qualify for a patent, an invention must be novel, useful, and not obvious to "a person having ordinary skill" in the subject matter relevant to the invention. An inventor awarded a patent has the legal right to prevent others from making, using, or selling the invention for twenty years from when the patent was filed. This includes the power to sell licenses to others authorizing them to engage in these activities. Patent holders and their licensees at all times remain subject to any applicable laws restricting the inventions, however. This means that holding a patent on an item or process does not exempt anyone from regulatory or other requirements governing the production, use, or sale of the invention.[12]

In exchange for the benefits accompanying the possession of a patent, the inventor must submit to the US Patent Office for public disclosure a description that would enable others in the field to duplicate the invention. By providing for financial rewards to individual inventors and open dissemination to others after the patent is granted, the patent system seeks to encourage new discoveries in science and technology. The goal is to enhance the discovery process so as to benefit society more broadly.[13]

Patents on Genetically Modified Organisms

The US patent system was first applied to genetically engineered life forms in 1980, when the Supreme Court decided the case of *Diamond v. Chakrabarty*. In ruling that genetically altered bacteria were patentable subject matter, the Court referred to documents indicating that Congress intended the federal patent provisions to cover "anything under the sun" that met the requirements for a patentable invention. According to the Court, the significant line to be drawn in determining whether the bacteria were patentable was "not between living and inanimate things, but between products of nature, whether living or not, and human-made inventions." If a person creates an organism through "human ingenuity and research," the Court held that the individual may be rewarded with patent rights under the same terms as any other inventor.[14]

Chakrabarty established that microorganisms such as bacteria could be patented. Seven years later, federal officials decided that multicellular organisms could be patented as well. After receiving an application for a patent on oysters with an extra set of chromosomes (designed to make them edible throughout the year), the commissioner of patents and trademarks announced that his office would henceforth give patent protection to "nonnaturally occurring nonhuman multicellular organisms, including animals" that met the legal qualifications for patentable inventions.[15] The oyster application was denied a patent, however, because it described a process that would have been obvious to others working in the area.[16] The oncomouse creators then became the first to obtain an animal patent.

Developments Subsequent to the Patent Office's Decision

Heated public debate followed the Patent Office's 1987 announcement that multicellular organisms could be patented. Four congressional hearings were conducted later that year, at which some speakers urged Congress to enact a variety of restrictions on animal patenting.[17] Since 1987, members of Congress have introduced numerous bills calling for a complete ban, a moratorium, and certain limitations on animal patents. None of these bills has been enacted into law. In the past, Congress has acted only once to restrict the subject matter of patentable inventions. The Atomic Energy Act prohibits the patenting of inventions whose sole usefulness involves atomic weaponry.[18]

Although Congress has not been persuaded to modify the decision to issue animal patents, the Patent Office itself may have been affected by the controversy that greeted its announcement and subsequent decision to issue the oncomouse patent. Whether they were apprehensive of congressional interference, or simply were slow to work through the complexities of processing animal patent applications, it took patent officials nearly five years to approve another animal patent.[19]

European officials have been more hesitant than their US counterparts to approve the oncomouse patent. Harvard filed its patent application with the European Patent Office (EPO) in 1985, but met strong resistance. The European patent examiners initially rejected the application on grounds that it conflicted with provisions of the European Patent Convention. Of major concern was the possibility that the mouse patent would violate a provision prohibiting patents on inventions whose use would be "contrary to public order or morality."[20] Harvard appealed this initial rejection, and the appeals board ordered the examiners to reconsider the application. The board instructed the examiners to weigh the research benefits to be gained from granting the patent against any pain and distress the mice could experience, as well as any possible environmental harm that could result from allowing the animals to be patented. The EPO subsequently agreed to issue the patent, but animal welfare and other interest groups appealed the decision.[21]

ETHICAL ISSUES

Transgenic animals exist only because of human interference in nature. They are novel creatures, never before present on earth. In the eyes of some observers, their extraordinary genetic composition makes these animals especially attractive for scientific research and livestock development. Because the animals are "unnatural," they provide novel opportunities to the public and may yield benefits unavailable from animals produced through usual breeding techniques. From this perspective, the patent system should be applied to enhance creation of transgenic "living inventions."

Yet it is the transgenic animal's novelty that triggers serious concern among opponents of animal patenting, who view the unprecedented genetic combinations in the animals as a threat. Instead of improving our lives and those of future generations, opponents suspect that genetically modified creatures will have a damaging effect on the earth and its occupants. Rather than encouraging the development of these new life forms through the patent system, opponents want the government to constrain or even prohibit this development.

The denial of patent protection would not stop all transgenic animal development, but the denial of this financial incentive would probably have an inhibiting effect on such work. Because patentability is likely to increase the number and variety of transgenic manipulations involving animals, it has become a target for those opposed to such manipulations. Thus, the debate over patenting animals turns on the ethics of creating genetically novel creatures.

Many of the ethical issues involve utilitarian balancing of harms, risk, and benefits: Will we be better or worse off as a result of this scientific work? Will harms to animals be compensated adequately by human benefits? Some of the issues, however, are not utilitarian. They concern the ethics of conducting such research on mice whether or not the harm-benefit ratio is favorable.

Issues about the Benefits of Patenting Transgenic Animals

Transgenic technology makes it possible to establish a genetically altered line of animals in a much briefer time than traditional breeding techniques allow. Traits may also be transferred to animals more precisely, because the technology allows small amounts of genetic material to be inserted. Transgenic techniques also enable researchers to transfer genes from distantly related species, while traditional breeding permits such transfers between only closely related species.[22]

It is predicted that transgenic animals will prove beneficial in three major areas: biomedical research, pharmaceutical manufacturing, and agriculture. The oncomouse exemplifies some of the traits biomedical researchers seek in transgenic laboratory animals: susceptibility to a human disease that inflicts death and suffering on many people, and, it is hoped, possession of similar physiological mechanisms involved in disease development and progression. Such an animal could be much more helpful than the normal laboratory mouse to scientists investigating causes of and potential treatments for breast cancer. Transgenic technology makes it possible for researchers to create nonhuman animals prone to developing various human afflictions that fail to affect biologically normal representatives of these species. Better animal models could hasten the arrival of ways to prevent and treat these afflictions.[23]

Molecular "pharming" is another target of transgenic animal development. The pharmaceutical industry is seeking to develop genetically altered animals whose bodies are able to "manufacture" drugs, veterinary biologics, and industrial enzymes. Patent applications have reportedly been filed for different transgenic animals that produce human growth hormone, insulin, and tissue plasminogen activator, a drug that helps minimize damage from heart attacks.[24] In some cases, these substances can be manufactured using other techniques, but at a higher cost and lesser quantity. Transgenic animals thus may offer a means of making the costly substances more accessible to those in need.[25]

An improved quality of livestock is the third goal cited by those seeking to promote transgenic animal technology. Researchers are attempting to create, for example, transgenic sheep that produce more wool, pigs that grow faster and have leaner meat, and livestock that are more resistant to disease than their biologically unaltered counterparts.[26] If these efforts come to fruition, people will benefit from the availability of cheaper and higher-quality animal products.

Applying the patent system to animal inventions is expected to yield the same benefit as it does regarding other types of inventions: promotion of scientific and technological progress. Giving those who develop novel transgenic creatures a property interest in their inventions enhances the financial rewards. As a result, more people are likely to channel their energies in this direction. Once the animal patent is obtained, inventors must reveal information that will enable others in the field to understand how the animal was created. Once the period of patent protection elapses, the animal invention may be freely used by anyone, provided of course, that any separate regulatory or other legal restrictions are observed. Extending patents to transgenic animals is expected to maximize the public's opportunity to obtain the benefits projected by researchers and analysts working in the field.[27]

However, some critics are unconvinced of these claims that transgenic animals will deliver the projected benefits. They question whether these animals will actually provide good human disease models, lower drug and food costs, or otherwise enhance human life in ways that cannot be achieved through alternative means. They point out, for example, that animals having the same genetic defect as humans often fail to develop the same disease as humans do. This reduces the value of what can be learned from such animals, they say.[28] If the proponents' projections about the benefits of transgenic technology are inflated and if the whole point of these benefit projections is to justify causing pain and suffering to animals, then the justification for exposing the animals to experiential burdens becomes suspect.[29]

Animal Welfare Issues

Some objections to uses of the oncomouse involve concerns about experimenting on genetically altered multicellular organisms. These concerns are independent of considerations of balancing risks, harms, and benefits. They have to do with whether we are morally obligated to recognize a threshold of pain, suffering, anxiety, fear, and distress for animals that cannot be exceeded, irrespective of the human benefits. Whether a threshold or upper limit of harm should be established as part of our network of protections of animal welfare is a pervasive issue about research with animal subjects. (See chapter 1)

The production and use of transgenic animals raise several novel issues. Some of the animals created to serve as biomedical research tools are, as one reporter put it, "genetically programmed to suffer."[30] Half of the female oncomice, for example, develop breast cancer before they are a year old.[31] Other transgenic mice are predisposed to develop AIDS, leukemia, and a condition similar to Alzheimer's disease.[32] Critics are dubious of the moral acceptability of this human quest to manipulate an animal's genetic structure for the purpose of making it vulnerable to human disease.[33] Moreover, although transgenic animals developed for use in pharmaceutical and agricultural production are not designed to become diseased, some of them experience unusual burdens because of the genetic changes they have undergone. Pigs given human growth hormone to reduce fat and speed growth, for instance, had arthritis so severe that they were unable to stand.[34]

Another issue involves the appropriate care and housing of newly created organisms. Some transgenic animals will have different needs than their component species. What constitutes humane treatment for an animal that has substantial genetic material from more than one species? If there is no wild or domestic predecessor to serve as a clear model for the new creature, how are its human caretakers to assess its well-being?[35] At minimum, the normal approach of assessing species-appropriate behavior in a natural or captive habitat will need to be refined to formulate humane treatment standards for such novel creatures.[36]

Advocates of transgenic technology dispute the charges that their activities have overwhelmingly negative effects on animal welfare. For instance, it is possible that improved transgenic animal models will reduce the overall number of laboratory animals needed to study human disease by adding precision to the studies that are conducted.[37] Transgenic research and farm animals could also be designed to resist some of the natural diseases and other conditions to which they normally are susceptible.[38] It has even been suggested that "genetic engineers could strive to create animals that suffer less in cages or confined pens, because their ability to learn, remember and perceive their environment has been genetically impaired."[39] This view is criticized by animal welfare advocates, who argue that it is the environment that should be modified to take the animals' needs into account, not the animals' genetic structure that should be modified to suit human utilitarian concerns.[40]

A few initial steps have been taken to address the special animal welfare issues arising in the care of transgenic animals. McGill University's Subcommittee on Ethics has proposed guidelines classifying all transgenic animal research in category "C," which includes interventions that cause "minor stress or pain of short duration." In light of current uncertainty regarding the effects of genetic manipulations on animals, the guidelines also require investigators to exercise "a high level of scrutiny" in monitoring transgenic animals for pain and distress, and to report to the subcommittee any painful or distressing abnormalities that are discovered.[41] Others have suggested that more frequent observations and enhanced care may be required to protect the welfare of transgenic animals.[42]

Thus far, the predominant response to concerns over the animal welfare issues raised by transgenic technology has been that these issues should be analyzed within the same framework as more traditional practices regarding animals. Pain, suffering, and distress should be reduced to the minimum necessary to achieve the results deemed to justify the animal use. Decisions on whether anticipated benefits to others justify imposing burdens on transgenic animals will presumably be made on a case-by-case basis, as opposed to an across-the-board judgment regarding all transgenic animal research. From this perspective, the customary ethical principles and regulatory provisions governing animal care and use should be applied to proposals to create and use transgenic animals.[43]

Issues about Interference with the Natural World

Other issues about creating and patenting transgenic animals, now to be considered, focus on broader social implications of the practice. These include potential negative consequences arising from human interventions in nature and from creating of human-animal hybrids. Other objections address animal patenting's potential negative effects on the advancement of science and the threats patenting poses to the family farm. Some of these issues turn on a balancing of risks and benefits, but again many parties do not see the issues as having anything to do with balancing.

Critics of transgenic animal biotechnology have voiced a variety of concerns about interfering with "the natural order." Transgenic manipulations exemplify the worrisome human tendency to tinker with the delicate natural balance millions of years of evolution have achieved. We have learned from past incidents that such tinkering can have disastrous consequences, such as the harmful effects the gypsy moth and kudzu vine have had in areas outside their normal habitats. Some varieties of transgenic animals might be capable of mating with wild species, perhaps leading to the extinction of some species.[44] Wide adoption of transgenic animals in agriculture could narrow genetic diversity among livestock, making the food supply more vulnerable to epidemics.[45]

Jeremy Rifkin uses the phrase "species integrity" to describe his concern over interference with the natural world. According to Rifkin, transgenic technology crosses species barriers, violating the right of every species "to exist as a separate, identifiable creature."[46] The result of this technology will be "genetic pollution," defined as the "unpredictable spread of DNA from genetically modified organisms with the potential to destroy the barriers between species."[47]

Critics are also troubled by the effect that treating animals as patentable inventions could have on religious and secular values. For some, creating transgenic animals is a disturbing indication of the lack of respect human beings have for the wonders of the natural world. The National Council of Churches has voiced its members' fear that developing and patenting genetically engineered animals could diminish "reverence for all life created by God."[48]

These critics see these interventions with nature as exemplifying a disturbing concept of the earth as a vehicle for human exploitation, as opposed to a precious resource worthy of our care and conservation. Living things become objectified, designed, and invented to suit our needs, as if they were computers or stereo equipment.[49] We humans lose the sense of ourselves as part of the animal kingdom, as "not the only center of the biosphere."[50] In a recent expression of these concerns, a coalition of more than eighty religious leaders issued a "Joint Appeal Against Human and Animal Patenting" and announced their intent to press for a congressional moratorium on patenting life forms.[51]

Supporters of transgenic technology respond to these concerns by noting that the same charges could be made about many human activities. The challenge posed by transgenic technology is similar to that posed by a number of modern human pursuits: to monitor and minimize environmental impacts through containment and other measures, to draw lines in specific cases when the manipulation goes "too far," and to maintain a healthy respect for the living things we use for our benefit. They also disagree with Rifkin's defense of species integrity, pointing out that the species classification system is simply a learning tool devised by human biologists, that species boundaries are commonly "violated" in nature, and that humans have interfered with these boundaries for thousands of years, using traditional breeding methods.[52]

Issues about the Possibility of Human-Animal Hybrids

According to many traditional beliefs, people occupy one moral category and nonhuman animals another. Moral standing is determined by the appropriate category—that is, status, grade, or rank of moral importance. In a *strong* sense, any creature that has standing has (at least some) rights. (See chapter 1.) But in which category do we put a mouse with a human growth hormone gene? Even if a relatively minor, single-gene insertion fails to disturb the traditional categorization and ranking scheme, how would we regard a chimpanzee that possessed a significant number of human genes, perhaps those genes that affect intelligence? Since chimpanzees and humans naturally share an estimated 99% of their genetic composition, the prospect of even greater genetic similarity could lead to uncertainty over the appropriate moral status to be assigned to a chimpanzee-human hybrid.

When the Patent Office announced that multicellular animals could be patented, officials cautioned that "[a] claim directed to or including within its scope a human being will not be considered to be patentable subject matter."[53] But officials failed to adopt a specific definition of genetic humanness in their statement. It is not clear how a chimpanzee-human hybrid would be classified.[54] Moreover, commentators have expressed doubt that the Patent Office has the proper legal authority to make this decision.[55]

Chimpanzee-human hybrids could serve as valuable biomedical research tools, for they would be much better models for studying human afflictions than any naturally occurring nonhuman species. An "oncochimp" would probably be a more superior animal model than an oncomouse. One can imagine other uses to which these creatures could be put, for example, performing low-level household chores and even serving as footsoldiers in military battles. But would it be morally defensible to use them in such ways? Indeed, would it be morally defensible even to create such hybrids? Although we humans are accustomed to creating new breeds and exploiting other species to serve our interests, such practices are deemed morally unacceptable when applied to our own species.

Chimpanzee-human hybrids would test the strength of this distinction, demand-ing a refined approach to analyzing the moral-status question.[56]

Those in favor of patenting transgenic animals agree that at some point there may be a need to address this issue. In the foreseeable future, however, they note that genetic alterations are likely to involve only single genes. Transfers of larger amounts of genetic material, including the genes controlling mental ca-pacities, probably will not be possible for many years.[57]

Issues about Negative Effects on Agriculture

Animal patent opponents also voice concern about the economic effects that animal patenting could have on farming. Farmers will face higher costs for transgenic animals in the form of licensing fees and royalties if the animals can be patented. Only large corporate farms will be able to afford the animals; family farmers will face yet another hurdle in their struggle to survive. Because the demise of the family farm would constitute the loss of a socially valuable institution, animal patents should be rejected. Opponents also are worried about the problem of monitoring offspring of patented animals. Will farmers be ex-pected to keep track of which offspring retain the gene alterations, and to pay patent holders fees on all such animals?[58]

Patenting supporters dispute these contentions. First, they predict that those who operate small farms will benefit from the availability of more productive transgenic livestock. Any increase in costs should be accompanied by an in-crease in the animal's value to the farmer. There is no obvious reason why family farmers will not be capable of obtaining the same benefits from purchas-ing patented animals as will larger agricultural operations.[59] Moreover, some disagree that the small farm deserves special moral consideration. If larger farms can produce the same quality food at less cost, they argue, then the public will benefit from the economic dominance of such farms.[60]

Those favoring animal patenting often concede that there are legitimate ques-tions regarding the appropriate way to handle the offspring of patented live-stock. Whether farmers should be required to monitor and pay royalties on such offspring is a complex question, as yet unresolved. Patent supporters are confi-dent, however, that the interested parties will eventually reach agreement on an arrangement that is fair to both farmers and patent holders.[61]

CONCLUSION

The Harvard oncomouse patent triggered a wide-ranging examination of issues concerning biotechnology and its potential effect on human and animal life. In many respects, the mouse patent created an opportunity for interest groups to raise questions on topics ranging far beyond the matter of animal patenting. The patent became a potent symbol for vast changes that the new scientific ability to engage in genetic manipulation could produce. A variety of "brave new world" fears were voiced about an event that in itself was a relatively trivial extension of existing activities and practices.

The debate over animal patenting is a debate over: (1) the risks and benefits of genetic engineering; (2) the role of religious and secular values in shaping the national scientific and economic policy of a pluralistic society; (3) the moral standing of animals; (4) the moral significance of animal pain and suffering; and (5) the proper economic conditions governing livestock production in the US.

Thus far, government officials have refused to restrict or ban animal patents in response to this debate. The predominant view has been that the Patent Office is not the appropriate setting in which to resolve such broad policy matters. Though it is conceded that the government and other policy-making entities have a responsibility to address all these areas, the general response has been that the proper place to do so is the legislative arena.

Unfortunately, there are few indications that policy makers are ready to engage in the broad-based inquiry that could be needed in this area. Instead, businesses and academic institutions are relatively free to pursue work involving transgenic animals, subject only to minimal federal oversight.[62] A more defensible approach would be for the government, business, and nonprofit organizations to create formal opportunities for discussion and debate among representatives of industry, agriculture, public health, the research community, environmental protection groups, animal welfare groups, and religious organizations. Also needed are formal efforts to educate the public and obtain their views on the issues raised by animal patenting. In the absence of a formal response to the broad ethical, social, and economic issues raised by animal biotechnology, the calls for caution and even prohibitions on animal patenting are likely to persist.

NOTES

1. Office of Technology Assessment, *New Developments in Biotechnology: Patenting Life* (Washington: Government Printing Office, 1989), p. 99.
2. Keith Schneider, "Harvard Gets Mouse Patent, a World First," *New York Times,* 12 April 1988, p. A1.
3. Office of Technology Assessment, *Patenting Life,* pp. 95–99; Council on Scientific Affairs, American Medical Association, "Biotechnology and the American Agriculture Industry," *Journal of the American Medical Association* 265 (1991): 1430, 1432.
4. Office of Technology Assessment, *Patenting Life,* p. 99; Schneider, "Mouse Patent"; Alex Kozlov, "Brave New Mouse," *Discover,* January 1989, p. 78.

5. Office of Technology Assessment, *Patenting Life,* p. 121.

6. Carl S. Kaplan, "Generations of Profits," *Newsday,* 29 October 1989, p. 62.

7. Gail Vines, "Guess What's Coming to Dinner?" *New Scientist,* 14 November 1992, p. 13.

8. Rivers Singleton, "Transgenic Organisms, Science, and Society," *Hastings Center Report* 24 (January/February 1994): S7.

9. Office of Technology Assessment, *Patenting Life,* p. 98.

10. US Const. art. I, sec. 8, cl. 8.

11. 35 USC sec. 101 (1988).

12. Rebecca Dresser, "Ethical and Legal Issues in Patenting New Animal Life," *Jurimetrics Journal* 28 (1988): 404.

13. Office of Technology Assessment, *Patenting Life,* pp. 37–43.

14. 447 US 303, 309, 313 (1980).

15. Commissioner's Notice, *Official Gazette of the Patent and Trademark Office* 1077 (21 April 1987): 24.

16. Ex parte Allen, 2 U.S.P.Q. 2d 1425 (Bd. Pat. App. & Int. 1987). Volume 2 of U.S. Patent Quarterly, second edition, page 1425; decision of Board of Patent Appeals and Interferences.

17. *Patents and the Constitution: Transgenic Animals: Hearings before the Subcommittee on Courts, Civil Liberties, and the Administration of Justice of the House Committee on the Judiciary,* 100th Cong., 1st Sess. (1987).

18. 35 USC sec. 181 (1988).

19. Edmund Andrews, "U.S. Resumes Granting Patents on Genetically Altered Animals," *New York Times,* 3 February 1993, p. A1. The patents were all granted on transgenic mice designed to serve as animal models for biomedical research. Lantz Miller, "Animal Patents Take Off," *Lab Animal* 22 (March 1993): 10.

20. "Patent for a Mouse," *Nature* 361 (21 January 1993): 192.

21. Nuala Moran, "EPO Caught in Mouse Maze," *Nature Medicine* 2 (1 January 1996): 12.

22. Office of Technology Assessment, *Patenting Life,* p. 97.

23. Lisa Raines, "Public Policy Aspects of Patenting Transgenic Animals," *Theriogenology* 33 (January 1990): 130.

24. Andrews, "U.S. Resumes Granting Patents," p. A1.

25. Vines, "Guess What's Coming," p. 14; Deborah Erickson, "Down on the Pharm," *Scientific American,* August 1990, p. 102.

26. Vines, "Guess What's Coming," p. 13; Office of Technology Assessment, *Patenting Life,* p. 98.

27. Office of Technology Assessment, *Patenting Life,* pp. 127–30; Paul B. Thompson, "Designing Animals: Ethical Issues for Genetic Engineers," *Journal of Dairy Science* 75 (1992): 2296–97.

28. Vines, "Guess What's Coming," p. 14.

29. British Union for the Abolition of Vivisection and Compassion in World Farming, "Opposition under Part V of the European Patent Convention to the Grant of a Patent for the Oncomouse," Case no. T 19/90–3.3.2, filing no. 85 304 490.7, pub. no. 0 169 672, 8 January 1993, pp. 8–18.

30. Andrews, "U.S. Resumes Granting Patents," p. A1.

31. Kozlov, "Brave New Mouse," p. 78.

32. Andrews, "U.S. Resumes Granting Patents," p. A1.

33. British Union for the Abolition of Vivisection and Compassion in World Farming, "Opposition," p. 22.

34. Vines, "Guess What's Coming," p. 14.

35. Henk Verhoog, "The Concept of Intrinsic Value and Transgenic Animals," *Journal of Agricultural and Environmental Ethics* (1992): 155.

36. Robert Wachbroit, "Eight Worries about Patenting Animals," *Philosophy and Public Policy* 8 (Summer 1988): 7–8.

37. Office of Technology Assessment, *Patenting Life,* p. 134; Jon Gordon, "Viewpoint: Transgenic Animals as 'Alternatives' to Animal Use," *Johns Hopkins Center for Alternatives to Animal Testing* 9 (Fall 1991): 8–9.

38. Office of Technology Assessment, *Patenting Life,* p. 134.

39. Vines, "Guess What's Coming," p. 14.

40. Verhoog, "Concept of Intrinsic Value," p. 155.

41. Ann McWilliams, "The Regulation of Transgenic Animals," *Canadian Council on Animal Care Resource* 17 (1992–93): 7, 12.

42. Charles McCarthy, "Developing Policies and Regulations for Animal Biotechnology and to Protect the Environment," *Hastings Center Report* 24 (January/February 1994): 526.

43. Office of Technology Assessment, *Patenting Life,* pp. 133–34.

44. Billy Goodman, "Debating the Use of Transgenic Predators," *Science* 262 (1993): 1507.

45. Office of Technology Assessment, *Patenting Life,* p. 136.

46. 49 Fed. Reg. 37,016 (20 September 1984) (letter from Jeremy Rifkin to William Gartland).

47. Vines, "Guess What's Coming," p. 13.

48. *Patents and the Constitution,* p. 401.

49. Claudia Wallis, "Should Animals Be Patented?" *Time,* 4 May 1987, p. 110.

50. Verhoog, "Concept of Intrinsic Value," p. 156.

51. Richard Stone, "Religious Leaders Oppose Patenting Genes and Animals," *Science* 268 (1995): 1126.

52. Office of Technology Assessment, *Patenting Life,* pp. 98–102, 136.

53. "Nonnaturally Occurring Non-human Animals," p. 664.

54. Rachel Fishman, "Patenting Human Beings: Do Sub-human Creatures Deserve Constitutional Protection?" *American Journal of Law & Medicine* 15 (1989): 461–82.

55. Michael D. Rivard, "Toward a General Theory of Constitutional Personhood: A Theory of Constitutional Personhood for Transgenic Humanoid Species," *UCLA Law Review* 39 (1992): 1440.

56. Wachbroit, "Eight Worries," p. 8; Samuel Gorovitz, "Will We Still Be 'Human' If We Have Engineered Genes and Animal Organs?" *Washington Post,* 9 December 1984, p. C1.

57. Office of Technology Assessment, *Patenting Life,* pp. 98, 132.

58. Office of Technology Assessment, *Patenting Life,* pp. 115–23, 136–37; Dresser, "Ethical and Legal Issues," pp. 417–18.

59. Raines, "Public Policy," p. 138.

60. Wachbroit, "Eight Worries," p. 8.

61. Raines, "Public Policy," pp. 137–38.

62. Office of Technology Assessment, *Patenting Life,* pp. 102–110; Dresser, "Ethical and Legal Issues," pp. 424–35.

5

WHAT DOES THE PUBLIC
HAVE A RIGHT TO KNOW?

The Progressive Animal Welfare Society (PAWS), a nonprofit organization in the state of Washington, and the University of Washington (UW), Seattle, have been at loggerheads over several issues: Does this activist animal welfare organization have a legal or a moral right to information about proposed animal experiments that the university does not want to divulge? Does PAWS have a legal right or a moral right to be present at oversight committee meetings where animal experiments are either approved or disapproved? Should animal protection groups be represented on committees that oversee animal experiments?

PAWS presents itself as representative of that segment of the community most concerned about the welfare and protection of laboratory animals, and it believes that it should have a voice in what is done to animals at the university. The university is partially funded by revenues from state taxes and therefore is publicly accountable. But the university disagrees with PAWS over questions of accountability. University officials view PAWS as an antivivisection group and as prone to distort information about animal experiments. John A. Coulter, executive director of Health Sciences Administration for the university, says that in general the university is not opposed to divulging information, but is opposed to giving certain types of information to PAWS and to having PAWS participate in university affairs. The university is concerned that PAWS might raise public opposition to already approved animal experiments, which might result in unwanted confrontation and, in an extreme case, stoppage of animal experiments and embarrassment to the university.

This conflict is representative of other battles in several states and countries between animal research facilities and animal protection organizations. PAWS, like other animal protection groups, believes that animal research should not be conducted behind closed doors.[1] But in Washington State, the issues have been pressed further than anywhere else in the United States and have attracted national attention.[2]

PAWS, like other animal advocates, has concentrated on the university's institutional oversight committee—the Animal Care Committee (ACC)—because this committee holds the legal power to approve or disapprove animal experiments conducted at that facility. (In general, these committees are called Institutional Animal Care and Use Committees, but institutions can select their own name and a number of names are in use.)

PAWS has pursued two major goals: it has sought information about records and meetings of the university's ACC and a voice in the decision making of this committee. These committees have a central role in the oversight of animal experiments. They are legally required to see, first, that anesthetics are administered where more than momentary pain exists (unless the anesthetic compromises justified research goals), that animals be humanely killed by prescribed methods, and, finally, that certain standards of animal husbandry be maintained.

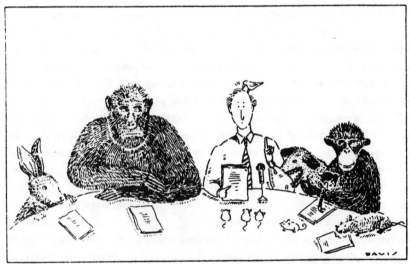

"What evidence is there that mistreatment of laboratory animals is a problem?"

This cartoon by Susan Davis appeared in The Washington Post. Credit: Susan Davis.

ISSUES ABOUT ACCESS TO MEETINGS

The Right to Attend Meetings

PAWS's first step was an attempt to obtain committee membership and therefore a vote on the ACC. The purpose was to gain the important right to vote on what animal experiments were approved or disapproved. Citing the legal requirement that ACCs must have at least three members, a scientist, a veterinarian, and a noninstitutional member, in 1987, PAWS applied to UW for the noninstitutional slot. But this petition was turned down. By law, committee membership is controlled by institutional officials, without rights of appeal granted to others.

After this effort failed, PAWS lowered its sights and applied for observer status on the ACC, which at least would give it access to information. This petition, too, was initially denied. At that point, PAWS sued the university under Washington State's Open Meeting Act, which permits public observers to attend certain decision-making meetings. In 1987 in the first of a succession of legal battles spanning seven years, PAWS won the legal right to observer status at ACC meetings. PAWS representatives then started attending the meetings as observers and have attended every meeting since. PAWS's Mitchell Fox has said that the committee "is our only window" into the research laboratories that house about 73,000 research animals a year.

UW officials have deplored the 1987 court ruling.[3] A prevalent view within the university has been that the review process of the ACC would be hampered if outside observers were present. John Lein, vice president for health sciences, said, "I fear mostly the harassment of our researchers and their families." His fears were well founded. For several weeks preceding the court ruling, some people picketed the homes of several UW scientists, including the chair of the ACC and an anesthesiologist whose work on dental pain had been particularly disturbing to some activists. These two scientists said they had received phone calls from people who harassed them and even threatened them with death. PAWS claimed it was not involved with these protests or death threats. The local press reported that the Northwest Animal Rights Network was responsible.

According to PAWS, during the eight months immediately following the first open ACC meeting, only "a handful" of projects were discussed. "The remaining [projects involving animal experimentation] have been summarily approved without even a mention. To the observer they are nonexistent: no title, no investigator, no purpose, no method. But in this void exist thousands of animals, unprotected by even the most cursory public scrutiny."[4] PAWS was of the opinion that the ACC's most meaningful deliberations were taking place behind closed doors.

Rights of Access to Protocol Review Forms

In a second suit, PAWS sought access to the ACC records under Washington State's Public Disclosure Law. After a contentious battle, later in 1987 PAWS successfully established a legal right to disclosure of the "protocol forms" used by ACCs in which investigators are required to describe their proposed animal experiments. At UW, these forms state the project title, the number and species of animal to be used, whether alternatives to animal use are available, the relevance of the project to human health or biology, the reason for using animals, and the care and treatment the animals will receive. At UW over six hundred protocol forms are processed each year that become part of the ACC's records.

According to court documents, UW officials contested this ruling on several grounds: that the forms are preliminary drafts and therefore exempt from the law; that the forms contain valuable research designs and formulae that are proprietary and could be stolen by competing researchers; and that disclosure would substantially and irreparably damage persons or vital government functions. In their written arguments, the university attorneys warned that the form's release would result in loss of research funds to UW, harm to its researchers' livelihood and careers, a decline in the quality of education in Washington State, and a decline in the university's ability to ensure the humane treatment of animals.

Sunshine Laws

The laws that PAWS used to achieve its goals of access to meetings are Washington State's so-called sunshine laws. These laws, also called open meeting and public disclosure laws, require that meetings of certain public agencies be open to the public and also that certain records be made public. These laws include state statutes (all states have sunshine laws) and the federal Freedom of Information Act, often used by watchdog organizations.

The underlying philosophy of these disclosure laws is that the public has a right to know what their government is doing and how their tax dollars are being spent. These laws help preserve central tenets of representative government. In her 1994 ruling on the *PAWS v. UW* case, Judge Barbara Durham wrote that without tools such as disclosure laws, "government of the people, by the people, for the people, risks becoming government of the people, by the bureaucrats, for the special interests."[5]

The federal Freedom of Information Act has been widely used by animal protection groups to obtain information about, for instance, the use of federal tax dollars by the NIH in support of animal experiments. On request, NIH is required to provide copies of funded grant applications to the public with certain deletions of confidential information. Releasable information includes: the project title, grantee institution, identity of principal investigator, and amount of award.[6]

The USDA is also required under the Freedom of Information Act to publicly disclose reports of its federally mandated inspections of animal research facilities. These reports include information about facilities' noncompliance with the Animal Welfare Act. Armed with this information, watchdog organizations can exert pressure to help ensure that federal agencies perform their mandated responsibilities.

A bill proposed in 1995 (but not passed into law) in the 104th Congress stated, "The Federal Government must bear the responsibility for making information about animal experimentation complete, coherent, and readily accessible to the American public."[7] A key provision of this bill was that a count be made of all laboratory animals of all species used. Currently, official government statistics include only about 10% of the total number of laboratory animals (rats and mice—the species most used—are excluded); under the proposed law, 100% of animals would be counted. For many years, these exclusions have aroused strong public protest by groups seeking increased access to information and meetings.

At the state level, sunshine laws vary in their impact, depending on the provisions of the law. Few universities have opened their meetings without a court ruling. The University of Florida in Gainesville is an exception. They recognized that the Florida sunshine laws (which are very broad) would cover their ACC. When activists—comprised heavily of faculty and students at the university—petitioned to sit in on the meetings, the university permitted them to do so in the belief that they would have no hope of winning a legal challenge. Since 1985 the ACC meetings have been open, and times and places of future meetings are always publicly announced. Although there have been some additional faculty protests, there apparently have been no ill-effects and the university has reached a mutually agreeable arrangement with those who sought increased access.

LEGAL REASONING IN TEST CASES

Inapplicable Laws

In the five states in the US in which closed Institutional Animal Care and Use Committee meetings are permitted by law, the specific legal reasoning in each case was as follows:[8]

- In 1989, the Virginia Supreme Court denied the group Students for Animals access to meetings of the University of Virginia's Animal Research

Committee. The law is written so that it applies only to meetings in which public policy is made; the Animal Research Committee did not meet this test. The court compared the Animal Research Committee to the university basketball or football coaching staff meetings. The court wrote, "To require meetings of such groups to be treated as public meetings would be to carry the idea of government in the 'sunshine' to an absurd extreme."

- In 1992 a Massachusetts State Appeals Court reversed lower-court decisions and found that since the Animal Care and Use Committee meetings are held to ensure compliance with state and federal animal care and use regulations and not to discuss public policy, they are exempt from the state open meeting laws. Again, the law is written so that sunshine is required only of meetings in which public-policy decisions are made.

- In 1991 a four-judge panel of the New York Supreme Court, Appellate Division, unanimously decided that the Laboratory Animal Use Committee of the State University of New York, Stony Brook, is not a "public body" as defined by the New York law. This committee acts only as an "advisory body" and is not involved in "deliberations and decisions that go into the making of public policy" and therefore does not perform a "government function." The meetings can therefore be closed.

- In 1989 an Alameda County Superior Court judge ruled that the University of California's ten campuses were not subject to the state's open-meeting law because the university system was exempt from the law's requirements. However, in a separate action brought under the Public Records Act, the court ruled in 1992 that the University of California must copy and turn over to an organization called In Defense of Animals uncensored autopsy reports on lab animals that had died in its care. Before this ruling, this animal rights group had been able to obtain only censored reports.

- In 1991 an Oregon Circuit Court judge ruled that People for the Ethical Treatment of Animals (PETA) lacked legal standing to seek judicial review of the University of Oregon's ban on public attendance at their Institutional Animal Care and Use Committee. To obtain standing—here meaning standing to sue—one must show that a legally protected interest of the party who complains of unlawful conduct has been invaded. Thus, PETA would have to show that it had been harmed.

Throughout these cases, the argument appears that the interests of universities would be invaded by public disclosure. For example, there are security risks in permitting the presence of animal rights sympathizers. If they are allowed to go on inspection tours of the animal facilities, which is a legally required activity of the committee, then knowledge would be gained of the locations of animal rooms that could potentially be used for future raids. Also, disclosure of names of ACC members could result in harassment or litigation against the members. Publicity about ACC discussions or records could stifle the review process and make ACC members more guarded in their comments— as appears to have happened at the University of Washington. Also, more-widespread knowledge about animal experiments could result in public protest and possible stoppage of experiments. This fallout might be unjust to individual investigators, because science is a competitive endeavor and creative ideas should not be usurped by premature disclosure.

Applicable Laws

In addition to Washington State, the states in which public disclosure laws have been tested and upheld are Florida, Texas, North Carolina, Vermont, and Kentucky. The fundamental rationale is that social value issues are a matter of concern for the whole of society. Scientists are not immune to public scrutiny; scientists and university officials have no standing as experts in social values. Therefore, they have no authority, by themselves, to determine what standards are to prevail regarding how animals are treated in the name of science. The universities and animal research facilities that accept public funding lack the independence of public scrutiny and parallel control that they would have with private funding. In publicly funded institutions, ethical standards of scientists need to conform to publicly acceptable standards, not just to scientifically acceptable standards. An assessment of what is socially acceptable can only be made if information is freely available and if the public is involved in decision making.

The case for opening ACC meetings to the public has been stated by counsel for the American Society for the Protection of Cruelty to Animals:

> True, the information learned at meetings may be distorted by some [members of the public] but few would argue that our press should be censored, or freedom of speech denied because some people in the media distort the truth now and then. The same reasoning should apply here. Furthermore, in the event this does occur, there are laws regarding defamation and harassment. . . . One can argue that to deny information merely gives the interested public few options, one being to break in and actually see what is going on. To deny access . . . could encourage the unlawful behavior that many scientists and administrators at research institutions are so concerned about.[9]

ETHICAL ISSUES

What Does the Public Have a Right to Know?

Sunshine laws establish a legal right of access for the public to certain types of information. It is easy to understand why these laws have been popular. If an activity is publicly funded (through state or federal tax dollars), then a level of public accountability is required. (If the activity is privately funded, however, information can often be withheld.) Without information, critics and persons with oversight responsibility have no basis for action; they cannot seek public support regarding specific allegations of wrongdoing but can merely complain about the secrecy of the activity. Lack of information can therefore be a death blow to the activities of watchdog organizations and reformers.

The University of Washington is publicly funded, and therefore legally and politically accountable. UW officials defended their position of refusing access in several ways. They believed there was no moral or legal obligation to give information about animal experiments to those whose ultimate objective is to terminate vital work by the institution. UW officials also argued their point on the grounds of academic freedom—a provision that historically arose more from moral than legal arguments. Academic freedom consists of the absence of, or protection from, restraints or pressures having the effect of inhibiting the freedom of scholars in studying, discussing, lecturing, or publishing ideas and opinions. Such freedom "implies protection from . . . attempts to intimidate, no matter whence they come."[10] UW lawyers commented after quoting this source: "Thus, the core values of academic freedom are unfettered inquiry and dissemination of knowledge."[11] So they went to court in order to defend what they consider an important social good, that is, scientific inquiry and dissemination of knowledge.

On a strong interpretation of this view, the value of unfettered scientific inquiry takes precedence over all other values. However, a compelling contrary perspective is that at least some animal experiments are morally wrong because the experiments infringe the rights of the animal or cause unwarranted animal pain and suffering (see chapter 1). PAWS supporters claim they are defending the rights and welfare of both animals and the public. Whatever the power of the moral values of academic freedom and privacy in universities, they maintain that protecting the interests of animals and of the public are moral values that are at least as powerful. From this perspective, the case of *PAWS v. UW* pits the rights and welfare of animals and the public against the rights of investigators and the value of academic freedom.

There are problems with any claim to have an absolute freedom—either to do research or to acquire information. Problems emerge in the present case because of the conflict among competing moral rights. Freedom of inquiry, for example, is a right that—like all moral rights—is constrained by other rights with which it may on occasion compete.

Scientists have a right to express beliefs and judgments about many matters, but if their statements or actions violate the moral rights of others (including animals), then the latter's right might override the investigator's right to freedom of inquiry and expression. The defenses of unrestrained freedom in science or in the university found in some contemporary writers and legal briefs do not consider the full range of moral rights and responsibilities that confront free expression.

Likewise, those who claim a right to information—the public's or their own—should be cognizant that competing values may, in certain circumstances, have moral weight equal to or greater than their rights.

Assessing Animal Pain and Suffering in Protocol Reviews

Any investigator or oversight committee has a responsibility to weigh and assess pain and suffering. Nationwide, ACC assessment of animal pain and suffering is far from uniform. Protocol forms may or may not provide much information, and the investigator's narrative description of the project often does not describe in detail the degree of animal pain or suffering. Typically, experimental methods are described from which a rough assessment can be made. The full protocol is not necessarily divulged to the full committee or to observers. (See chapter 1.)

Animal research facilities in the US must report to the government whether an anesthetic is used in experiments involving certain species of animals. This information is reported to the USDA annually as part of the provisions of the Animal Welfare Act. But this system is an inadequate method of reporting animal pain, because it provides no information about whether the animal harms are minor, moderate, or major. The current reporting system also does not capture information on sensory or social deprivation of the animal, nor on the debilitating effect of infections, nor whether surgery is minor or major.

Some people consider that the most informative system of assessing the degree of animal pain and suffering is to categorize experiments according to a ranked order of minor, moderate, or severe. This system is used by the University of Washington and several other American universities. The system is national policy in several countries, including the UK, Canada, and the Netherlands, and has been found to work well.[12] According to University of Washington documents, ACC personnel categorize each submitted protocol according to potential discomfort or pain to the animal on a 1 to 4 scale of increasing severity of the procedure. Category 1 projects involve "little or no discomfort"; Category 2 projects involve "some distress or discomfort"; Category 3 projects involve "significant distress or discomfort"; and Category 4 projects involve "severe pain."

Not all projects at the university receive full committee review. Projects falling within Categories 1 and 2 are automatically exempt from full committee review unless it is specially requested by a committee member, which rarely if ever happens. Category 3 projects are "studied by a review group" which makes recommendations to the full committee. Projects falling within Category 4 are the only ones that automatically receive full committee review.

In 1995, after years of observation of ACC meetings, PAWS publicly charged that the ACC was underestimating animal pain for some protocols. This lower estimate meant that review for these projects was conducted out of the public eye, without any real scrutiny. PAWS contends that, in some cases, full committee review is circumvented by unjustifiable designation of a lower pain category. In 1994, seven years after being granted observer status and access to ACC documents, PAWS analyzed the committee procedures and concluded some projects involving cats and dogs had been incorrectly ranked so that the degree of animal pain was underestimated. Because of the ranking, these projects had avoided full committee review at the open session. PAWS believed that, for cat and dog projects, a higher ranking of animal pain should have been given to five projects and that these projects should have been discussed openly at ACC meetings, and not approved without full committee review. The university conceded that the ranking of one project was too low, but held that others were accurately ranked.

Community Representation in Decision Making

Another contentious issue is the degree to which representatives of animal protection groups should be allowed a voice in decision making about animal research. PAWS failed to achieve its objective of membership and a vote on UW's Animal Care Committee. But is such representation socially justified?

Within the scientific community, opinions are mixed regarding the degree to which the public, let alone animal advocates, should participate in day-to-day decision making on animal experiments. This was the single most contentious issue in the passage of the 1985 amendments to the Animal Welfare Act. In the end, Congress decreed that a nonaffiliated member (variously called community or noninstitutional member) must be appointed to each committee to represent "general community interests in the proper care and treatment of animals." Congress made no stipulation about who that member should be. Since appointment to ACC membership is made by the institution's chief executive office or other designated official, the community has no say in who will represent the public's interest.

Although ACC's are required to appoint a community member, few have appointed representatives from the animal protection movement.[13] As a general rule, animal rights advocates and antivivisectionists are automatically excluded. A 1996 article in *The Physiologist* voices fairly typical perspectives within the animal research community.[14] The author advises that universities "must not give in to animal activists' demands to sit on [institutional committees] that review research proposals. Activists must not be given access to any research activities because . . . their goal is destruction of animal-based biomedical research." But, exclusion of opponents' points of view means that public review is diminished.

One of the deepest moral problems about review of research involving animals is *conflict of interest.* Many relationships encountered in biomedical research involve problems of conflict of interest. A conflict of interest is present whenever the researcher's role-obligation or personal interest in accommodating an institution, in job security, in personal goals, and the like compromises or threatens to compromise obligations to others who have a right to expect objectivity and fairness. In the present case, having investigators and university administrators decide about either the welfare of animals or the legitimacy of the interests of animal welfarists seems to involve a conflict of interest. But, similarly, animal welfarists opposed to much if not all scientific research involving animals would be involved in a conflict of interest if they were to review protocols. Is there a solution to the review of animal research that is relatively free of bias and conflict of interest?

Perhaps the person appointed for the community slot—or even for a much larger role on these committees—should be a more independent person, for example, a lawyer, teacher of ethics, or businessperson. Since proportional representation is not required, usually animal researchers both chair and control the committees; as long as there is one noninstitutional member, the committee is legally constituted. This system has kept the public voice at a minimal level on many committees and again risks the problem of conflict of interest.

Even though animal advocates are usually not welcome on ACCs, there is now a general recognition among ACC members that having some sort of community representative is beneficial. Community members are often free of conflict of interest, bring credibility to committee deliberations, and bring different perspectives and can stimulate discussion. An outsider can keep the scientists alert to community concerns and remind investigators to explain in laypersons' terms what they are doing and why—possibly even making scientists more introspective about their work.

The ACC's legal charge is to ensure compliance with federally established national standards. The US law does not specifically mention that *ethical* considerations are involved in this review, only that *legal* requirements be satisfied. In the deliberations of ACCs, animal researchers may raise ethical questions, but it is not surprising that community members who represent the animal protection movement tend to raise ethical concerns more often. For example, they see that animals, being unable to consent to the research, are vulnerable and in need of someone to represent their interests.

The risks present in appointing committee members from the community is that they often have no special expertise in either animal welfare or the science involved in the protocol being reviewed. One could argue that assessment of biomedical research, like treatment at the hands of a veterinarian, is a task that belongs to persons with a certain professional expertise and commitment— including, many would claim, a commitment to the welfare of animal subjects. From this perspective, expertise in the relevant profession will alone eventuate in a discerning review of both the science and the comfort of the animals, which is the immediate business at hand. If one believes that animal researchers can both be unbiased in their scientific expertise and morally sensitive in their use of the animals, this can be an argument to allow scientists to be sole reviewers. But if doubts exist, as is suggested by the congressional requirement to have a community member, then wider representation is desirable.

Nonetheless, the need for a thoroughly impartial review is morally attractive. In contrast to the United States, several countries explicitly provide for participation of animal welfare groups in decision making about animal experimentation. As examples:

- The 1991 Swiss Law on Animal Welfare (article 18, enacted 21 March) requires that cantons (equivalent to states) institute commissions for review and approval of animal experiments; each commission must include representatives from animal protection organizations.
- Under the 1986 German First Amendment to Animal Protection Law, 25 April, the national oversight committee has twelve members, of whom one-third are experts from national animal welfare organizations. This one-third is chosen by the federal ministry from lists put forward by animal protection groups.
- The 1987 Danish Law on Animal Experimentation mandates a ten-person national oversight committee which must include four persons proposed by animal welfare organizations.

A few American ACCs have voluntarily appointed representatives of animal protection organizations and occasionally even antivivisectionists. For instance, the Wisconsin Regional Primate Research Center's policy states, "Advocates of animal rights, along with scientific peers, will be appointed by the Director to participate with full voice and vote,"[15] and the University of Southern California's policy requires a committee "composed of an inter-disciplinary group of faculty most of whom are not in animal research, the Vivaria Director, a public member representing the animal advocate community, a public member representing the community-at-large, and at least one graduate student."[16]

Does Public Sanction Indicate Moral Acceptability?

Public opinion polls repeatedly show that there is public support for animal research, although the approval rate has been falling in recent years. For instance, the Science Indicators survey commissioned by the National Science Board in the US has asked a question on animal research since 1985. Survey participants were asked to express their level of agreement or disagreement with the statement: "Scientists should be allowed to do research that causes pain and injury to animals like dogs and chimpanzees if it produces new information about human health problems." Over the last decade, from 1985 to 1995, the level of agreement has dropped from 63% in agreement to 50% in agreement.[17] In 1995, 45% of those surveyed stated they disagreed with the statement, and 5% said they did not know.

What moral weight, if any, does this public opinion carry? Here is a situation in which public opinion appears to be split fairly evenly between those who approve of painful animal research and those who disapprove of it. Does public sanction carry with it moral acceptability?

Defensible Tactics in Protesting the Policies of Institutions

Many tactics are available to protest the policies of institutions. Protestors often start with the mildest tactic and work through increasingly more aggressive means to achieve their end. The mildest tactic is to document complaints and present them to institutional officials with recommendations for correction. More forceful tactics include street demonstrations, political action to curb certain practices, legal challenge, harassment, public ridicule or embarrassment, harm to an individual or to the institution by bringing discredit, destruction of property, efforts to put the institution out of business, and threats to life.

Any aggressive act might be countered by retaliatory aggression. If an employee protests, even mildly, against a policy of an institution, there is also some risk of retribution. A whistle-blower is often at serious risk of harassment by co-workers and the institution can threaten the whistle-blower with loss of employment, financial loss, and marking this person as a "troublemaker," thus lessening chances of future employment. There are laws to protect whistle-blowers, but even so, the penalties can be severe.

CONCLUSION

Opinions vary on the effect that open meetings have had on the protocol review process. PAWS officials believe that the review procedure has moved from being "a mockery" to being more professional. For PAWS, Fox claims that "the unrelenting sunshine the UW committee has had to endure" has benefited both the animals and the university; ACC discussion is "more serious, spirited and substantive."[18] Fox also applauds some changes that have been made in committee membership.

However, university official John A. Coulter expressed the view that committee review procedures have remained unchanged by the court rulings and that tensions between PAWS and the university have not been diminished. In fact, the situation is now more politicized, since not only do critics of animal research attend the university's ACC meeting but, at the invitation of the university, so do advocates from a group called the "Incurably Ill for Animal Research." This helps to ensure that the ACC will receive favorable comment to help counter the criticisms from PAWS.

During the several years since the ACC meetings have been open, some barriers have been crossed though not broken down. At the ACC meetings, scientists and animal advocates meet on a regular basis and, to some extent, get to know each other, which they had not done before. This interaction may increase the possibility of greater mutual understanding and respect, though it undoubtedly will also increase some tensions. The challenge is how to establish an environment in which more responsible and fairer decisions can be made that will win greater public support and confidence.

NOTES

1. For instance, the Physicians Committee for Responsible Medicine, in Washington, DC, circulates a publication, *Your Right to Know: Animal Experiments in Your Community,* which instructs animal activists on how to obtain information about animal experiments.

2. This legal case has been reported on in (1) A. Anderson, "US University Told to Reveal Unfunded NIH Application," *Nature* 359 (September 1992): 98; and (2) T. Adler, "APA Files Amicus Brief in Grant Application Case," *Monitor* (American Psychological Association) 24 (September 1993): 26.

3. Sally Macdonald, "Animal-Rights Group Wins Order Opening UW Research Meetings," *Seattle Times,* 20 March 1987, p. B1.

4. "Suit Concluded, Dispute Drags On," *PAWS News,* February 1988, p. 40.

5. Judge Barbara Durham, Acting Chief Justice of the Supreme Court of the State of Washington, *PAWS v. University of Washington,* 22 November 1994, no. 59714–6, p. 7.

6. The Federal Advisory Committee Act, another statute promoting public access has also been used to challenge the procedures of the committees which establish national policy. A recent court case challenged the lack of public access to the meetings of the committee that prepares the NIH *Guide for the Care and Use of Laboratory Animals.* This manual sets national policy for handling and monitoring the treatment of laboratory animals by NIH grantees. On 10 January 1997, the United States Court of Appeals for the District of Columbia Circuit ruled in favor of the animal rights groups who had brought the case (the Animal Legal Defense Fund and others). In future such committees may not work in secrecy. In 1993 the NIH had contracted with the National Academy of Sciences (NAS), a quasi-public organization, to prepare a seventh edition of the *Guide.* At that point, several animal rights groups sought access to the *Guide* committee's deliberative meetings and to any minutes, transcripts, or records. The NAS denied this access, and a legal challenge ensued. At issue was the applicability of the Federal Advisory

Committee Act to this committee. The seventh edition of the *Guide* was issued in 1996, before the appeals court ruling was made, but future committees to revise the *Guide* and other NAS committees advising federal agencies will be affected. On a related issue, the Animal Legal Defense Fund is intent on gaining representation for persons from the animal protection movement on future NAS committees to revise the *Guide*. The first seven editions of the *Guide* were prepared by committees overwhelmingly composed of members who are animal researchers, and there has never been any formal representation from the animal protection movement.

7. "Animal Experimentation Right to Know Act," HR 1547, introduced by Robert G. Torricelli and others, 2 May 1995, in the 104th Congress.

8. For more details, see F. Barbara Orlans, *In the Name of Science: Issues in Responsible Animal Experimentation* (New York: Oxford University Press 1993), pp. 173–74, 257–60.

9. Elinor Molbegott, counsel for ASPCA, New York. Transcript of a speech given in October 1989 at Rockefeller University.

10. Fritz Machlup, "On Some Misconceptions Concerning Academic Freedom," in *Academic Freedom and Tenure: A Handbook of the American Association of University Professors,* ed. Louis Joughlin (Madison: University of Wisconsin, 1967): p. 184, app. B at 178.

11. Tammy L. Lewis and Lisa A. Vincler, "Storming the Ivory Tower: The Competing Interests of the Public's Right to Know and Protecting the Integrity of University Research," *Journal of College and University Law* 20 (Spring 1994): 440.

12. Orlans, *In the Name of Science,* pp. 86–89, 119–21.

13. Ibid., pp. 99–104.

14. Michael E. Carey, "Lessons Learned from a Scientist's Personal Confrontation with Animal Zealots," *Physiologist* 39, no. 1 (1996): 9.

15. Wisconsin Regional Primate Research Center, "Policy Statement on Principles for the Ethical Use of Animals," *American Journal of Primatology* 3 (1982): 345–47.

16. University of Southern California, Los Angeles. *Policies Governing the Use of Live Vertebrate Animals.* Revised 1 July 1991.

17. J. D. Miller and Linda K. Pifer, *Public Attitudes toward Science and Technology, 1979–1995, Integrated Codebook* (Chicago: International Center for the Advancement of Scientific Literacy, Chicago Academy of Sciences, 1995); and National Science Board, *Science and Engineering Indicators: 1989* (Washington: Government Printing Office, 1989).

18. Mitchell Fox, animal issues director, Progressive Animal Welfare Society. Public statement made at the University of Washington Animal Care Committee, 26 May 1994.

III

COSMETIC SAFETY
TESTING

6

BEAUTY WITHOUT THE BEAST

> We have produced a range of products which are 'cruelty-free,'
> non-toxic and environmentally safe with ingredients which are
> not animal tested
>
> Homecare Technology Ltd
>
> Organic Product Company skin care products are based on tradi-
> tional herbal remedies that have been tried and tested on people
> not animals[1]

The production of new cosmetics is now considered by many persons to be unjustified if animals suffer pain, distress, or death during premarketing safety testing. When the campaign against cosmetic testing reached significant dimensions in the 1970s and 1980s, animal tests commonly caused blindness, pain, and death to rabbits, rats, and other animals. Many improvements have been made to alleviate these problems, but animal welfare groups as well as some cosmetics manufacturers remain active in pressing for a ban on testing the safety of cosmetics that involves animals.

One of many examples was found in a June 1996 national animal rights demonstration in Washington, DC. Some three thousand signs with the message "Against Animal Testing" were distributed to demonstrators by the Body Shop, a cosmetic retailer and a major sponsor of the demonstration. The Body Shop has tried to build a reputation in both the United Kingdom and the United States based on its condemnation of animal testing.

The Body Shop's policy is that the company does not conduct animal tests and will only purchase cosmetic ingredients that suppliers have either never tested on animals for cosmetic purposes or at least not tested nor retested since December 31, 1990.[2] They have established a monitoring system to enforce this policy with suppliers. This policy is noted in its marketing, and products carry the label "Against Animal Testing." This label is a statement of philosophy, not a claim that their products have never been tested on animals—a claim that is still made by various companies.

According to Jon Entine, the Body Shop's purchasing manager, in 1992 46.5% of its ingredients had been tested on animals for some purpose at some time.[3] The policy does limit the Body Shop from using any newly developed ingredient (a dye or other substance) that has been tested on animals, even if this places them at a disadvantage with competitors.

Other product labels in common use are "Cruelty Free" and "Never Tested on Animals." People for the Ethical Treatment of Animals publishes an annual shopping guide, which includes companies such as Revlon, John Mitchell Systems, and Estee Lauder, and more than five hundred other companies. These companies assure PETA that they and their suppliers do not test on animals; they can then use PETA's "caring consumer" logo on their products, a rabbit in a box that says, "Not Tested on Animals. No Animal Ingredients."

These assurances make claims that companies using these labels are prepared to assert that the finished product contains no ingredients tested on animals by the distributor, supplier, or anyone else. Nonetheless, some consumer protection organizations and animal protection groups[4] argue that "No Animal Testing" claims are misleading and deceive consumers, because almost all ingredients in

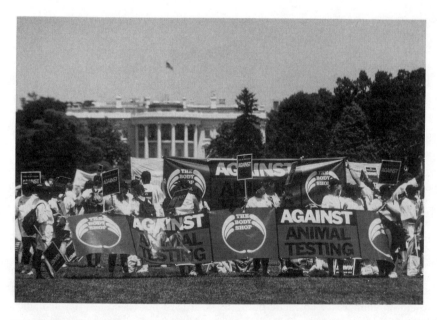

Marchers carrying placards announcing The Body Shop's opposition to animal testing at the animal rights parade in Washington, D.C., June 23, 1996. Credit: Marilyn Kazmers/ Sharksong.

use today in health and beauty aids have been-safety tested on animals at some time by some company.

In November 1995, in efforts to secure stringent product labeling standards, the National Consumers' League recommended to the US Federal Trade Commission that a ban be placed on the use of product labels such as "Against Animal Testing," "No Animal Testing," or "Not Tested on Animals."[5] The league believes that these labels should not be allowed because they do not convey specific information that is meaningful to consumers in making choices. However, in July 1996, the Federal Trade Commission responded to the league, stating that they would take no action on this matter on grounds that no consumer injury results from these product labels.[6]

THE NATURE AND JUSTIFICATION OF TESTING

Just about every item made by humans that we touch, smell, taste, or are exposed to has been tested on animals at some time, because synthetic chemicals will have been used in the production or preservation of these products. We now assume the safety of such products to an extraordinary degree. For example, we do not stop to consider that the chemicals in the colored clothes that we wear might lead to cancer of the skin, where it has been in direct contact with our bodies. Similarly, we use deodorants, antiperspirants, shaving creams, suntan and sunblock lotions, toothpastes, and household products such as washing powders and liquids, polishes, disinfectants, cleaners of various goods (for example, silver, brass, oven, window, floor) without fear, although some carry warning labels. Thousands of similar examples could be listed.

Reasons for Safety Testing

Apart from safeguarding the health of the consumer, there are several reasons to implement safety testing. There is a need to protect workers in the factories producing the chemicals, a need to protect the environment from inadvertent pollution, a need to protect the user of the chemicals in agriculture, at work, in industry, or in the backyard, and a need to know what to do when a person has been accidentally exposed to a significant amount of a substance, such as children swallowing a bottle of herbicide, or spilling a household chemical on themselves (that is, the need to identify organs that may be affected and the treatment of poisoning). Finally, there is a need to label a chemical either for marketing with suitable warnings on the packaging or for bulk transport when large amounts are being moved around the country on trucks or railways.

These, then, are the reasons for testing, but what should be tested, and how should it be tested? New chemicals, new substances, and new "improved" products are generally required by law to be tested before being marketed. The new product may use ingredients with well-known toxic or nontoxic safety profiles. Questions of risk then turn on whether there may be some unsuspected synergistic actions between the calculated "safe levels" of ingredients. New chemicals are safety-tested by giving them to animals in single and multiple doses of varying size and by various routes, intended to mimic approximated human exposures. The effects on the animals are noted, such as whether the compound is an irritant (for example, to the eye or skin) and by what route (for example, oral or inhaled), and the dose at which a single dose of compound causes signs of toxicity or kills the animals (for example, Lethal Dose 50% known as the LD50 Test).[7]

The Animals Used in Safety Testing

Detailed figures on the use of animals in safety testing have been kept in the United Kingdom for decades: In 1994, 7.6% of all vertebrates used in research were used for safety testing (see Table 1).

Andrew Rowan[8] estimated that in the US in 1980 some 14 million animals were used in the safety testing of cosmetics and household products, but no official statistics are kept in the US, and it is impossible to obtain accurate information.

Cosmetic Testing

The federal Food, Drug, and Cosmetic Act (US) defines "cosmetics" as articles intended to be applied to the human body for cleansing, beautifying, promoting attractiveness, or altering the appearance without affecting the body's structure or functions.[10] The European Directive 93/35/EEC is more explicit and defines a "cosmetic product" as "any substance or preparation intended to be placed in contact with the various external parts of the human body (epidermis, hair system, nails, lips, and external genital organs) or with the teeth and the mucous membranes of the oral cavity with a view exclusively or mainly to cleaning them, perfuming them, changing their appearance, and/or correcting body odors and/or protecting them or keeping them in good condition."[11]

Included in these definitions are "vanity products"—although it might be argued that some of these products are beneficial and even therapeutic—such as skin creams, lotions, sunblocks or sunscreens, suntan creams, aftershaves, perfumes, lipsticks, fingernail polishes, hardeners and enamels, eye and facial makeup, depilatories, hair straighteners, preparations, shower gels, bubble baths, shampoos, conditioners, permanent waves, hair dyes, rinses and sprays, toothpastes, mouthwashes, deodorants, talcum powders and soaps.

Safety testing involves a range of in vitro and in vivo[12] assessments, and is

TABLE 1. Numbers of different substances tested on various kinds of animals in the UK in 1994.[9]

Species of animal	Environmental pollution	Substances used in agriculture	Substances used in industry	Substances used in the household	Food additives	Cosmetics and toiletries	Total substances
Mouse	4,718	7,475	9,281	0	228	498	22,200
Rat	2,182	43,285	34,389	1,037	7,520	1,490	89,903
Guinea pig	33	5,717	15,557	168	376	1,430	23,281
Hamster	8	0	43	0	0	0	51
Other rodent	383	0	0	0	0	0	383
Rabbit	2	2,780	4,808	147	24	83	7,844
Beagle	34	470	103	0	18	0	625
Other carnivore	0	0	0	0	0	19	19
Pig	14	0	0	0	0	0	14
Goat	9	16	0	0	0	0	25
Sheep	132	0	0	0	0	0	132
Cattle	0	84	0	0	0	0	84
Other mammal	10	0	0	0	0	0	10
Bird	4	4,914	24	0	60	0	5,002
Reptile	0	0	0	0	0	0	0
Amphibian	25	118	0	0	0	0	143
Fish	44,245	3,756	1,679	0	0	0	49,680
Totals	51,799	68,615	65,884	1,352	8,226	3,520	199,396

considered necessary only for new cosmetic substances or new combinations of ingredients that need to be more carefully evaluated. The tests are designed mainly to look for skin irritation, absorption, phototoxicity (in response to ultra-violet radiation) and sensitization; eye and mucous membrane irritation; acute oral or inhalation toxicity; and any long-term effects such as carcinogenicity (cancer inducing), or teratogenicity (inducing defects in the unborn). New cosmetic *products* or formulations are examined for a No Effect Level (NOEL), or a No Adverse Effect Level (NOAEL) at a dosage similar to the calculated human exposure. Cosmetic *ingredients,* on the other hand, will be tested for their safety to protect the industrial chemical worker. In these tests the doses given will be increased until signs of toxicity are seen in order to obtain an idea of the level at which the substance is hazardous.

The Draize Skin-Irritancy Test and the Draize Eye Irritancy Test, developed in 1944, have acquired notoriety over the past fifty years because of the damaging effects on the animals, causing them pain, distress, and, in the early days of the test, blindness. In the skin test, the fur of the animal's trunk is clipped and the skin may then be abraded before a sleeve or semi-occlusive patch containing the test substance is applied for 24 hours. The animal and the skin are then examined at varying intervals for signs of toxicity and local injury. The skin test is used to predict sensitization of the skin, and phototoxic effects (sensitization in response to light). In the past decade, these tests have been considerably modified in Europe through strategic and humane experimental designs so that the animals suffer far less than before.

The eye test in the United States involves placing a small volume of diluted test substance in the eye of six[13] albino rabbits and observing them for signs of irritation for up to 3 days. If damage has occurred, animals will be followed up for 21 days to see if the damage is repaired, and if little or no repair occurs, the substance will be classified as corrosive. The eye test has been criticized because the rabbit's eye is significantly different from the human eye on several counts. For example, rabbits have a third eyelid, unlike humans; rabbits also have a slower blink reflex, a thinner cornea, and produce fewer tears than humans. Furthermore, the test has given inconsistent results between laboratories.[14] Nevertheless, the US Food and Drug Administration (FDA) and the European Scientific Committee on Cosmetology[15] still consider the test to be useful to understand and predict injury to or around the eye.

Acute toxicity tests are usually carried out on white rats to determine safe exposure levels. The LD50 test, as described more than seventy years ago,[16] involved causing at least 50% of the animals to die (often a slow, painful death) from a single dose of the test substance, but this approach has now been superseded by requiring that fewer animals be used. The test normally performed today accepts estimated data on lethality (for example, by using data from other structurally related chemicals).

Human data, if available, are used in all safety evaluations. However, it often takes several years for such evidence to accumulate from reports of routine use as well as accidental exposures.

STAKEHOLDERS IN CONTROVERSIES
OVER THE USE OF ANIMALS

The cosmetics industry is still expanding. In the seven major European cosmetics markets, the value of the industry was around $32 billion in 1993[17] with an annual growth rate of 6% per year. In the United States, Avon, Revlon, and Fabergé rank first, second, and fourth with 1988 sales of $2.1 billion, $1.79 billion and $1.2 billion, respectively.[18] The market is currently expanding into Asia and South America.

It has become increasingly apparent that the public does not want products that have been tested on laboratory animals, and therefore many companies have ended their testing. Some cosmetic manufacturers are so opposed to animal testing they have formed the Cosmetics Industry Coalition for Animal Welfare (CICAW). CICAW members agree not to use any ingredient that has been tested since 1976, that is, they adhere to a fixed-cutoff-date criterion; by so doing they risk going out of business. Furthermore, a number of their key cosmetic ingredients have been superseded.[19] Other companies choose to roll a five-year cutoff date forward each year.

The general public is undoubtedly concerned about the use of animals to test cosmetic products. Polls have shown between 85% and 96% of the public are against animal testing of beauty, vanity, and household products.[20]

Legislation in Europe is somewhat at odds with itself as, on the one hand, it requires animal testing of ingredients for the purpose of health and safety, but on the other, requires that animal testing should be reduced.[21] However, legislation has now been passed in Europe for the industry to phase out animal testing to help meet consumer demands but without endangering human health.[22] In the United States the FDA now states that it does *not* require LD50 test data to establish toxicity, and, furthermore, it advocates the use of validated non-whole animal techniques.[23]

Animal rights and antivivisection organizations demand an immediate end to all animal experimentation and have campaigned for a ban on animal testing of cosmetics, in particular, since cosmetics testing is viewed as a relatively easy target. The moderate animal welfare organizations, who typically promote the "Three Rs" concept are insistent in their claims that the use of animals for testing cosmetics is unnecessary. Even the pro-animal-research groups, established to defend the use of animals in biomedical research, now accept the claim that animals should not be used for testing cosmetics and certain other types of consumer products. Many of the products are now often tested on employees of cosmetics companies.

ETHICAL ISSUES

Harms and Benefits in New Product Testing

It is generally accepted that new *chemicals* should be tested, but not everyone agrees that all new *products* should be tested, especially cosmetic products. It has been suggested that the benefits to be gained from cosmetics are so trivial that the use of animals for the purpose of ensuring safety is immoral and not to be condoned because the harms done to the animals do not compensate for the relatively small benefits to humans. Typically, animal protection organizations state that there are enough products available already, and that new ones should not be developed if it involves animal experimentation.

However, if we had taken this view in 1960 and consistently practiced it, we might not have various hair conditioners, sunblock lotions, fluoride toothpastes, antiperspirants, and so on that we have today. Nor would they be available in their present range and quality. The failure to test not only runs risks of harms for humans, but also results in lost opportunities for industries and their consumers. If rules are overly stringent, whole areas of research can be brought to a standstill, with consequent loss of the benefits of that line of research.

Where does one draw the line regarding what will be tested as well as the harms that will be permitted in the testing? How are permitted harms to be balanced against possible benefits? (See chapter 1) In assessing such questions, we need to take account of the many types of harm and benefit that might come into consideration. For example, would pressure not to use animals to test cosmetic products preclude the safety testing of the chemical ingredients that are used to make up those same cosmetics as well as many noncosmetic products?

A related question is, how hard should we try to use animals to mimic extreme misuses or abuses of substances by humans in order to prevent harm? Should our research be done on the basis that someone somewhere may ignore all the warnings and take in a dose that would not normally occur if the product was used properly? Accidental ingestion and exposure by children does occasionally occur, and toxicity data *may* provide some information on what organs are affected and how to treat such persons, depending on whether the animal absorbs, metabolizes, and excretes the chemical in a similar fashion.

This problem exists with all toxicity testing in animals, because species extrapolation is an unavoidable aspect of human safety testing. However, do manufacturers go beyond what would normally be possible in dosage rates—that is, do they unjustifiably give animals dose levels that no human could possibly reach?[24] Evidence suggests they have done so on occasion, which may add weight to the thesis that scientists should carry out more limited tests, as described below.

Two ways forward might be to try to make animal tests more humane or to replace them altogether with in vitro methods. But is our science currently good enough to warrant this replacement?

The Alternative of Human Volunteers

Alternatives to the use of animals are often suggested as a way around moral problems in their use. The Three Rs first put forward by Russell and Burch in 1959[25] include *replacement alternatives* as a major moral responsibility in planning for new research. (See chapter 1)

Human volunteers are now increasingly being used to test cosmetic products, just as they have long been used in biomedical research. An essential element of carrying out research on humans is not only that they should be adequately aware of the risks involved, but also that they not be manipulated or coerced into participating. It is debatable whether an employee of a cosmetics company can take part free of manipulation by the implicit structure of rewards and punishments (salary increases, job transfers, and the like). The employee may feel that it will stand him or her in good stead for promotion or a wage increase, or keeping his or her job in times of redundancy, even though this may be explicitly disclaimed in any contract by the employer. For a similar reason it is not acceptable for prisoners to be used in research in the United States and United Kingdom (except for research on prison conditions).

The essence of manipulation is swaying people to do what the manipulator wants by means other than persuasion. For purposes of decision making when volunteering for tests, the key forms of manipulation are not punishment and threat, but the effect of rewards, offers, and encouragement. When an offer is made in a setting in which it is abnormally attractive—for example, an offer of a promotion (or freedom for destitute prisoners), it may be manipulative. It is especially vital to ensure that conditions permitting resistance to control are preserved in institutions where it might be exerted.

This shows how moral problems can arise from reflection on alternatives to our use of animals that are not specifically about the morality of *animal* use. However, associated and more general questions arise about our obligations to both humans and animals. The chief question is, are we obligated to seek human volunteers to replace animals in cosmetic testing; and, if the risk is similar for both, are we obligated to use humans first or animals first?

Alternatives to Using Whole Animals in Safety Tests

The US Public Health Service policy on protocol review by institutional animal care and use committees states that in vitro biological systems to replace animals should be considered in testing. A similar approach urging scientists to "consider alternatives" has been adopted in the United Kingdom in the Animals (Scientific Procedures) Act of 1986. The European Directive is more explicit and states, "An experiment shall not be performed if another scientifically satisfactory method of obtaining the result sought, not entailing the use of an animals, is reasonably and practicably available."[26]

Alternatives to the use of whole animals are currently being developed.[27] Cell culture, tissue slices, organ culture, computer modeling, use of lower organisms, and so forth can all provide useful information in research and safety testing, but to date cannot entirely replace whole animal tests, because whole animals are made up of body systems, that is, interacting body organs, and not just cells. In vitro methods can reveal useful information about a chemical and its interactions with specific cell types (the scientific discipline of toxicology). For example, they can expose overt toxicity as it kills cells or alters a cellular function. What in vitro methods cannot do is replace the complex interactions within a whole animal. That is why such methods are often referred to as "adjuncts" rather than "replacements."

Although animal protection organizations tend to overstate the availability and current applicability of alternative tests, some alternatives can provide useful screening techniques. For example, substances that are toxic to cells in culture may well be toxic to whole animals and so need not be tested further. Studies are being carried out to seek alternatives to the Draize Eye-Irritancy Test, but such alternatives are still at an early stage of development and evaluation. They include the use of isolated eyes (rabbit, chicken, bovine); complex artificial skin mixtures and skin slices, chicken egg membranes, and cell cultures. These tests still have to be fully validated for a large range of chemicals for the toxicities that we presently investigate such as irritancy and sensitization, before being widely accepted.[28]

Humane Endpoints When Using Whole Animals in Safety Tests

The Three Rs of Russell and Burch include not only the replacement alternatives outlined above, but also *refinement alternatives,* which are means by which animal suffering can be *reduced to a minimum.* (See chapter 1.) In the past decade the Draize eye and skin tests have been considerably modified through strategic and humane experimental designs so that the animals suffer far less than before. In many cases suffering may be quite slight and far less severe than one might see daily in an average veterinarian's clinic. Unlike the past, when animals were restrained in stocks, the animals are now allowed free mobility, and have continual access to food and water.

However, the amount of skin exposed to the test substance can be large, and adverse effects such as irritation and inflammation can be significant during the 24-hour period. The potential for the eye test to cause pain is considerable, and this test, like the skin test, has been modified over the past decade or so. The mucous membranes of the eye may now be anesthetized with local anesthetic before the test substance is introduced. Solutions of extreme acidity or alkalinity are not tested in the eye, as they will be assumed to be irritant, and substances that have been shown to be skin irritants do not go on to be used in the eye (skin irritation studies precede eye tests in the tiered systems of testing now being used).[29]

Acute toxicity tests, as described more than fifty years ago, involved large numbers of animals and required death as an integral part of the test. These tests have now been superseded. The test normally performed today accepts *estimated data* on lethality, and a major advance has been that in some countries regulatory authorities accept signs of toxicity rather than death as a valid endpoint.[30] The test has been further refined so that a maximum dose level is laid down, the so-called Limit Test, in which a maximum single dose rate of 2 g/kg (in Europe) or 5 g/kg (in the United States) is given. If the substance shows no toxicity at that level (interpreted as one or no animal(s) dying out of ten dosed after 14 days) the substance will be classified as nontoxic. If two or more animals die, then a second group will be tested at a lower dose. The complete test normally requires ten to twenty rats.

Michael Balls and Julia Fentem have compared the various acute toxicity tests available today, as summarized in Table 2.[31] The data show that since 1927 significant changes have been made for various tests. In addition, the tests themselves have been refined so that they cause less pain for the animals.

TABLE 2. Comparison of single oral dose acute toxicity test procedures.

Name of test	Minimum number of animals used	Maximum number of animals used	Death as the endpoint	Time taken (days)
Classical (1927)	60	80	yes	> 14
OECD (1981)	30	30	yes	> 14
Up and Down (1985)	6	10	yes	< 25
ATC-BGA (1985)	6	18	yes	28
OECD (1987)	20	20	yes	> 28
FDP-BTS (1987)	10	20	no	> 14

The tests referred to in the left column are the Classical LD50 Test (Classical); the Organization for Economic Cooperation and Development recommended standards in the years cited (OECD); the Up and Down Test (Up and Down); the Acute Toxic Class–Bundesgesundheitsamt (ATC-BGA); and the Fixed Dose Procedure–British Toxicology Society (FDP-BTS).

Desensitization of Animal Researchers

The vast scale on which animals are used in safety testing often desensitizes those connected with the practice. Such desensitization presents many moral problems. (See chapter 1) A duty of care extends to all animals, but discharging this obligation to the large number of animals involved in safety testing is plainly very difficult.

Desensitization may occur as a consequence of being continually exposed to animal suffering, as in acute toxicity testing. "Once you've been here a few days, you lose respect for all living things."[32] "Oversensitization" of employees toward animals may be seen by some as sentimentality, but today's animal concerns were, perhaps, yesterday's sentimentality.

Management has reacted to this "sentimentality" in some laboratories by discouraging the naming of animals. Such distancing of the researcher from the animal may encourage poorer care and fewer questions as to why animals are being used than in other laboratories where such concerns are more openly discussed.

Ill-Gotten Gains

Because the humaneness of safety testing has increased over the past five to ten years, ingredients tested during this period are likely to have caused far less animal suffering than ingredients tested before 1986. Therefore, from the perspective of ill-gotten gains, there is a moral obligation to use newer over old ingredients.

The argument of ill-gotten gains could also be applied to the importation of cosmetic products from those countries whose standards of testing are less humane. At what point should a government or a corporation decide not to import goods that have been produced by means that would be unethical or illegal in their own country? Are governments obligated to abide by such a standard in a way that corporations are not? Are individual consumers bound to the logic of ill-gotten gains in their purchases?

Mislabeling and the Ethics of Advertising

Labeling of products and advertising claims can teeter on the border of the misleading. Can credibility be retained if the relevant facts are not revealed? In theory, advertising should be limited to the dissemination of information from which consumers are able to make an informed choice. If they are misled in the attempt to make an intelligent choice or are enticed into the choice by deception, the advertising has an enormous burden of justification. If advertisements are not designed to be rationally persuasive, but rather manipulative, we will almost surely judge them morally inappropriate.

For many large and diversified companies, it is virtually impossible to claim that products and ingredients have not been tested on animals. What standards of disclosure, then, are appropriate in advertising their products in order that they not be deceptive? The FTC and other regulatory institutions in the United States hold that if consumers are misled by deception, the advertising cannot be justified—morally or legally. The FTC has therefore placed strict regulations on industries that produce products that are potentially harmful to humans.

Typically, both the government and consumer protection groups focus on consumer *response* to advertising and its social effects, rather than on the *intention* of the creators of that advertising. By contrast, those who defend controversial advertising often focus more on the intentions of advertising agencies and manufacturers in marketing a product, namely, the intent to sell a good product. These different emphases complicate the issues, because a product marketed with good intentions can nonetheless be advertised in a misleading way or otherwise have negative consequences. One could view the ethics of cosmetics advertisements by responsible companies as falling into this domain.

A different perspective is that of quality control. If products like cosmetics had to be certified by an independent agency as both safe and free of animal testing to be allowed on the market, we might care much less about the messages of advertisements or sales representatives. Taking this view amounts to a call for higher qualitative standards in industry and regulatory branches of government as a means to resolve consumer protection issues.

Too stringent a standard of either disclosure or quality control could thwart the efforts of companies that currently are not doing animal testing, thereby frustrating goals of preventing unnecessary animal testing. Too weak a standard runs the risks already noted, allowing fraud and causing consumers to lose any meaningful opportunity to select appropriate products.

A coalition of animal protection groups including the Humane Society of the United States, PETA, the Doris Day Animal League, and others, began in 1996 to prepare an "animal testing standard" that is to be proposed to all cosmetic manufacturers to attempt to bring clarity to the terminology used on cosmetic products. The standard defines what is meant by "animal," "nonanimal," and "in vitro testing." Individual cosmetic companies are asked to make a commitment to abide by the standard not to conduct or commission animal testing or purchase ingredients from a supplier that conducted animal testing on the company's behalf after the date of agreement. The coalition plans to publicize the names of companies so committed and to identify its products. The standard permits all companies to adopt this policy and to benefit in its marketing from this commitment. In this way, the coalition hopes to exert pressure to end animal testing on cosmetics in the future.

CONCLUSION

Professor Michael Balls, director of the European Center for the Validation of Alternative Methods (ECVAM), suggests that the goal in cosmetic testing should be the manufacture and marketing of new, better, and safer cosmetic products containing new, better, and safer ingredients. This goal can presumably be achieved using sound cosmetic science and reliable safety assessment, and without using toxicity test procedures on laboratory animals. Balls asserts that action must be taken now, to ensure that some progress toward this goal is made before the status of alternatives to animal testing for cosmetics is reviewed and a decision taken about postponing the proposed ban on cosmetic testing.

In reality the ban is not likely to be accepted. To minimize the criticism from animal protection organizations that will inevitably follow from postponement, the cosmetics industry and the European Community (EC) must be able to provide strong evidence that they are continuing to support the development, evaluation, and validation of alternative methods of testing. That alternative tests are playing a major role during "in-house" development and testing of new formulation will, however, not be morally sufficient in the eyes of animal protection organizations—not in the EC or in other developed countries. There is certain to be renewed pressure for moral progress in actually replacing animal tests for cosmetics with validated alternatives.

NOTES

1. Royal Society for the Prevention of Cruelty to Animals, Think Before You Shop . . . Cruelty-Free Shopping Guide. (London: UK RSPCA, 1995), pp. 22–26.

2. The Body Shop Animal Protection Statement 95 (Watermead, West Sussex, England: The Body Shop International PLC, 1996), p. 21.

3. Quoted in: Jon Entine, "Shattered Image," Business Ethics (September/October 1994): 26.

4. Michael Balls, "Comments on Labelling Related to the Animal Testing of Cosmetic Ingredients and Products Manufactured and/or Marketed within the European Economic Community," Alternatives to Laboratory Animals 19 (1991): 302–7.

5. Letter from Karin L. Bolte of the National Consumers League to the Honorable Robert Pitofsky, chairman, US Federal Trade Commission, Washington, DC, p. 9. November 5, 1995.

6. Letter from Jodie Bernstein, director, US Federal Trade Commission to Linda F. Golodner, president, National Consumers League, 9 July 1996.

7. The formal or "classified" LD50 test subjected animals to increasing doses until a significant number of them died, so that it was possible to compute a Lethal Dose 50% by extrapolation. Normally more than 50% of animals died.

8. A. N. Rowan, Of Mice, Models and Men: A Critical Evaluation of Animal Research (Albany: State University of New York Press, 1984). Since 1984 Rowan has

reestimated the number to be nearer 4 million, but because of poor and inadequate data in the United States it is impossible to be precise.

9. HMSO 1994 Statistics of Scientific Procedures on Living Animals in Great Britain. Cm. 3012

10. FDA, *Cosmetics Handbook* (Washington: US Department of Health and Human Services, Public Health Service, Food and Drug Administration, 1992).

11. Council Directive 93/35/EEC, amending for the sixth time Directive 76/768/EEC, Article 1(1).

12. *In vitro,* literally meaning "in glass," is used to describe those tests which can be carried out without the use of living animals, although for some tests an animal may have to be killed to provide tissue. In vivo tests, on the other hand, require whole living animals to be used.

13. The OECD test, with which the United States has agreed to comply under the Mutual Acceptance of Data agreement, requires only three rabbits to be used, but the US Environmental Protection Agency appears to request that six animals be routinely used.

14. "The Draize Eye-Irritancy Test," *Fact Sheet* (Humane Society of the United States), 1993.

15. The SCC was established by the European Commission to assist in examining the complex scientific and technical problems surrounding cosmetics composition, manufacture, packaging, and labeling.

16. J. W. Trevan, "The Error of Determination of Toxicity," *Proceedings of the Royal Society of London,* series B (1927): 101, 483–514.

17. A. J. Suckling, "The RSPCA, Cosmetics and Animal Testing," *International Conference on Animal Welfare in the Cosmetics and Toiletries Industry* (Cosmetic Industry Coalition for Animal Welfare Ltd., 1995), p. 1. Available from RSPCA, Causeway, Horsham, West Sussex RH12 1HG, UK.

18. "Cosmetics Companies Quietly Ending Animal Tests," *New York Times,* 2 August 1989, pp. A1, D22.

19. J. Piccioni, "Welcome Address," *International Conference on Animal Welfare in the Cosmetics and Toiletries Industry"* (Cosmetics Industry Coalition for Animal Welfare Ltd., 1995), p. 1.

20. Virginia Mathews, "Putting Cruelty to the Test," *Marketing Week,* 14 May 1993, p. 21. BUAV found 85% and the RSPCA 96% were against animal testing of beauty and household products. The *Daily Mirror* (United Kingdom), October 29, 1992, reported a MORI poll giving the figure of 87% not wanting cosmetics tested on animals.

21. D. W. Straughan, "The EU Target for a 50% Reduction in the Use of Experimental Animals by the Year 2000: What Does It Mean?" *ATLA* 23, no. 2 (1995): 262.

22. European Council Directive 93/35/EEC amending for the sixth time Directive 76/768/EEC on the approximation of laws of the Member States relating to cosmetic products states that testing on animals of ingredients or combinations of ingredients should be banned from 1st January 1998, but only if alternative methods of testing have been scientifically validated. If this does not happen then the end date can be postponed, which is most likely to happen. *Official Journal of the European Communities* L.151 (23 June 1993): 32–36.

23. FDA position paper on "Animal Use in Testing FDA-Regulated Products," October 1992; see also *Scientists Center for Animal Welfare (SCAW) Newsletter* 11, no. 3 (Fall 1989): 12.

24. "Beauty Without Cruelty Cosmetic Guide" (November 1990). Leslie Fain witnessed rats being placed in an airtight chamber and having hair spray sprayed in. This

was apparently equivalent to sealing oneself in the bathroom and spraying hair spray for one hour. The rats died from poisoning by the solvent rather than the chemicals in the hair spray. Leaflet BWC, PO Box 97, Newlands 7725 S. Africa.

25. William M. S. Russell and Rex L. Burch, *The Principles of Humane Experimental Technique* (London: Methuen, 1959).

26. European Council Directive 86/609/EEC on the approximation of laws, regulations, and administrative provisions of the Member States regarding the protection of animals used for other scientific purposes. Article 7.2. *Official Journal of the European Communities* 29, L.358 (18 December 1986): 1–29.

27. L. H. Bruner, "Alternatives to the Use of Animals in Household Products and Cosmetic Testing," *Journal of the American Veterinary Medical Association* 200 (1992): 669–673.

28. See European Council Directive 93/35/EEC.

29. R. J. Fielder, I. F. Gaunt, C. Rhodes, F. M. Sullivan, and D. W. Swanston, "A Hierarchical Approach to the Assessment of Dermal and Ocular Irritancy: A Report by the British Toxicology Society Working Party on Irritancy," *Human Toxicology* 6 (1987): 269–78; *Federal Register* 49, no. 105 (1984): 2252; Home Office Guidelines on Eye Irritation Tests (1995), Report of the Animals Procedures Committee for 1994, HMSO Cm, 2996, 12–14. In the United Kingdom, the Home Office is the government department responsible for animal research. In the United States it is the USDA, which does not issue experimental guidelines.

30. M. J. van den Heuvel, D. G. Clark, R. J. Fielder, P. P. Koundakjian, G. J. A. Oliver, D. Pelling, N. J. Tomlinson, and A. P. Walker, "The International Validation of a Fixed Dose Procedure as an Alternative to the Classical LD50 Test," *Food Chemical Toxicology* 28 (1990): 469–82; OECD Revised Guideline 401 (OECD 1987) for acute oral toxicity testing; R. D. Bruce, "An Up-and-Down Procedure for Acute Toxicity Testing," *Fundamental & Applied Toxicology* 6 (1985): 151–57.

31. Taken from M. Balls and J. H. Fentem, "The On-Going Process to Replace the LD50 Test," *Humane Innovations & Alternatives* 7 (1993): 544–47.

32. People for the Ethical Treatment of Animals, "Undercover Investigator," quoting an employee at Biosearch Laboratories, USA, in 1988, in *The PETA Guide to Compassionate Living,* (Washington, D.C.: PETA, no date), p. 9.

IV

BEHAVIORAL RESEARCH

7

APES AND LANGUAGE:
WASHOE AND HER SUCCESSORS

Washoe is a chimpanzee who was the first great ape—a classification that includes chimpanzees, gorillas, and orangutans—to be taught American Sign Language (ASL), a gestural language used by deaf people to communicate.[1] Washoe's history is as remarkable as the moral problems raised by that history.

WASHOE'S HISTORY

Washoe spent her early years in the household of R. Allen and Beatrix T. Gardner, who were part of an ape language research project sponsored by the University of Nevada.

The Gardners provided Washoe with an environment and routine quite similar to that given a typical human child. Under natural conditions, chimpanzees rely on their mothers for most needs until they are between two and three years old. When she came to the Gardner house, Washoe was only a baby: "She did not have her first canines or molars, her eye-hand coordination was rudimentary, she could only crawl about, and she slept a good deal."[2] She was taught to eat and drink with human utensils, as well as to dress and use the toilet. She was given typical children's toys, and exhibited a special affinity for dolls and picture books. She became accustomed to being cared for by the same group of people, and she was left alone only when sleeping.[3]

Prior to Washoe's experience, other chimpanzees had been brought up in circumstances similar to hers, a process called "cross-fostering." In addition, several attempts had been made to teach cross-fostered chimpanzees spoken language, without notable success. Eventually, scientists concluded that verbal speech was ill-suited to the chimpanzee's anatomical structure.[4] Proposals then emerged to teach chimpanzees alternative forms of symbolic communication that did not require speech. Besides ASL, chimpanzees have been taught specially improvised languages, in which plastic tokens or computer keys symbolize various objects and actions.[5]

In their time with Washoe, the Gardners and other members of Washoe's foster family used only ASL to communicate with her and among themselves, on the assumption that this would provide the least confusing learning situation for Washoe.[6] Their teaching methods resembled those used to teach language to human children. They signed frequently to each other and to Washoe. They used simple words and gestures repetitively, complimented Washoe's correct usage, and tried to comply with her requests.

At first, they used operant-conditioning techniques, in which certain naturally

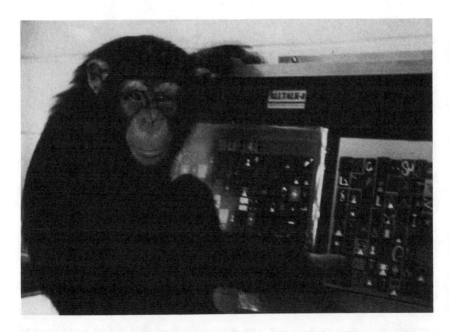

This chimpanzee, at the Language Research Center of Georgia State University, sits at a computerized instrument panel learning sign language. Credit: Professor Duane Rumbaugh, Language Research Center, Georgia State University, Atlanta.

occurring chimpanzee gestures were modified into ASL signs, and then reinforced. They found, however, that this process was less efficient than direct teaching, in which they simply told Washoe, "This is a ____," "You are now ____ing," and so forth. Following the methods of parents and teachers of deaf children, they would take Washoe's hands and put them in the correct position for the sign that was being taught. They responded to Washoe's signing behavior "by smiling or frowning, by nodding or shaking [their] heads, and by praising or scolding [Washoe] in ASL, just as human adults normally respond to the verbal behavior of human children."[7] The outcome of these efforts was four-year-old Washoe's apparent ability to recognize and use at least 132 ASL signs.[8]

When she was five years old, Washoe was moved to the Institute for Primate Studies, at the University of Oklahoma. The move was initiated by Roger Fouts, a researcher who began working with Washoe in Reno. Fouts had obtained financial support from the university to extend his study of Washoe's language abilities.[9] Although she was still involved in sign language research, Washoe's life at the Primate Institute was very different. For the first time, she was living with other chimpanzees and spending part of her time in a cage. She left confinement less often, and then on a leash. Roger Fouts maintained a close relationship with her, but she no longer received the intense human attention she had been given in her early years.[10]

Fouts began a new series of studies involving Washoe. Other chimpanzees at the Primate Institute were taught ASL, and communication among the animals was observed. In 1979, a few weeks after her own infant died, Washoe was given a baby chimpanzee with the hope that she would begin to treat it as her own. She did so, and a new experiment was initiated. The goal was to determine whether Washoe would teach ASL to the infant, who was named Loulis. Her human caregivers stopped signing to Washoe whenever Loulis was present. The other chimpanzees continued to sign as they interacted with Washoe and Loulis.

A year later, Fouts moved Washoe and Loulis to new housing at Central Washington University, where they were eventually joined by three other signing chimpanzees who had been raised in the Gardners' home. After about five years, Loulis appeared to have knowledge of 51 signs. At that point, "the restriction on human signing in Loulis' presence was ended, because, in essence, it was a form of deprivation for Loulis as well as for the other chimpanzees."[11]

Washoe, Loulis, and the other three chimpanzees continue to live in a facility at Central Washington University. Their living quarters, recently improved and expanded, include both indoor and outdoor exercise rooms, as well as sleeping quarters and a human-observation area. An organization called Friends of Washoe provides financial support and produces a newsletter describing ongoing research projects and reporting on the daily lives of Washoe and the rest of the group. In 1992 Roger and Deborah Fouts established the Chimpanzee and

Human Communication Institute, which is "dedicated to the better understanding of communications, both human and chimpanzee."[12]

Through programs offered by the university and this institute, many graduate and undergraduate students conduct observational and other noninvasive studies of the chimpanzees' language use and other behavior. Volunteer docents conduct public education sessions on the signing chimpanzees and issues relevant to the species in general.[13] The animals continue to use signs in their interactions among themselves and with the humans who work with and care for them. Washoe is the oldest member of the group, and she is "perhaps best known for her ability to comfort and reassure chimps and humans alike."[14]

Some of the other signing chimpanzees at the Primate Institute have been less fortunate than Washoe. When the University of Oklahoma decided to withdraw its financial support, the institute closed. One of the chimpanzees (Nim Chimpsky, whose case is discussed below) was sent to a wildlife rehabilitation center, where he was the sole chimpanzee on the premises, and others went to biomedical research facilities, where little attention was given to their signing abilities.[15]

DID WASHOE LEARN A LANGUAGE?

The seeming language abilities of Washoe and other subjects in the ape language experiments remain controversial. Critics of the research have raised a number of doubts about these abilities. Two recurring questions are whether the researchers, who often develop personal ties to their subjects, are unconsciously biased toward seeing correct responses, or alternatively, tend inadvertently to signal the correct response to the subjects, a phenomenon called "cueing."

To avoid the problems of interpreter bias and cueing, the Gardners set up an elaborate procedure to assess Washoe's knowledge of words. In random order, slides showing various objects were projected onto a screen facing Washoe. Two human observers recorded her responses; because neither was able to see the projection screen, they did not know the identities of the objects in the slides. One observer was in the room with Washoe, and asked her to identify the object if she did not do so spontaneously. The other observer watched through a one-way window. Both observers recorded the sign they believed Washoe made in response to each slide. The two observers could not see each other, so each was unaware of the sign recorded by the other until a full test (of either 64 or 128 slides) was completed.

In the first test, interobserver agreement on the specific signs Washoe used was 95% and in the second test, agreement was 86%. In the first test, one observer recorded 86% correct responses, the other observer found 88% correct. In the second, the scores were 72% and 71% correct. These figures are higher than would be expected by chance. The findings are particularly interesting in that each slide represented a different exemplar of the object in question. For example, the "shoe" category was represented by a woman's high-heeled shoe, a winter boot, a tie shoe, and a loafer. No slide was shown more than once. Washoe was apparently able to recognize that objects with different appearances belonged to the same general language category.[16] Some commentators believe that Washoe possessed general concepts or abstract ideas.

Even with the Gardners' testing method, however, there is a small chance that the human observers might have guessed what was on the later slides in the test series, based on Washoe's prior responses and their knowledge that she would be shown the same number of exemplars for each language category investigated. As a result, they might have been biased in favor of interpreting Washoe's sign as the correct one, and the observer in the same room might somehow have indicated to Washoe the sign she should make.[17]

LANGUAGE ACQUISITION IN OTHER PRIMATES

To reduce even this small possibility of interpreter bias and inadvertent cueing, a separate group of investigators at Yerkes Primate Center in Georgia adopted a different testing procedure, which involved two chimpanzees communicating to each other out of the presence of any human observers. Sherman and Austin were taught a language involving symbols on a computer board. This approach removes the possibility of interpreter bias, since the responses are unambiguously clear and can easily be recorded for later study. In one of the many studies conducted by the Yerkes group, Sherman and Austin were taught to share foods with each other. Both were seated at a table that contained two portions of from 7 to 13 of a possible 20 desirable foods. The chimpanzee seated closest to the computer keyboard was designated the "requester." The requester could use the keyboard to ask for a specific food; the other chimpanzee would then be expected to hand one portion of that food to the requester and to eat the remaining portion himself.

According to the Yerkes researchers, "sharing was an accepted and comfortable means of dealing with food, and using the keyboard to request foods was easy for [Sherman and Austin] to do."[18] The activity could be monitored by videocamera, dispensing with the need for human observers who might inadvertently signal correct responses. Of 255 exchanges, 92% were fully correct in that the requested food was present on the tray and the food item delivered to the requester was the same as the one indicated on the computer keyboard.[19]

The above methods, as well as others devised by ape language researchers, substantially reduce the possibility that interpreter bias and human cueing account for the animals' correct responses in various tests.[20] Other challenges to the research findings are more difficult to address, however. These include arguments that evidence of the apes' ability to use signs and symbols to request desired items and activities and to respond to simple questions does not demonstrate that they have acquired a language.[21]

The debate over whether ape study subjects really learn language occurs in part because there is disagreement over what constitutes a language and consequently what it means to be a true language user. In the early years of the ape language studies, many scientists and linguists emphasized the importance of grammar, or syntax, which is concerned with the order in which words occur. Facility with grammatical rules enables language users to convey many more meaningful phrases and sentences than would be possible if word order had no effect on meaning.[22] To many language analysts, syntax is the fundamental characteristic of language.[23] Those holding this view refuse to confer the title of language user on individuals who can use words, but cannot create sentences that have different meanings due to their different word order.

At first, it seemed that apes could learn some basic rules governing sentence construction. For example, when Washoe was asked the identity of a swan, she responded with the signs for "water bird," which was for her a novel combination of words presented in the appropriate descriptive order. She also was able to combine several items in her vocabulary into longer utterances.[24]

However, the significance of this behavior was severely challenged in the late seventies, by the investigator in a language study involving a chimpanzee named Nim Chimpsky (named after the linguist Noam Chomsky). Herbert Terrace, a scientist at Columbia University, obtained Nim shortly after the animal's birth at the Primate Institute in Oklahoma. More than sixty people participated in the effort to teach Nim ASL.[25] He received training in a formal, very structured classroom setting, as well as in the home of the human family where he spent his earliest years. When he was almost four years old, Nim was sent back to the Primate Institute.[26] At that point, Terrace began in-depth analysis of his data.

Terrace's primary interest was in Nim's ability to create sentences. After examining his written and videotaped records, Terrace concluded, "[T]he fact that Nim's utterances were less spontaneous and less original than those of a child, and that his utterances did not become longer, both as he learned new signs and as he acquired more experience in using sign language, suggests that much of the structure and meaning of his [word] combinations was determined, or at least suggested, by his teachers."[27] Terrace also found that rather than engaging in conversational exchanges, Nim frequently interrupted other signers. Moreover, he appeared to Terrace to sign only as much as was necessary to obtain the desired object or action. Finally, Terrace asserted that the signs made by Nim and other chimpanzees he had observed were often mere imitations of signs their teachers had recently made.[28]

Terrace qualified his claims by noting that problems caused by his project's training procedures and number of teachers, and not Nim's lack of linguistic abilities, might have accounted for the negative findings. Furthermore, other researchers have criticized various aspects of Terrace's study, and challenged many of his assertions.[29] Nevertheless, Terrace's report substantially diminished the scientific interest in and financial support for ape language studies.[30]

RECENT ASSESSMENTS IN APE LANGUAGE STUDIES

In recent years, a more balanced assessment of the ape language studies has emerged. This is due largely to work conducted by Sue Savage-Rumbaugh and her colleagues at Yerkes Primate Center. Their research with Sherman and Austin, together with another project involving a bonobo, or pygmy chimpanzee, named Kanzi, provides a careful and detailed picture of ape language capacities.

Savage-Rumbaugh has shifted the focus of her research from syntax to other dimensions of language use. Like many psychologists studying language development in young children, she is most interested in the communicative function of language, in how her research subjects put their knowledge of the world around them into words to convey to others. Although they have begun to look more extensively into grammatical structure, Savage-Rumbaugh and her colleagues have primarily studied how their subjects use words to exchange meaning with others.[31] Savage-Rumbaugh also believes that possession of language ought not be viewed as an all-or-nothing characteristic: "[M]ore profitable in the case of both child and ape is to ask what elements of language are present and what elements are absent at a particular point in development."[32]

Besides the food-sharing activity described above, Sherman and Austin have learned to use the symbols on their computer keyboards to request from each other specific tools needed to open different types of food containers. They demonstrate this skill in carefully designed experimental conditions in which computer language is the sole means available for communication.[33] According to ethologist Donald Griffin, these and other examinations "make it absolutely clear that these two apes were intentionally communicating by means of the Yerkes keyboard as well as by gesturing, and that they not only understood but often enjoyed what they were doing."[34] Terrace himself has commented, "Savage-Rumbaugh's program of research shows how other projects missed a wealth of important issues about symbol use by pursuing the unrealistically ambitious goals of demonstrating grammatical competence."[35]

Further support for the belief that apes are capable of significant linguistic achievement comes from a study that arose after an unforeseen development at Yerkes. Savage-Rumbaugh and her colleagues were attempting to teach the

Yerkes computer language to a female bonobo (the pygmy chimpanzee), who at the time was also caring for her six-month-old infant, Kanzi. Though his mother did not do well at learning language (which may indicate that the age of exposure to language is important), Kanzi apparently learned some of the symbols and spontaneously began to use the keyboard when he was two-and-a-half years old. The researchers began to encourage his symbolic utterances, and to provide communicative modeling, but did not initiate formal training.[36] His skills quickly improved, and he surpassed other subjects in the ape language studies.

In carefully designed tests, Kanzi has demonstrated a relatively high level of language comprehension. When presented with over seven hundred different novel commands, he responded correctly over 90% of the time.[37] Based on extensive recording of Kanzi's two- and three-element symbol and gestural combinations, Savage-Rumbaugh and her colleagues believe that Kanzi has also learned simple grammatical rules and has even created some rules himself.[38] According to Griffin, "[t]he versatility and spontaneity with which Kanzi does this, together with the behavioral concordance between what he asks for and what he does subsequently, make it abundantly clear that he can voluntarily communicate simple desires and intentions. His communication certainly serves as an effective 'window' on what he is feeling and thinking."[39]

Although the Yerkes researchers thought that Kanzi's success was due to the bonobo's greater natural propensity for language acquisition, they also believed that changes in their teaching methods were responsible for his improved performance. Instead of the usual restricted environment, Kanzi lives in a facility that includes fifty-five wooded acres. He spends his time in the forest and in five large living spaces. At least one human member of the project team is with him every hour of every day.[40] His more complex and natural surroundings appear to stimulate Kanzi's language use. In addition, by the time Kanzi began using language, the researchers had attached a voice synthesizer to the computer, which produced spoken words to correspond with the symbols on the keyboard. They also had designed a portable keyboard for use in the forest. Savage-Rumbaugh and her colleagues have applied these new approaches to improve the language abilities of chimpanzees, yet they continue to believe that the innate language abilities of the bonobo are superior.[41]

Many questions remain concerning the degree to which nonhumans can learn to use language. Debate continues about the nature of true language use, as well as the extent to which ape language subjects have exhibited various dimensions of the activity.[42] The ape language research as a whole suggests that Washoe and her successors are capable of learning significant, albeit limited, language skills. In some respects, their achievements appear to resemble those of young human children learning to talk. In other respects the apes' capabilities appear more limited than those of young children.[43] The findings may be interpreted to reinforce the notion that humans are vastly superior in their linguistic abilities. Yet one might also interpret the data in the following way: "It is not surprising that chimps should be different from humans. What is remarkable is not how much bonobos and chimpanzees differ from human infants, but how similar they are when appropriate methods are developed to create an environment for learning language."[44]

ETHICAL ISSUES

The ape language studies raise a variety of ethical issues. Unlike many cases in which risks and benefits are central to ethical evaluation of the case, the moral standing of the apes and its implications is the central consideration in this case.

Cognitive Capacity and Moral Standing

Some writers have suggested that the scientific controversies surrounding this research are grounded in concern about challenges the findings could pose to the traditional moral hierarchy. According to the traditional view (see chapter 1), humans are qualitatively unique in their intellectual capacities and, hence, occupy a category of moral standing above that of any other species. Sue Savage-Rumbaugh makes the following observation:

> Many scientists are not certain that they wish to share a sense of mental identity with apes. Consequently they tend to erect impossible standards that apes must meet before they can be considered "language users." Moreover, it is implicitly suggested that all behavior which does not meet these standards is to be explained by basic conditioning principles. Such views serve to maintain the comfortable conception that all animals, apart from man, are simple, irrational creatures.[45]

The conclusion that members of another species are able to use language to communicate, albeit in a relatively rudimentary fashion, would seem to support the view that some nonhumans are capable of mental processes that are relevantly similar to human mental processes.[46] (Other researchers have found that chimpanzees can perform rudimentary mathematical tasks.[47]) Although Savage-Rumbaugh's comment may improperly conflate *rationality* and *language ability,* a reevaluation of the moral standing of apes would be in order in light of significant reevaluations of either their rationality or their linguistic capacity. If apes are language users, it is difficult to defend the position that humans possess such unique intellectual talents that they merit distinctly higher moral value and standing than any other sort of creature.

Improved Access to Nonhuman Experience

Another ethically relevant feature of the ape language studies is the opportunity they create for achieving a better understanding of a nonhuman animal's mental and emotional life. (See chapter 1.) Although behavior, appearance, and physiological data can provide strong evidence of a nonspeaking creature's mental experiences, the ability to communicate using language opens a new "window," as Griffin puts it, for examining the creature's mind.

The ethical relevance of this window is illustrated in Patterson and Gordon's account of an event in the life of Koko, a signing gorilla. A few years ago, Koko was given a pet kitten, All Ball, to whom she became very attached. All Ball was later killed by a car. In the months following the accident, Patterson periodically asked Koko about All Ball. In response, Koko would make the signs for "cry," "sorry," "sad," "trouble," and so forth. She also made these signs spontaneously upon seeing a picture of a cat that resembled All Ball. Three years after the kitten's death, when she saw a photograph of herself and All Ball, Koko signed "that bad frown sorry inattention."

Patterson and Gordon make reference to ethicist Arthur Caplan's argument that the human being's greater emotional and cognitive complexity supports attributing greater moral significance to human interests than to the interests of other species. In defense of his view, Caplan cites the example of the powerful and long-standing grief a human mother feels at the loss of her baby. In contrast, he notes, "[I]f you kill the baby of a baboon the mother may spend many weeks looking for her baby [but this] behavior soon passes and the baboon will go on to resume her normal life."[48]

Patterson and Gordon contend that this assertion rests in part on our current inability to investigate the nature and duration of the baboon mother's grief—for example, its intensity and whether it persists for months or years. If an observer were unable to communicate with a human mother, the observer might infer that the human mother's grief was over when she resumed her ordinary life. With conversation, however, that impression would be corrected. With the ability to communicate, the human observer can learn more about the nonhuman mother's emotions as well. Based on Koko's responses, Patterson and Gordon note, "[W]hile we cannot make any claims here about the emotional life of baboons, we have considerable evidence that Koko continues to mourn the loss of her adopted 'baby,' All Ball, even years after his death."[49]

If some animals can tell us how they feel about events in their lives, their messages could also clarify the extent to which various human actions produce subjective burdens and benefits in those animals. In turn, it could become more difficult to justify the harm conferred by, for example, confinement, separation from conspecifics, capture, killing, or biomedical research interventions. Of course, the animals' reports could also point to novel, even unexpected, measures by which to improve their well-being in various settings.[50]

Language and Moral Agency

Some language researchers claim that their subjects use language not only to describe their emotions, but also to reveal their empathy for other creatures, both human and animal, and to express a rudimentary sense of what constitutes acceptable and unacceptable behavior. If this claim is correct, does it follow that language-using apes can be assigned a level of responsibility—moral or otherwise—for their conduct? Based on her extensive interactions with and observations of the orangutan Chantek, researcher Lyn White Miles concluded that Chantek "used his signs deceptively to gain social advantage in games, to divert attention in social interactions, and to avoid testing situations and coming home after walks on campus."[51] Chantek also "labelled his own disapproved behaviour as BAD, and even on occasion signed BAD to himself."[52]

Chantek's conduct indicated to Miles that he had developed a childlike understanding of the morality of the human culture in which he was raised. What are the implications of Chantek's knowledge? Would it be morally appropriate to blame him for behavior he apparently realizes is wrong? Should he be praised when he performs a morally admirable action? If so, would the praise be moral praise? Washoe has reportedly engaged in such "culpable" behavior as biting a visiting scientist and possibly killing the infant that Loulis replaced (although this matter is in dispute).[53] Yet according to Roger and Deborah Fouts, she also has exhibited extremely altruistic behavior. For example, she once jumped an electric fence and saved another chimpanzee from drowning.[54] Does she deserve something resembling the blame and praise that the analogous conduct in humans would produce?

Although we might properly view the cross-fostered, language-trained apes as capable of respecting the basic moral values of their "foster culture," Miles argues that we should not extend this view to their conspecifics who have never been exposed to a human moral system.[55] Her point raises the broader ethical question of whether the language-trained apes should be assigned a different moral status than other members of their species who lack such training.

The argument in favor of conferring special moral standing on the "talking apes" is supported by two different rationales. One is that their knowledge of language gives certain apes cognitive skills beyond those they would otherwise possess. This enhanced intellectual prowess makes them at least seem "more human" than other members of their species, which implies to some that they should receive a corresponding elevation in their moral status.

An alternative rationale for elevating the moral status of the ape language study subjects is based on the researchers' decisions to remove the animals from their customary settings, raise them in human homes, and establish close relationships with them. One could argue that the scientists' participation in these events provides the moral foundation for making an extraordinary commitment to the lives and welfare of these research subjects. In a sense, Washoe, Nim, Kanzi, and the other apes taught language became part of the scientists' families. Roger Fouts's establishment of a long-term home for Washoe and the other chimpanzees in her group indicates that he has made such a commitment.

In light of this possible moral commitment, the fates of some of the other signing chimpanzees, including Nim, raise related moral questions. Animals accustomed to relatively intense interaction and communication with humans were suddenly, and to them inexplicably, removed from their homes and put in comparatively sterile surroundings. One might reasonably believe that these animals experienced greater deprivation as a result of this transition than the deprivation experienced by those who spend their entire lives in such surroundings.

However, a case can also be made against the idea of a special moral standing for the language users. Bernard Rollin argues that "language is . . . morally irrelevant to being a rights-bearer."[56] Rollin agrees that publicizing the achievements of the signing chimpanzees could be a powerful political tool for convincing the human community to elevate the moral and legal status of nonhuman animals. But he argues that this elevated status should be extended to all great apes, based on their natural capacities for emotion, personality, individuality, reason, and intelligence, which exist apart from any human language skills they may acquire. Indeed, one could argue that it is anthropocentric to consider language use in particular as bestowing moral status. Why should language skills be more relevant to a creature's moral status than other abilities possessed by apes?

Similarly, in concluding his extensive account of the aftermath of several ape language studies, Eugene Linden states, "[T]he basic difference between the language-taught chimp and any other chimp is simply a matter of education."[57] Though the human ability to empathize increases when a chimpanzee is equipped with language skills, Linden believes this emotional response is not relevant to the decision, for example, whether to use a particular chimpanzee in biomedical research. In his view, special treatment for the language-users would constitute unjustified discrimination against those who happened not to be chosen to participate in the language research.

There is also an intermediate position on the relative moral responsibilities humans have toward language-using and non-language-using apes. This position resembles one commonly adopted by writers considering the special moral obligations we humans owe to our families and other people with whom we have especially close relationships. The individual apes participating in the language studies can be seen as analogous to the friends and relatives to whom we owe extraordinary care and protection. On this view, there could be special obligations to ensure that these apes remain in an environment presenting opportunities for communication and interaction.

At the same time, subscribers to this view could support the existence of certain fundamental responsibilities owed to all great apes. Consistent with the latter position, supporters of the recently launched "Great Ape Project" contend that established moral rules on the right to life, protection of individual liberty, and prohibition of torture should govern our behavior toward "all great apes: human beings, chimpanzees, gorillas, and orang-utans."[58] (See chapter 1.)

The Moral Status of Nonhuman Species

Whether the ape language subjects ought to be regarded as having special moral significance is relevant to a broader question regarding the relative moral standing of many other nonhuman species. Some analysts believe that characteristics such as sentience or conscious awareness constitute the basis for admission to the moral community. All mammals and many other nonhuman species appear to possess these characteristics. On this view, it is unjustified discrimination to treat one species with the relevant moral characteristic as having higher moral value than another species that possesses the same (or a relevantly similar) characteristic.

Do the great apes' apparently exceptional capacities for thought and emotion justify conferring higher moral value on them than on other nonhuman species? One response is that the richness of the apes' mental lives makes them more aware of and more distressed by the pain, suffering, or discomfort they experience from being confined in a sterile environment or deprived of opportunities to form relationships than is experienced by less cognitively complex creatures kept in such conditions. Members of the US Congress seemed to rely on a version of this position when they enacted a statutory provision that laboratory primates (and no other species) must be given "a physical environment adequate to promote [their] psychological well-being."[59]

The moral relevance of cognitive complexity is an issue that merits extensive scientific, conceptual, and ethical analysis.[60] Some have argued that it is "speciesist" (See chapter 1) to ignore the interests that many other species have in receiving housing that permits them to exercise various dimensions of species-appropriate complex behavior. Any conclusions reached on these issues will affect questions of the moral permissibility of using, for example, dogs or rats to replace primates in biomedical research studies.

Practical Effects of an Elevated Moral Status

A final ethical question concerns the practical effect of a decision to elevate the moral standing of either language-trained or all great apes. Significant upgrading would necessitate the adoption of new legal and moral rules governing human conduct toward the relevant group of apes. For example, subscribers to the Great Ape Project argue that the extension of certain basic rights to apes would require that they be removed from zoos, circuses, and laboratories and released to an expanded array of natural sanctuaries.[61] As part of this plan, humans would be hired to supervise formerly captive animals and to promote the apes' comfort and survival. Yet many captive apes, especially those cross-fostered in human homes, would need extensive protection and rehabilitation to survive in the wild.[62] It might be impossible to teach them the survival skills they would otherwise have learned in the forest. Given these constraints, what setting should be provided for the formerly captive apes?

Constraints on the apes' use in scientific research might also follow from an upgrading in moral standing. If constraints were adopted similar to those governing research on human children and other people incapable of making decisions for themselves, chimpanzees could no longer be used as research subjects in many currently accepted scientific studies. It might even be questioned whether it is permissible to place them in captivity, thereby depriving them of the opportunity to learn their normal social and survival skills.

As scientific understanding of the great apes' cognitive capacities increases, political pressure could emerge in favor of adjusting many human attitudes and practices affecting these creatures. Some signs of modification are already evident, including the creation of retirement housing for some laboratory chimpanzees and the legislative requirement that research primates be provided with enriched environments. A hundred years from now, will human society regard the great apes as moral cousins, or will they remain distant moral strangers?

NOTES

1. Subsequently, researchers have also reported on efforts to teach ASL to other chimps, as well as to lowland gorillas and an orangutan. Charles T. Snowden, "Language Capacities of Nonhuman Animals," *Yearbook of Physical Anthropology* 33 (1990): 219.

2. R. Allen Gardner and Beatrix T. Gardner, "A Cross-Fostering Laboratory," in *Teaching Sign Language to Chimpanzees,* ed. R. Allen Gardner, Beatrix T. Gardner and Thomas E. Van Cantfort, (Albany: State University of New York Press, 1989), p. 5.

3. Gardner and Gardner, "Cross-Fostering Laboratory," pp. 1, 8.

4. E. Sue Savage-Rumbaugh, *Ape Language: From Conditioned Response to Symbol* (New York: Columbia University Press, 1986), p. 6.

5. Donald R. Griffin, *Animal Minds* (Chicago: University of Chicago Press, 1992), p. 221.

6. Gardner and Gardner, "Cross-Fostering Laboratory," pp. 6–7.

7. Ibid., p. 19.

8. Ibid., pp. 5–6.

9. Roger S. Fouts, Deborah H. Fouts, and Thomas E. Van Cantfort, "The Infant Loulis Learns Signs from Cross-Fostered Chimpanzees," in *Teaching Sign Language to Chimpanzees,* pp. 280–92.

10. Roger S. Fouts and Deborah H. Fouts, "Chimpanzees' Use of Sign Language," in *The Great Ape Project,* ed. Peter Singer and Paola Cavalieri (New York: St. Martin's Press, 1993), pp. 28–41; Eugene Linden, *Silent Partners: The Legacy of the Ape Language Experiments* (New York: Times Books, 1986), p. 53.

11. Fouts, Fouts, and Van Cantfort, "Infant Loulis," p. 285.

12. Debbi Fouts, "Backslaps, Footstamps and Pant Hoots," *Friends of Washoe* 15 (Winter/Spring 1994): 13, 24.

13. Kathleen Beach, "Chimposiums and the Docent Program," *Friends of Washoe* 15 (Winter/Spring 1994): 7–8.

14. Jennifer Beaucher, "Secondary Emotions in Chimpanzees," *Friends of Washoe* 15 (Winter/Spring 1994): 15.

15. Linden, *Silent Partners,* pp. 139–62, 225–32.

16. Beatrix T. Gardner and R. Allen Gardner, "A Test of Communication," in *Teaching Sign Language to Chimpanzees,* pp. 181–97.

17. Ibid., pp. 189–92.

18. Savage-Rumbaugh, *Ape Language,* p. 211.

19. Ibid., p. 214.

20. Griffin, *Animal Minds,* p. 220.

21. Ibid., p. 222.

22. George Miller, *The Psychology of Communication* (New York: Basic Books, 1967), pp. 70–92.

23. Noam Chomsky, *Aspects of the Theory of Syntax* (Cambridge, MA: MIT Press, 1965).

24. Herbert S. Terrace, *Nim* (New York: Knopf, 1979), pp. 10–13.

25. Ibid., p. 137.

26. Ibid., pp. 192–207.

27. Ibid., p. 221.

28. Savage-Rumbaugh, *Ape Language,* pp. 377–79.

29. Ibid., pp. 377–79; Chris O'Sullivan and Carey P. Yeager, "Communicative Context and Linguistic Competence: The Effects of Social Setting on a Chimpanzee's Conversational Skill," in *Teaching Sign Language to Chimpanzees,* pp. 269–79.

30. Griffin, *Animal Minds,* p. 223; Savage-Rumbaugh, *Ape Language,* pp. 9–10.

31. Savage-Rumbaugh, *Ape Language,* p. 17

32. Patricia M. Greenfield and Sue Savage-Rumbaugh, "Grammatical Combination in *Pan Paniscus*: Processes of Learning and Invention in the Evolution and Development of Language," in *"Language" and Intelligence in Monkeys and Apes,* ed. Sue T. Parker and Kathleen R. Gibson (Cambridge: Cambridge University Press, 1990), p. 543.

33. Savage-Rumbaugh, *Ape Language,* pp. 174–205.

34. Griffin, *Animal Minds,* p. 229.

35. Herbert S. Terrace, "Foreword," in Savage-Rumbaugh, *Ape Language,* p. 16.

36. Savage-Rumbaugh, *Ape Language,* pp. 395–97.

37. Snowden, "Language Capacities," p. 221.

38. Greenfield and Savage-Rumbaugh, "Grammatical Combination in *Pan Paniscus,*" p. 543.

39. Griffin, *Animal Minds*, p. 231.

40. Savage-Rumbaugh, *Ape Language*, p. 386. A recent book describes in detail Kanzi's life and Savage-Rumbaugh's language studies with him. Sue Savage-Rumbaugh and Roger Lewin, *Kanzi: The Ape at the Brink of the Human Mind* (New York: John Wiley & Sons, 1994).

41. Duane M. Rumbaugh and E. Sue Savage-Rumbaugh, "Language and Apes," *Psychology Teacher Network* 4 (January/February 1994): 4.

42. Griffin, *Animal Minds*, p. 226.

43. For extensive discussion of these issues, see E. Sue Savage-Rumbaugh, Jeannine Murphy, Rose Sevcik, et al., *Language Comprehension in Ape and Child*, Monographs of the Society for Research in Child Development, Serial number 233 (Chicago: University of Chicago Press, 1993).

44. Snowden, "Language Capacities," p. 222.

45. Savage-Rumbaugh, *Ape Language*, p. 21.

46. Ibid.; Griffin, *Animal Minds*, p. 231.

47. Sarah T. Boysen and Gary G. Berntson, "The Development of Numerical Skills in the Chimpanzee *(Pan Troglodytes)*," in *"Language" and Intelligence*, pp. 435–50.

48. Arthur Caplan, "Moral Community and the Responsibility of Scientists," *Acta Physiologica Scandinavica* 128 (Supplement 1986): 87–88.

49. Francine Patterson and Wendy Gordon, "The Case for the Personhood of Gorillas," in *Great Ape Project*, p. 68.

50. Griffin, *Animal Minds*, p. 252.

51. H. Lyn White Miles, "Language and the Orang-utan: The Old 'Person' of the Forest," in *Great Ape Project*, p. 48; H. Lyn White Miles, "The Cognitive Foundations for Reference in a Signing Orangutan," in *"Language" and Intelligence*, p. 529.

52. Miles, "Language and the Orang-utan," p. 52.

53. Linden, *Silent Partners*, pp. 85–113.

54. Fouts and Fouts, "Chimpanzees' Use of Sign Language," p. 29.

55. Miles, "Language and the Orang-utan," pp. 52–53.

56. Bernard Rollin, "The Ascent of Apes: Broadening the Moral Community," in *Great Ape Project*, p. 217.

57. Linden, *Silent Partners*, p. 208.

58. Editors and Contributors, "A Declaration on Great Apes," in *Great Ape Project*, pp. 4–7. In a separate development, some members of the scientific community appear to endorse the view that humans have certain responsibilities toward all chimps used in biomedical research. These individuals have created a retirement facility in which chimpanzees used in nonterminal AIDS and other biomedical research studies may live out their natural lifespan of forty-to-fifty years in a relatively comfortable environment that provides them with opportunities for interaction with other chimpanzees. This program implicitly supports the view that laboratory chimpanzees as a group are owed at least this level of care.

59. Animal Welfare Act, 7 USC sec. 2143(a)(2)(B) (1988).

60. Marc Bekoff, "Cognitive Ethology and the Treatment of Non-Human Animals: How Matters of Mind Inform Matters of Welfare," *Animal Welfare* 3 (1994): 82–87.

61. Paola Cavalieri and Peter Singer, "The Great Ape Project—and Beyond," in *Great Ape Project*, p. 311.

62. Gail Vines, "Planet of the Free Apes?" *New Scientist*, 5 June 1993, p. 42.

8

CAN ANIMAL AGGRESSION BE
STUDIED IN AN ETHICAL MANNER?

Aggression is a behavior found almost universally in the animal kingdom. It is an unprovoked, hostile act that poses a threat to the victim. It is shown in many ways, including threatening body movements, vocalization, fighting, wounding and infliction of pain, sexual attack, and killing. Commonly, animals act aggressively to exclude others from their territory, to capture food, and to control populations. Displays of aggression are influenced by age (newborns and infants below a certain age do not fight), by the physical environment, by previous social experience, and by the aggression level in a particular community.

One manifestation of aggression is infanticide—the killing of young by adults. It occurs in several species of animal. Human infanticide is practiced in several cultures to control population, to favor the birth of a particular sex, usually male, and in waging war. In nonhuman animals, infanticidal behavior has been described as a type of social pathology induced by overcrowding and by intense competition for scarce resources. Some investigators have suggested that infanticide may be a genetically influenced aspect of an animal's "normal" behavioral repertory—an adaptive strategy in circumstances of shortage of food, for example. It could be interpreted as a normal maternal culling of the litter under those conditions.

In the eighteenth and nineteenth centuries, biologists reported anecdotal observations of infanticide by wild animals (such as lions, monkeys, rodents), but the many biological variables that remained uncontrolled in field studies made it difficult to state unequivocally that the observed infanticide was attributable to a particular underlying mechanism. It was not until the 1970s that infanticide among animals began to receive systematic study. The investigations moved to laboratory-based studies, where conditions could be more readily controlled. Rodents became a commonly used species because they breed readily in the laboratory and individuals or entire litters of neonates could be introduced to male or female test subjects with or without their mothers present. Infanticide continues to attract scientific investigation of many poorly understood aspects of the phenomena.

In the 1970s and 1980s, studies of aggressive encounters of many kinds, not only infanticide, but also fighting and predation, developed a significant scientific literature.[1] At first, the studies were of naturally occurring events among free-living animals. But then some animal behavior researchers turned to laboratory-based studies. These studies provoked criticism because they were human-manipulated. *Animal Behaviour* was one of several journals publishing research results about animal aggression, and out of a total of about 120 articles published in 1984, *Animal Behaviour* published approximately ten articles on artificially staged aggressive encounters of captive animals.[2] At this time, the

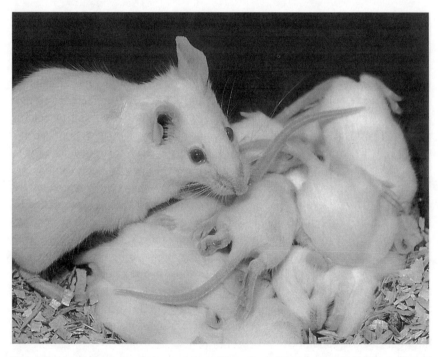

This laboratory mouse tends her newborn litter. Credit: Alexis Wenski-Roberts, Cornell University.

focus of the research was on understanding more about the subject animal, but as time passed, the purpose shifted to possible application to human aggressive behavior, as will be recounted later.

THE ELWOOD-OSTERMEYER PROJECT

In the early 1980s, animal behaviorists Robert W. Elwood and Malcomb C. Ostermeyer became interested in factors that influence male animals to kill the young of their own species. Previous work had shown that adult male rodents of many species killed infants unrelated to them and that this behavior seemed to confer some reproductive advantage to the adult. For example, the male, after removing the babies, is then able to mate with the mother, becoming the father of his own litter. Of course, if an adult male is to perpetuate his genotype, it is imperative that his infanticidal tendencies be inhibited prior to the birth of his own offspring. It was known that male laboratory mice do not usually harm their own litters, even though they may kill many other infants prior to mating.

Some researchers had linked the inhibition of infanticide with copulation, but Elwood and Ostermeyer were skeptical and wanted to test this hypothesis. Accordingly, in their laboratory at Queen's University of Belfast, in Northern Ireland, Elwood and Ostermeyer conducted studies on the development of infanticide in male mice. Their method was to repeatedly place live newborns into the cage of sexually naive (never mated) adult mice for 36 hours and record the number of kills. There was no possibility of escape for the newborns. Adult animals were preselected for their killing tendencies in some initial screening tests. "Killers," who repeatedly and consistently killed the pups that were presented to them, were identified and used for the main experiment. Adults who did not repeatedly kill were "nonkillers" and not used further.

Initially, killers and nonkillers were individually housed. They were then subjected to various regimens including mating and subsequent cohabitation with the female, or mating followed immediately by single housing again. The investigators wanted to see whether it was copulation with a female or cohabitation with the pregnant mother that caused inhibition of infanticide. Animals were tested for infanticidal behavior at three time intervals: preexperimentally, on the day of mating, and 18 days after mating. The results showed that copulation had no effect on inhibiting infanticidal behavior, but that cohabitation with the female did. The results were published in an article entitled "Does Copulation Inhibit Infanticide in Male Rodents?" which appeared in 1984 in *Animal Behaviour.*[3] For this study, at least 87 newborn pups were killed by the adult males.

The experimental method engendered a controversy. When the manuscript of the article was being considered for publication, the journal's Ethics Committee deliberated on how to proceed. Eventually the committee decided to approve publication subject to the condition that it be accompanied by an editorial note stating that the killing of the pups was instantaneous and no suffering was involved. This note from an Ethics Committee was unprecedented. It marked the first pronouncement that studies published in this journal were being formally reviewed for ethical concerns.

The Ethics Committee's note attached to the Elwood and Ostermeyer paper demonstrated that a professional body of animal behaviorists were enforcing certain standards. This note turned out to be an event of historical importance in ethical review, and its publication opened the door to additional debate on what a researcher should or should not do regarding studies of infanticide, aggression, and predator-prey relationships, and what should or should not be published.

THE EVOLUTION OF ETHICAL CONCERN

The Elwood and Ostermeyer project aroused some ethical concern, but other studies of staged infanticide generate stronger criticism. Yet these other studies had not been subject to editorial scrutiny or official sanction on ethical grounds. Among the methods used by researchers to stimulate animal aggression were administration of electric shocks to the potential aggressor,[4] injecting hormones,[5] disturbing the newborn by surgically lesioning their brains,[6] and artificially increasing the litter size to well beyond normal range so that the mother could not provide enough milk.[7] One study of the effects of social status and prior sexual experience on infanticidal behavior involved killing 795 newborn mice.[8] Many of these experiments were conducted by highly respected investigators and, at that time, were considered acceptable among animal behaviorists.

Ethically questionable aspects of experimental procedures had not gone unnoticed by a number of animal behaviorists. Growing concern about methods used to study aggression, predator-prey relationships, cannibalism, and infanticide had resulted in the formulation of first-ever guidelines jointly endorsed by the UK and US professional associations of animal behaviorists. They were published in 1981.[9] An ethics committee was charged with seeing that these guidelines were followed and, as necessary, enforced. Among professional associations, the animal behaviorists are unusual in establishing methods of enforcement of their guidelines.

Ethical debate on aggression research still goes on today, but many new ideas have emerged since the early 1980s. Several researchers, including Elwood, have contributed to this discussion.[10] Several significant papers were reprinted in a booklet entitled *Ethics in Research on Animal Behaviour*[11] by the two professional associations (in the United States and United Kingdom) that jointly publish the journal *Animal Behaviour;* and several important papers have been published that address ethical standards of animal behavior research.[12] Some manuscripts describing infanticide have also been rejected by *Animal Behaviour.*

In 1994 the Animal Behavior Society (ABS) issued revised guidelines updating its earlier versions.[13] All versions state that laboratory studies should involve the smallest number of animals necessary to accomplish the research goals and that careful thought should be given to the design of an experiment in this context. The advice of a biostatistician is required. Elwood and Ostermeyer address this point: "The numbers used were kept to the minimum consistent with scientific validity." They also ran statistical analyses of the results. Although it is not explicitly stated, it can be calculated from the reported results that at least 87 newborn pups were killed (test animals were given the opportunity to kill pups at least four times).

However, it has often been noted that researchers are frequently not careful to state the methods of their conformity to the ethical obligation to reduce the numbers of animals to the minimum necessary. According to geneticist Michael Festing,[14] it is still relatively rare for investigators to state specifically that they have considered this point. For instance, in one survey of published articles, Festing found that about a third of the experiments may have been unnecessarily large for statistical validity. Failure to conform to existing guidelines has led to proposals for a more demanding and explicit body of guidelines.

SCIENTIFIC ISSUES

Discussion of the Elwood and Ostermeyer paper among animal behaviorists also raised a number of methodological issues in science that have ethical implications. The main question is, are studies of caged animals scientifically valid and representative of normal behavior? Or does the caging itself so influence behavior that there is no scientific value to such studies, therefore making them unethical.

The basic purpose of studying animal behavior is to learn more about the life history and social interactions of an individual or species. The results should be generalizable to other animals. Most animal behavioral studies are conducted in the field and are observational in nature. Investigators do not normally introduce intentional harm to the animals they study. Field studies of aggression in free-living animals generally have fewer problems of scientific validity and are more representative of the species as a whole than laboratory-based studies.

However, field studies have their limitations. Unlike laboratory studies, they cannot be standardized—often a crippling methodological problem. Furthermore, manipulation of the environment is often not possible; nor is it desirable since human interference may alter an animal's natural behavior. Laboratory studies make it possible both to regulate the experimental situation, by controlling potentially relevant variables, and to replicate the experiment. Thus, the underlying mechanisms can be understood more precisely.

Elwood and Ostermeyer chose to do the infanticide study in the laboratory because they could manipulate the animals and standardize the tests in ways that would be impossible in the field. Yet, their ultimate objective was to understand normally occurring infanticidal behavior that would be relevant to the species. The implication of their paper is that the results are generalizable to other mice and their wild counterparts, but is this assumption supported by a wider body of scientific evidence?

Animals that are singly caged throughout their lives do not necessarily behave like free-living animals, thus the results of experiments may sometimes be questionable. Is an encounter between two animals in the environment of a cage a fair duplication of naturally occurring conditions? Also, was an "abnormal" population selected since Elwood and Ostermeyer selected their test animals for superaggressive traits? Did this selection invalidate the generalizability of this study to other mice?

Psychologist Lewis Petrinovich has stated: "The essential artificiality of the laboratory and the usual lack of any essential relationship of the laboratory setting to an organism's adaptive capacities do violence to the integrity of behavioral [studies]. . . . If the situations are not representative . . . then no analytical method is of much value."[15] It is a matter of judgment whether staged infanticide is representative of normal behavior, but the controversial character of such judgments has often been noted in evaluations of both the science and the ethics of studies of aggression.

Finally, it has been argued that if the purpose of an experiment is trivial, then no infliction of harms on animals whatever is justified.[16] This point shows how valid methodology in science is closely connected to justification in ethics.

ETHICAL ISSUES

The Justification of the Experiments

Does basic zoological research, in which there is no known application of the knowledge that would provide benefits to the animals or to human health, provide a sufficient justification for killing animals? The researchers do not discuss the significance of their results, but they do claim a contribution to knowledge about inhibition of infanticide. For example, they maintain that infanticide is a matter of basic interest in understanding the social structure of a group and the dynamics of the individual male's paternal behavior. Is such a contribution sufficient to justify the research?

It has never been entirely clear in the evaluation of this kind of research which criteria should be used for judging the significance of experimental results. A provision of the 1981 ABS guidelines states: "If animals are confined, constrained, harmed or stressed in any way, the investigator must consider whether the knowledge that may be gained justifies the procedures. Some knowledge is trivial, and experiments must not be done simply because it is possible to do them." So, in permitting publication, the Ethics Committee's opinion was that these staged infanticide studies were not trivial and the knowledge gained justified the harms to the animals. Was this judgment correct?

It is always possible that some specific knowledge of animal behavior could be put to use to help protect a species or its environment—such as human understanding about migratory instincts or preferred routes. We often do not see the utility in scientific experiments until some time well after their completion. The key question seems to be, when knowledge gained contributes to an understanding of the animal world, without any clear application or rationale for use of the information, should we declare the information trivial or should we say that we rarely understand exactly how future scientists will use information and must not judge science on the basis of immediate benefit?

In some cases, investigators in laboratory studies of rodent and nonhuman primate aggression claim that their work is intended to shed light on *human* aggression. Good work in this area might go a long way toward strengthening the justification for the research. However, the relevance of nonhuman animal studies to an understanding of human behavior has long been a matter of substantial moral and scientific controversy—as has some research involving humans that attempts to study human aggression in an artificial environment.

According to a 1994 report,[17] the National Institute of Health (NIH) has in the past supported much animal aggression research that attempts to connect animal and human behaviors. Federal funding for these studies reached a peak in 1975 when the Division of Neuroscience and Behavioral Science of NIH funded 27 studies at a total cost of $900,000. These studies showed that among the factors that influence aggression are genetics (it is possible to selectively breed for aggressive strains) and various hormones such as testosterone. The report continues, "Funding for this area steadily declined due to waning interest, because exact causal relationships were difficult to prove."

The usefulness of studies of animal behavior for understanding parallel forms of human behavior is open to question. Some psychologists who engage in this research have questioned the clinical value of laboratory research on animals. Among them is J. A. Kelly, who examined the 1984 volume of *Behavior Therapy,* a journal specializing in behavioral intervention and therefore likely to report human studies that draw on prior animal studies.[18] He found that of 1,132 citations in *Behavior Therapy,* only 2.0% referred to animal studies. Similarly, the results of a large-scale 1996 survey of psychologists conducted by S. Plous, show that mental-health workers rarely or never use findings from psychological research on animals.[19] Nearly 95% of these psychologists indicated they would not be seriously hampered by a ban on animal research, the study found.

That stress induces aggressive behavior has been demonstrated repeatedly in both animal and human studies. For instance, isolation in the mouse, and sleep deprivation or immobilization in the rat can induce marked increase in affective aggression. Critics argue that these studies merely confirm observations that are available from humans and add little if anything to these observations.

Animal studies have also successfully demonstrated that aggressive behavior may be modulated through neuroanatomic sites and through the modulation of neurotransmitter systems, including serotonin and norepinephrine. The application of this information to regulating aggression in humans is still under study.

According to one view, animal studies have limitations in contributing to our understanding of human violence. Human aggression involves complicated social and environmental factors that are not and cannot be duplicated by animal studies. Aggression is mediated by cultures that are not duplicated in captive, nonhuman animals. Furthermore, the unpredictable and sometimes explosive manner in which the trait of human aggression is displayed provides little basis for trying to replicate these situations in nonhuman, captive animals.

According to another view, animal experimentation may suggest *research methods* for studies involving human subjects. Burr Eichelman holds that animal studies of aggression have provided a strong conceptual base for approaching the study of human aggressive behavior.[20] He cites past animal studies that have searched for an "aggressive center" in the brain. The search failed, but he believes it yielded valuable information. Studies of animal models of aggression are also strongly defended by Huntingford as being of theoretical importance, even if not as yet of clear practical importance. She thinks they can contribute to our understanding of the adaptive significance of group life: "I cannot accept the most radical solution to the ethical problems raised by [animal aggression] studies, namely that this area of research be abandoned entirely."[21]

Despite these hopes for solid scientific results and applications, it has been difficult to demonstrate practical application or to develop therapeutic interventions that might help in the relief of human antisocial behaviors.

Adequacy of Review

In the Elwood and Ostermeyer case, both *Animal Behaviour*'s Ethics Committee (which was comprised of animal behaviorists) and the researchers themselves (also animal behaviorists) believed there was value in answering the hypotheses posed in the study. But was the review sufficient?

Those outside the animal behavior discipline are more likely than those within it to raise questions about the rationale for such a study. The 1981 ABS guidelines encouraged review by those who are "in a different discipline" as being especially likely to be helpful since they "will not share all the investigator's assumptions." Similarly, Huntingford recommends that, since it is not easy for investigators to judge for themselves whether or not their experiments are trivial, the opinion of colleagues from other disciplines should be sought.[22]

Some of the often-remarked inadequacies of ethical review of animal research by researchers in the field was demonstrated in a recent survey conducted by Frans R. Stafleu.[23] The survey was of all licensed biomedical animal researchers in the Netherlands. They were asked about the justification of several protocols, some of which involved significant animal pain. The results showed that respondents always assumed that the experiment was justified; even those procedures involving considerable harm to monkeys were not challenged. According to this report, respondents, all of whom were animal researchers, accepted the goal of the research as an "incontestable fact."

Nevertheless, it would be too quick to dismiss committee review by peers as so contaminated by conflict of interest as to be worthless. The fairness of the review appears to depend heavily on the persons involved, the resources and training given to the committee, and the environment in which it operates. The committee review conducted by *Animal Behaviour* was of some value even though the reviewers were all from the same discipline. In all likelihood, committee members had an intimate understanding of the purpose and significance of the work under review and had been chosen because they were professional leaders with ethical sensitivity. But would review that included persons outside the discipline have been even more valuable? (See the survey of ethical issues about both the justification of research and review committees in chapter 1, pp. 31–41.)

Extent of Animal Suffering

Ethical considerations require that animal pain and suffering be kept to a minimum, commensurate with valid experimental design (see chapter 1, pp. 000–00). This requirement is a cornerstone for policies on humane animal experimentation. In written accounts of experiments, the extent of animal pain or suffering should be specifically described in order to assess the justifiability of the work.

In much of the scientific literature, there has been a tendency to magnify certain potential benefits of research, while downplaying the animal harm resulting from experimental procedures.[24] This one-sided view has the effect of making the research seem clearly justified, even though a more measured approach might find that the data on animal harm recorded by scientists is inadequate. The inclusion of more information about the condition of experimental animals, the severity and duration of their pain or distress, and how adverse states are to be alleviated should produce better forms of review than those that often occur.

The Elwood and Ostermeyer paper did address the issue of pain but gave an incomplete account of the potential sources of animal pain or suffering. Only one potential source was addressed, the manner of death at the moment when an adult kills a pup. The researchers reported that death "usually" came about from a swift bite to the newborn pups' head or chest. Elwood defended the use of day-old pups on the grounds that older pups have greater perception of discomfort and pain.[25] Without elaboration, the Ethics Committee judged the deaths to be "instantaneous and that no suffering was involved." It was not reported whether, in some unusual instances, there was greater pain or that the death was not instantaneous.

Harms potentially came from sources in addition to the pups' deaths. For instance, questions could be asked about what happened to the pups who were not killed but were left in the males' cages for 36 hours. Did they die of lack of maternal care? Were they alive when the researchers removed them? The investigators did not report whether they attempted to return these pups to their mothers, or whether and by what method the pups were humanely killed. Questions might also be raised about whether the mothers suffered from the loss of their newborn pups. Affirmative answers to these questions would not automatically render the research unjustified, but they would presumably make impartial reviewers more informed and less certain to find the research justified.

Some scientists have judged their own work ethically unacceptable because the animal harms were too great. For instance, in the late 1970s, ethologist Marc Bekoff gave up his studies of predatory behavior in captive coyotes because he considered the work impossible to justify.[26] His decision came as a result of his own evaluation of the psychological pain and suffering to which the prey (mice and young chickens) were subjected by being placed in a small arena with the coyotes. There were no possibilities for the prey animals to escape; they suffered the physical consequences of being stalked, chased, caught, maimed, and killed. Bekoff acknowledged that by abandoning this line of research, scientific knowledge would be lost, because other ways of designing the experiments using free-living coyotes were not available. He believed that pursuit of the scientific information could not be justified in light of the harms that befell the subject animals.

Bekoff has also raised objections to what he regards as unjustifiable methods used by other researchers.[27] He questioned the purpose of a 1993 study that tested whether infanticidal behavior in birds could be induced under specific field conditions. The experimental method was to shoot and kill two resident female birds who were caring for nests of chicks. This disturbance caused neighboring female birds to move into this territory and attack the chicks. Seven chicks in total were maimed and killed. Bekoff objected that the nests had been disturbed and that efforts were not made to save the chicks.

In response, the researcher, Stephen T. Emlen, defended his experiment on the grounds that: (1) this experimental design had provided clear answers to the research questions he had posed; (2) there was scientific importance in the questions and hypotheses being studied; and (3) he had limited animal harm by calling off the study after killing only two females.[28] He believed that this methodology was restrained and brought the study into compliance with professional requirements. Emlen did not, however, specifically consider the balancing question of whether the knowledge gained was worth the price paid by the animals.

One possible difference between Bekoff and Emlen may be the seriousness with which each treats the issue of human responsibility for creating situations that bring about suffering and death for animals. This issue is also raised by the Elwood and Ostermeyer project, in that the infanticidal events were contrived and did not occur naturally as they would in field studies. In staged encounters in a laboratory or interventions in field studies, the researcher is responsible for creating the conditions that bring about the acts of infanticide. When infanticide and predation occur naturally among free-living wild animals, by contrast, human beings are not causally responsible. Bekoff appears to think that causal responsibility for bringing about death bears a heavier burden of justification than many in the animal research community seem to have thought.

Alternatives

In recent years, several new ideas have been put forward either to refine the procedure to reduce animal harms or to reduce the numbers of animal used, or to replace the subject species with less sentient species or with nonanimal models (see chapter 1 on obligations to seek alternatives). Familiarity with these so-called Three-R alternatives is a responsibility of researchers planning aggression studies and those performing committee review. Some alternatives applicable to aggression studies merit attention.

Observing natural interactions in the wild

Observational field studies of naturally occurring events of aggression have been recommended repeatedly in guidelines addressing the ethical dilemmas of studies of aggression. If no interference by the observer would affect the animals' behavior, field encounters are valid and representative of behavior within a normal range. Field studies are ethically more defensible because the researcher does not contribute to animal harm or death. However, field studies may involve extra time and expense for the researcher because it is difficult to anticipate when and where an aggressive encounter will take place.

Protecting the prey from injury

In 1989 Glenn Perrigo and his associates commented on the "escalating public and scientific concern" about studies of infanticide where live pups are used to measure behavior.[29] At that time, the standard research procedure was still to place a newborn pup at the end of the home cage of an adult mouse and wait for the attack and death. But these authors developed a wire-mesh tube in which the pups are effectively protected from serious injury. Afterwards, all pups are returned safe and uninjured to their mothers. An alternative to the wire mesh could be to place an intervening transparent partition between the aggressor and victim. These methods have been used with success in several studies by Perrigo and others.

Another way of protecting prey from injury is simply by human intervention to remove the prey before the onslaught of attack. In situations where there is a long latency before an attack, there may be time for the researcher to recognize an imminent attack (by the animal's posture and behavior) and rescue the victim. Robert Elwood states that with gerbils and certain other species, intervention is essential because otherwise adults will cannibalize a pup even before it has been killed.[30] In these cases, Elwood removes the pups in his experiments and "immediately" and humanely kills them. In this setting and using this methodology rescue is impossible: To return the pup to its original litter after human handling and interference would probably result in rejection of the pup by its mother.

Using less sentient species

According to Huntingford, aggression experiments should be conducted with invertebrates rather than vertebrates, and among vertebrates, with fish rather than birds or mammals.[31] These preferences pose fewer ethical problems because the simpler the nervous system an animal has, the less it is likely to experience suffering. Huntingford's recommendation follows the guidelines on replacement in the alternatives movement; however, the recommendation does not appear to have been influential in the aggression literature, which is still dominated by studies of mammals, including primates. Are such studies needed in order to reach useful results about aggression?

Other possibilities

Among other alternatives recommended by Huntingford are extracting the maximum information from each aggressive encounter by careful experimental design and by producing descriptions of the encounter that are as detailed as possible; reducing sample size; reducing the numbers of encounters; reducing the duration of encounters; and using models rather than live predators. She and her colleagues have used an artificial model pike (a species of fish) in experiments to test antipredatory behavior in sticklebacks, a small fish that pike eat. The fish models elicit physiological and behavioral responses in the sticklebacks that resemble those elicited by the pike itself.[32]

The Problem of Retrospective Moral Judgment

It is widely believed that it is morally inappropriate to judge people or institutions based on today's standards or knowledge for actions taken many years ago. The claim is that people cannot be judged or held responsible for research practices that were common and rarely challenged until more recently. However, this thesis cannot be sustained when moral wrongs are so egregious that persons in any place or time should have known that they were wrong. In the case of aggression studies, should researchers have known that particularly vicious attacks staged by humans that caused other animals to suffer were morally dubious, or is such thinking purely a product of recent moral reflection?

In looking back on studies conducted before, say, 1985, and attempting to evaluate their moral acceptability, we need to take into consideration the assumptions of the period in which the work was done, especially the kinds of ethical standards that were relevant to the evaluation of experiments involving animals, such as basic principles, government policies, and rules of professional ethics. In 1984—to consider a single year—the newly devised ABS professional guidelines were still untested; institutional committee review was not common (it was not mandated until 1985); and professional journals rarely subjected manuscripts to ethical review for animal welfare concerns prior to publication. The ethics of animal behavior research was still an emerging field, and indeed the profession showed itself to be comparatively more responsive to ethical concerns than many other disciplines.

Today's professional standards and climate are clearly different. There is more professional-society involvement and an increased awareness throughout the relevant professions of the Three-R alternatives. If relevant standards and duties were largely or even entirely undeveloped at the time, this lamentable circumstance becomes exculpatory for persons accused of wrongdoing. Such circumstances would be very different from a situation in which there existed well developed and officially endorsed policies for research involving animals.

In making these judgments, it is useful to evaluate the moral quality—in particular, the *wrongness*—of actions, practices, policies, and institutions by contrast to the blameworthiness (culpability) of agents. This distinction is of the highest significance when engaging in retrospective moral judgments. Sometimes officials and investigators are blameworthy for not having had policies and practices in place to protect subjects in research, but sometimes there are mitigating conditions that shield them from blame, even though we recognize moral deficiencies. For example, the scientific culture of the time may have fostered certain forms of moral ignorance or moral blindness, or a research institution's division of labor and designation of responsibility may have been diffuse. These mitigating conditions might exculpate the persons involved even though wrongdoing occurred. (See additional discussion of these questions of retrospective moral judgement in the cases of chapter 9 "Monkeys Without Mothers," and chapter 3, "Head Injury Experiments on Primates.")

CONCLUSION

Interest in studies of infanticide, *per se,* as opposed to other studies of aggression, has waned since the Elwood and Ostermeyer paper was published in 1984. But in 1996 NIH funded a number of studies of aggression among nonhuman primates. Scientific interest in aggression has been stimulated by efforts to place laboratory animals in paired or group houses instead of keeping them alone in small cages that offered no opportunities for social contact with other animals. Group housing has been tried with varying degrees of success in an effort to comply with the 1985 amendment to the Animal Welfare Act that requires that the "psychological well-being" of primates be addressed. Also, monkeys are used as models for human antisocial behavioral states, such as the increased aggression resulting from substance abuse of cocaine or alcohol. Scientists also use nonhuman primates to study the biobehavioral effects of drugs used clinically to treat violent aggression in humans. Since researchers continue to study aggression and violence among animals and humans, the challenge remains to design experiments that are ethically sound.

NOTES

1. A. F. Dixson, "Sexual and Aggressive Behaviors of Adult Male Marmosets *(Callithrix jacchus)* Castrated Neonatally, Prepubertally, or in Adulthood," *Physiology and Behavior* 54 (1993): 301–7.
2. Felicity A. Huntingford, "Some Ethical Issues Raised by Studies of Predation and Aggression," *Animal Behaviour* 32 (1984): 210–15.
3. Robert W. Elwood and Malcolm C. Ostermeyer, "Does Copulation Inhibit Infanticide in Male Rodents?" *Animal Behaviour* 32 (1984): 293–94.
4. R. Ulrich and N. H. Azrin, "Reflexive Fighting in Response to Aversive Stimulation," *Journal of Experimental Analysis of Behavior* 5 (1962): 511–20.
5. O. Samuels, G. Jason, M. Mann, and B. Svare, "Pup-Killing Behavior in Mice: Suppression by Early Androgen Exposure," *Physiological Behavior* 26 (1981): 473–77.
6. Darlene T. DeSantis and Leonard W. Schmaltz, "The Mother-Litter Relationship in Developmental Rat Studies: Cannibalism vs. Caring," *Developmental Psychobiology* 17 (1984): 255–62.
7. Ronald Gandelman and Neal G. Simon, "Spontaneous Pup-Killing by Mice in Response to Large Litters," *Developmental Psychobiology* 11 (1987): 235–41.
8. U. William Huck, Robin L. Soltis, Carol B. Coopersmith, "Infanticide in Male Laboratory Mice: Effects of Social Status, Prior Sexual Experience, and Basis for Discrimination Between Related and Unrelated Young," *Animal Behaviour* 30 (1982): 1158–65.

9. "Guidelines for the Use of Animals in Research," *Animal Behaviour* 29 (1981): 1–2.

10. Robert W. Elwood, "Ethical Implications of Studies on Infanticide and Maternal Aggression in Rodents," *Animal Behaviour* 42 (1991): 841–49; Robert W. Elwood and Stefano Parmigiani, "Ethical Recommendations for Workers on Aggression and Predation in Animals," *Aggressive Behavior* 18 (1992): 139–42.

11. Marian Stamp Dawkins and Morris Gosling, eds., *Ethics in Research on Animal Behaviour* (Association for the Study of Animal Behaviour and the Animal Behavior Society, 1992). Copies of 'Ethics in Research on Animal Bahaviour' can be obtained from: Dr L. M. Gosling, Secretary, ASAB Ethical Committee, Central Science Laboratory, MAFF, London Road, Slough SL3 7HJ, U.K.

12. Felicity A. Huntingford, "Some Ethical Issues Raised by Studies of Predation and Aggression"; Paul Frederic Brain, "Comments on Laboratory- Based 'Aggression' Tests," *Animal Behaviour* 32 (1984): 1256–57; Glenn Perrigo, W. Cully Bryant, Lee Belvin, and Frederick S. vom Saal, "The Use of Live Pups in a Humane, Injury-Free Test for Infanticidal Behaviour in Male Mice," *Animal Behaviour* 38 (1989): 897–98; Elwood, "Ethical Implications of Studies on Infanticide," pp. 841–49.

13. "Guidelines for the Treatment of Animals in Behavioural Research and Teaching," *Animal Behaviour* 47 (1994): 245–50. Previous versions had been published in *Animal Behaviour* 34 (1986): 314–17 and *Animal Behaviour* 29 (1981): 1–2.

14. Michael F. W. Festing, "Reduction of Animal Use: Experimental Design and Quality of Experiments," *Laboratory Animals* 28 (1994): 212–21.

15. Lewis Petrinovich, "Probabilistic Functionalism: A Conception of Research Method," *American Psychologist* 34 (1979): 383, 388.

16. See, for example, Patrick Bateson, "When to Experiment on Animals," *New Scientist* 109 (20 February 1986): 30–32.

17. *Report of the Panel on NIH Research on Anti-Social, Aggressive, and Violence-Related Behaviors and Their Consequences.* (Bethesda, MD: National Institutes of Health, 1994).

18. J. A. Kelly, "Psychological Research and the Rights of Animals: Disagreement with Miller," *American Psychologist* 41 (1986): 839–41.

19. S. Plous, "Attitudes toward the Use of Animals in Psychological Research and Education: Results from a National Survey of Psychologists." *American Psychologist* 51 (November 1996): 1167–80.

20. Burr Eichelman, "Aggressive Behavior: From Laboratory to Clinic. Quo Vadit?" *Archives of General Psychiatry* 49 (June 1992): 488–92; "Animal Models: Their Role in the Study of Aggressive Behavior in Humans," *Neuro-Psychopharmacology* 2 (1978): 633–43.

21. Huntingford, "Some Ethical Issues," pp. 210–11.

22. Ibid., p. 211.

23. Frans R. Stafleu, "The Ethical Acceptability of Animal Experiments as Judged by Researchers," Ph.D. thesis, University of Utrecht, the Netherlands, 1994, p. 83.

24. David B. Morton, "A Fair Press for Animals," *New Scientist* 1816 (1992): 28–30; Lynda Birke and Jane Smith, "Animals in Experimental Reports: The Rhetoric of Science," *Society and Animals* 3 (1995): 23–42; F. Barbara Orlans, *In the Name of Science* (New York: Oxford University Press, 1993), pp. 221–39.

25. Elwood, "Ethical Implications of Studies on Infanticide."

26. Marc Bekoff and Dale Jamieson, *Reflective Ethology, Applied Philosophy, and the Moral Status of Animals,* Perspectives in Ethology, ed. P. P. G. Bateson and Peter H. Klopfer, vol. 9 (New York: Plenum Press, 1991), p. 26, note 20.

27. Marc Bekoff, "Experimentally Induced Infanticide: The Removal of Birds and Its Ramifications," *The Auk* 110 (1993): 404–6.

28. Stephen T. Emlen, "Ethics and Experimentation: Hard Choices for the Field Ornithologist," *The Auk* 110 (1993): 406–9.

29. Perrigo et al., "The Use of Live Pups in a Humane, Injury-Free Test."

30. Elwood, "Ethical Implications of Studies on Infanticide," pp. 841–49.

31. Huntingford, "Some Ethical Issues," p. 212.

32. William M. S. Russell and Rex L. Burch, *The Principles of Humane Experimental Technique* (London: Methuen, 1959), p. 64.

9

MONKEYS WITHOUT MOTHERS

Following approximately a six-month gestational period, a pregnant female rhesus monkey *(Macaca mulatta)* begins to show evidence of the imminent birth of her infant. If she lives in a natural environment like a forest in southeast Asia, she starts to change her usual activity patterns and may move away from the typical social pathways of her group to more secluded and quieter parts of the environment. Her group will likely be comprised of many other adult females, males, and immature animals of varying ages and temperaments. As the time of birth nears, she shows evidence of labor by hunching, squatting, leaning on vertical surfaces, and touching her vagina frequently.

As the labor progresses, the placental sac ruptures and the head of the infant eventually emerges from the birth canal. The mother then reaches between her legs with both hands, carefully grasps the head of the baby with her fingertips, makes a gentle bending movement to the right or left and then firmly pulls the infant free. She immediately places the newborn on her chest.[1] The rhesus monkey infant is born equipped with strong grasping, rooting, and sucking reflexes which help to secure it to the mother and help it to locate the nipples and to suckle.

Once the infant is in place, the mother fastidiously cleans the infant, removing all traces of the blood, soil, and amniotic fluid that remain. Once the coat of the infant is dry, active grooming begins. At this time she closes her body around the infant in a warm and protective posture with her pale flesh, hands, and brown-gray fur constantly in contact with the infant. The infant reciprocates by grasping the mother's flesh and fur with its hands and feet.

Under field conditions the infant stays in this close physical bond with the mother for weeks before the loosening grasp of the mother and the emerging curiosity of the infant combine to allow it to make brief excursions, first to other parts of the mother's body and then to other parts of the physical and social environment barely inches away. By three to five months the infant may cautiously start to move brief distances away from the actual grasp of the mother. Here it begins to encounter other animals, including other infants.[2]

Though the infant does not go far during these excursions, the attention of the mother remains riveted on the infant. Similarly, the infant completely depends on the presence of the mother as a base of security from which these tentative expressions of independence can be safely launched. Infants are actively protected by their mothers from overly rambunctious play partners and

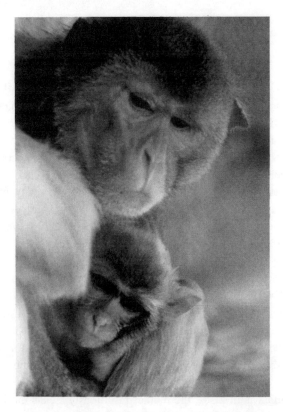

A rhesus monkey mother with her child. Credit: Professor John P. Gluck, University of New Mexico.

from more aggressive and less tolerant group members; there is an absolute certainty of direct intervention should it be required. The mother responds with haste and patience to the demands of her infant. Her ministrations, more often than not, bring ease and relief to a frightened or hungry infant. Breaks in this responsiveness result in intense emotional distress and behavioral disruption on the part of the infant. Should the mother disappear or die during this early period of development, the infant, if not adopted by another female, would certainly die.

As its first year progresses, the infant spends more and more time away from the direct physical control of the mother. The infant becomes involved in the work of play and bonding with other infants and group members. Yet the connection between the mother and infant remains obvious and enduring. Rest, protection, nutrition, play, and sleep are sought in the comfort of the mother's proximity and embrace. The explicitness of this attachment relationship continues at least until the birth of the next infant, which requires a more active process of weaning. Even then, and perhaps for the rest of the life of the mother, her offspring, both male and female, maintain a lifelong recognition and deference for her, and she for them.[3]

It is clear that for a rhesus monkey infant in the field to lose or be separated from its mother early in life is a natural and unfortunate tragedy whose consequences are played out with Darwinian directness. Because of the stark and predictable consequences of such a separation, biological mechanisms have evolved to prevent this loss and separation. Therefore, raising monkeys without mothers is virtually certain to produce profound confusion, disorientation, and behavioral changes in the infants.

Yet, purposely raising monkeys without access to mothers and peers has a long history in the research on the experimental psychology of development. Monkeys have been raised without or separated from mothers for various scientific reasons: to test theories of attachment, to create models of a variety of human behavioral disorders, and to test the effect of certain medications proposed to treat those human disorders, to name just a few.

HARLOW AND HIS MONKEYS

Perhaps most notable among those researchers who have used this rearing procedure as a central part of their work was the late Harry F. Harlow (1905–1981) of the University of Wisconsin. While other researchers have also separated monkeys from their mothers for research purposes, Harlow has perhaps received the greatest amount of attention from the animal protection community, at least in part because of the acclaim he received from many of his scientific peers.[4] Harlow's motives for using this procedure have been characterized by elements of the animal protection community as expressions of sadism or at least extreme indifference, and his research has been declared redundant and irrelevant.[5] Others have staunchly defended his character and his work and have pointed out its major and enduring significance. It is fair to say that both the man and the work have been at the vortex of ethical debate since at least the mid-1970s.

Any discussion of the science and the ethics of Harlow's work must begin by acknowledging that he was a most productive and professionally acclaimed psychologist. He published over three hundred articles and books and graduated 36 Ph.D. students over an active research career that spanned nearly fifty years. Along the way he received virtually every significant prize for scientific achievement available. For example, he received the Gold Medal from the American Psychological Association in 1973, became a member in the American Philosophical Society, and was the first psychologist to be elected a member of the National Academy of Sciences. He received the National Medal of Science from President Lyndon Johnson in 1967 and the Kittay Award from the psychiatric community in 1975.

The historical context in which Harlow's work proceeded is also important. He was an early soldier in the profession of experimental psychology's campaign to be acknowledged as a natural science. This acknowledgement was judged to require the adoption and application of a strictly scientific methodology, then widely interpreted to mean the explicit use of experiment and controlled observation.[6] Inference from uncontrolled observation was not sufficient.

Harlow's work has been extensively chronicled in scientific journals, the popular press, and TV documentaries. He traveled and spoke constantly to large and small audiences at scientific meetings, interest groups, and thousands of introductory psychology students who attended the University of Wisconsin. He rarely turned down any serious group who made a request for him to discuss his ideas. He was proud of his work and actively exposed the form, structure, and proposed implications of his research to the scientific and lay public.

Soon after he joined the faculty of the University of Wisconsin, he initiated a research program concerned with learning abilities of nonhuman primates. In this program he adapted for animal use some of the evaluation techniques of the human intelligence testing movement. As the results of this research program proved successful, he found it necessary to establish his own facilities where he could specify more precisely the conditions of housing and testing.

The Mind of the Rhesus Monkey

Harlow's work on the process and manner by which monkeys learn to solve discrimination problems began to attract interested attention in the 1940s. The attention came as he began to defend an unpopular theoretical position. He proposed that monkeys solve discrimination problems by developing various hypotheses about the solution and then by testing them; the process of learning occurs as incorrect hypotheses are steadily eliminated in favor of the correct approach.

In some of these experiments, monkeys were tested in an apparatus in which they were presented with two three-dimensional objects that differed from one another in a variety of ways (e.g. color, shape, and size). One of the objects was randomly selected as "correct." The objects were presented to the monkey on a sliding tray, which was moved to within its reach when the trial was to begin. The monkeys were trained to make their choice by pushing the object to one side. If the monkey chose the correct object, a small piece of food would be revealed beneath it in a small, shallow well. The food was then quickly eaten or stored in the monkey's large-capacity cheek pouches to be consumed at another time. The position of the correct object would be changed at random from one side of the tray to the other. Each separate problem would be presented for a fixed number of trials, usually six.

The monkeys were tested on literally hundreds of these problems over the course of several months. As the monkeys' experience proceeded, it was observed that their performance improved to the point where they eventually made errors on only the first trial of a new problem. In Harlow's words, the monkeys had "learned how to learn" by applying a "win-stay, lose-shift" strategy: If on the first trial of a new problem the monkey "won," that is, was rewarded for its choice, he should "stay" with that object in whatever position the object appeared on the tray during the following trials. If, on the other hand, the monkey "lost" on the first trial, it learned to shift to the other object on all succeeding trials.[7]

Harlow's hypothesis was controversial for a number of reasons. First, it flew in the face of the rather mechanistic explanations of animal learning then favored by the dominant behavioristic school. This mechanistic perspective tried to explain the changes seen during learning as the result of the connection or disconnection of small response units to specific stimuli through the processes of contiguity, reward, nonreward, and punishment—not as the development of cognitive strategies. In addition, a substantial portion of the learning process was thought to be motivated by the need of animals to maintain physiological homeostasis. This drive reduction theory claimed that an imbalance in physiological equilibrium creates a psychological state called a drive, which prompts the animal to take action. Those behaviors that facilitate a return to equilibrium become part of the animal's behavioral repertoire. It was assumed that if there were no such imbalance an animal will not be motivated to learn. Therefore, the typical learning experiment required that the animals be placed on some form of deprivation (e.g. food or water) so that learning would take place.[8]

Clearly Harlow's notions painted a very different picture of primate learning and the "mind" of the monkey. He described monkeys as having complex cognitive abilities that involved the existence of intentions, curiosity, and solution plans. This was not a description of the insensate automata implied by the behavioristic explanations. As for the drive reduction theory of motivation, Harlow revealed that he fed the animals in his experiments their normal day's ration of food *before* he tested them on his discrimination problems. He described the monkeys as participating in these problems with their cheek pouches full of food, swallowing bits of that food after having made either correct or incorrect responses.[9] This picture was devastating to purely behavioristic interpretations, which depended on differential drive reduction to account for behavior change and correct responding.

Harlow encountered strong criticisms of his interpretations on methodological grounds as well. One of the foundational criticisms was that since the monkeys in Harlow's experiments had been captured and imported as adults from the forests and cities of southern Asia, one could not be certain that the responses observed during the laboratory experiments were not acquired previously in the complex natural environments from which these animals had been snatched.

Harlow reasoned that in order to respond to the criticism he had to establish experimentally the ontogeny (course of development in the individual) of learning abilities in rhesus monkeys. He would then be able to empirically determine the point in time when various learning abilities emerged. Together with A. J. Blomquist, Harlow developed a protocol[10] where infant rhesus monkeys could be separated from their mothers at or soon after birth and raised in a nursery where their life experiences could be tightly controlled for as long as required by the experimental design.[11] At this point ethical problems began to be discernible in Harlow's work.

The Motherless Monkey as Experimental Control

The first step required a procedure in which the gestational stage of pregnant females could be known. With this information the experimenters would know when to be present to separate the infant from the mother as soon after birth as possible. Once the infants were separated, they would be housed alone in small wire-mesh cages where they could be fed and cared for according to strict schedules. During the first months after birth, the singly housed infants were placed in a setting modeled after a human nursery. The cages, with Plexiglas and wire-mesh walls, were arranged so that the monkeys could see and hear other infants but could not contact one another physically. A staff of technicians prepared formula and bottle-fed the infants around the clock.

During the initial feedings the small infants were wrapped snugly in a gauze cheesecloth which restrained the monkeys firmly without injury while they were hand-held and trained to drink from a bottle. This human-infant contact was maintained only for the minimum amount of time required to complete the feedings. Once the feedings were completed, the infant was placed back into its individual wire cage with a clean cloth provided as insulation against the bare metal of the cage floor. The monkeys tended to wrap themselves in this cloth while they were alone in their cage, a fact that would change the course and purpose of raising monkeys without mothers at a later time.

Once the infants had gained strength and mobility, the formula was presented to the monkeys on a small inclined rack. The rack mimicked the feeding position of mother-reared infants. The rack provided the infants with an apparatus that would support their weight and climbing abilities and that further reduced the amount of necessary contact with human handlers. Once the monkeys were old enough they were weaned to a cup and then to solid food. They were moved to larger individual cages and into standard holding rooms. There the animals stayed from months to years until they were assigned to a learning experiment. They were removed from their "home" cages for weekly weighing, cage cleaning, occasional health checks, and regular TB testing. The monkeys could see and hear other monkeys but could not physically contact them.

At this point in history, rearing monkeys without access to mothers and without physical access to peers was considered by Harlow to be a procedure whose main purpose was to standardize the pre-experimental ages and histories of the monkeys to be used in his experiments on learning. These procedures were viewed as a legitimate and sound way for an experimentalist to control the effects of variables that potentially confound the interpretation of an experiment. From an experimental perspective, the procedures proved useful. Harlow and his associates detailed the learning capacities of rhesus monkeys beginning within the first week after birth until sexual maturity. The results supported his earlier descriptions of monkey learning.[12]

Harlow did not intend to "do" anything to the monkeys in this work in order to change them. Nor did he want to produce a defect or injury in them, since this would only serve to further complicate the results of experiments that the procedure was intended to clarify. Less clear, however, is whether Harlow believed that raising monkeys in the prescribed manner would produce distress and discomfort, and whether this risk mattered to him. The only hint of an answer to this question is that in his writing he takes pride in the fact that the mortality rates of his nursery-reared animals were lower than that seen in the wild as well as in infants reared by their own mothers in the laboratory environment. He almost seems to be boasting that he and his staff were better monkey mothers than were monkey mothers.[13]

RAISING MONKEYS WITHOUT MOTHERS AS AN INVESTIGATIVE PROCEDURE

The initial reason Harlow raised monkeys without mothers was to standardize life histories and ages of animals in experiments in order to eliminate potential problems in his research. However, a significant shift occurred in this intention: Harlow began to use the motherless rearing protocol as a way to learn something about the psychological makeup of the animals. Harlow now wanted to discover what factors contributed to the attachment bond that so obviously exists between a mother and her infant. Clearly human and nonhuman offspring alike maintain proximity to the mother and seek out her protection at times of stress and danger. But what mechanisms account for the connection? Pursuit of this question became a turning point in Harlow's research career that moved him from the ranks of the respected psychological researchers to the rarefied atmosphere of the famous—and, to some, the infamous.

In the 1950s, explanations of the basis of development of the early attachment bond between human mothers and caretakers and their infants consisted of four positions:

1. The theory of secondary drive. According to this perspective, the infant becomes attached to the mother because the mother's actions meet the infants's pressing physiological needs.
2. The theory of primary object sucking. Here the infants are considered to possess an inborn need to relate to the breast and to suck it.
3. The theory of primary object clinging. Under this explanation, the infant is believed to possess an inborn need to touch and to cling.
4. The theory of primary return-to-womb craving. Here the infant is seen as resenting its expulsion from the womb and then seeking to return there. Therefore, the infant stays in close proximity to the mother.

The first two explanations stress the importance of the early feeding situation. The act of feeding the dependent infant, thereby reducing its hunger drive, establishes through reinforcement the behaviors of approach, contact, and maintenance of proximity by the infant. These attachment behaviors are then considered to be "derived" from the more basic and essential action of drive reduction. Elements of these explanations were favored by proponents of both the behavioristic perspective and certain psychoanalytic traditions, two groups who tended to agree on nothing. On the other hand, members of the psychoanalytic tradition called the British Middle Group believed in the third alternative and the innate importance of contact and clinging in the development of attachment. Prominent among these theorists was psychoanalyst John Bowlby.[14] The fourth position also had prominent adherents.

To test these differing conceptualizations in the format of a traditional experiment would require an approach that could determine the effect of feeding independently from these other factors. One obvious complicating factor was that a living mother or caretaker could not easily be created that could feed an infant without also holding it. The act of holding an infant to the breast or cradling the infant during bottle feeding automatically exposed the infant to a host of other factors. Prominent among these factors were body heat, skin, surface texture, heart sounds, and vocalizations. Thus, an experiment that was to test the feeding explanation of early attachment would require that feeding occur in the absence of all or most of those other factors. If such a situation could be created, one then could assess whether attachment developed or not. But how could such an experimental arrangement be created?

The Development of the Mother Surrogate

According to Harlow's own description of the development of the experimental approach, the solution to the problem came to him in a vision: in late 1957 Harlow was returning to Madison, Wisconsin, from a business trip to Detroit. He was still in need of a topic for his presidential address to the American Psychological Association which he would deliver during the next year. He wanted something strong, dramatic, and critical of drive reduction theorists who remained very influential in psychology. The hour was late and he had consumed a fair amount of complimentary airline champagne. As he turned to look out the window above Lake Michigan, he visualized in the empty seat next to him a fully formed mechanical mother surrogate: "As I turned to look out the window, I saw the cloth surrogate sitting in the seat beside me with all her bold and barren charms."[15] The mother in the vision had a cylindrical body that leaned back at approximately a 45-degree angle. In the upper third of her chest was an aperture where a feeding bottle could be inserted. It was also clear that the cylindrical body could accommodate coverings of various textures from soft and warm to cold and rough.

The visualized model seemed to contain all the attributes necessary to test the nutritional theory of early attachment in monkeys. Contact comfort could be presented with or without feeding, and rough-textured "mothers" could be made to be the source of nutrition. Harlow already had an idea that the monkeys would attach to soft textured mothers. As mentioned earlier, the basic nursery-rearing protocol included presenting a soft cheesecloth gauze pad to the newly born infants which were held in individual wire-mesh cages. The monkeys invariably wrapped themselves up in those cloths and showed clear signs of disturbance when the cloths were removed; the monkeys grabbed them tightly, resisting the technicians' attempts to take them away. Once removed, the infant monkeys screeched and jerked convulsively in protest. When a clean cloth was returned, the disturbance calmed immediately as they recontacted the cloth.

These observations were powerful but were certainly not definitive; and they did not meet the requirements of a "true" experiment, which requires specificity and controlled comparisons. Casual observations in an uncontrolled setting like a nursery would not do, especially for a presidential address to the American

Psychological Association, an association deeply involved in the continuing struggle for recognition as a "hard" science.

The Initial Mother Surrogate Experiments

After his vision, Harlow soon commenced conducting a series of mother surrogate experiments designed to test the central controversies. The present discussion will focus on the report published in the journal *Science* in 1959.[16] *Science,* the oldest American scientific publication, has been devoted to the dissemination of new, provocative findings; it has been said that publication in this journal can make a research career. Therefore, competition for publication in this periodical is fierce. For a psychologist like Harry Harlow to have a paper accepted for publication in *Science* would indicate the potential significance of the experiments; further, it would show that psychology was in reality a scientific enterprise in the same way that biology, physiology, and chemistry were legitimate scientific enterprises.

The paper in *Science* reports the result of fourteen distinguishable experimental tests. The experiments divide into the core demonstration of the effect of nutrition on the preference for an inanimate surrogate, fear challenge tests designed to determine the initial existence of an attachment, and whether the attachments maintained their strength over time. The article reports that the cloth mother was constructed from a cylinder of wood covered with a sheath of terry cloth, whereas a wire surrogate mother was constructed of hardware-cloth cylinder. The cylinders were mounted on an aluminum base situated at a 45-degree angle. Each surrogate had a distinctively different wooden head.

Dual surrogates

In the initial experiment, eight newborn rhesus monkeys were separated from their mothers and were placed individually in standard laboratory cages. Attached to each cage were two booths containing a cloth surrogate and a wire surrogate. For half of the monkeys their total nutrition was obtained from bottles available on the cloth surrogate while the nutritional allotment for the remaining monkeys was available from the wire mother. A gauze-covered heating pad was also available to all the monkeys on the floor of their cages positioned away from the surrogates during the first 14 days of the experiment. The mean number of hours each monkey spent in contact with the two different surrogates was recorded for a minimum of 165 days.

Results showed that by day 25, all the monkeys chose to spend nearly 18 hours a day in direct physical contact with the cloth surrogate regardless of the surrogate from which the monkey received its feedings. Contact with the wire mother was minimal throughout the experiment, stabilizing at about one and one-half hours per day with no difference between the monkeys fed on the wire surrogates or those fed on the cloth surrogates. On the surface, it appeared that the nutritional theory of attachment had been defeated by this rather simple demonstration. However, Harlow recognized that the observed differential contact time between the cloth and the wire mothers might simply reflect the fact that the cloth mothers were a more comfortable "nest" and not that an actual psychological bond had been established. In other words, attachment and comfort explanations both fit the data.

Fear-challenge tests

In order to eliminate this ambiguity, Harlow arranged a series of challenges in which the monkeys were exposed to stimuli and situations known to produce fear in infant monkeys. The kind of fear that would, under normal rearing situations, drive an infant to seek protection and contact from an attachment object like a "real" mother, but not from another object. What would these surrogate-reared monkeys do when faced with these circumstances?

Fear-challenge tests involved introducing fear-provoking objects (e.g., a mechanical toy bear) into the home cage of the infant monkeys living with the cloth and the wire surrogates and observing their response. The introductions occurred three times during the first 22 days of age and then every 20 days afterward. Two types of data were recorded: first, the type of the surrogate to which the monkey retreated when first exposed to the intruder; and second, the quality of the response made once the chosen surrogate was contacted. Results showed that when the infant monkeys were exposed to a fear stimulus they strongly tended to retreat to the cloth surrogate regardless of the feeding arrangements they had experienced. In addition, once the monkeys were in contact with the cloth surrogates their fear responses rapidly reduced, to the point that some of them ventured back toward the stimulus and explored it.

Single surrogates

Other experiments involved animals that were raised with experience of only one surrogate. One group of four monkeys was raised with and bottle-fed from a single wire surrogate. A second group of four monkeys lived with a cloth mother who did not provide nutrition. By raising monkeys with only a feeding wire surrogate, Harlow was attempting to determine whether a bond could be nutritionally created with a wire surrogate if the infant was provided no opportunities to experience a cloth surrogate providing contact comfort.

Results showed that, consistent with the previous experiments, monkeys raised with nonfeeding cloth surrogates spent nearly 18 hours per day in contact with the surrogate. Monkeys raised with feeding wire surrogates only increased their time in contact with the surrogate from 6 to 12 hours per day over the course of 165 days. These findings suggested that under certain circumstances an attachment bond could be derived from a feeding relationship. The nutritional theory once again had to be reconsidered.

Did this nutritionally based relationship confer the kind of protections or reassurances that had been observed for the cloth surrogate monkeys? Home cage challenge tests showed that though the wire-surrogate infants retreated from the fear objects in the direction of their surrogates, the monkeys did not embrace them. Nor did they show a reduction in fear that had been seen for the cloth surrogate groups. Instead, these animals clutched themselves, body-rocked, called out, and screamed until the fear object was removed.

In other challenge tests, dual- and single-surrogate-raised monkeys were introduced. They again showed that the wire surrogate failed to relieve fear. These findings were interpreted as further evidence against the nutritional theory of attachment. In still other tests, it was found that monkeys reared in the dual- or single-cloth-surrogate conditions worked to gain visual access to their cloth surrogates and to a live monkey to an equivalent degree. Single-wire-reared monkeys strongly preferred to view the live monkey.

Open-field challenge and attachment retention tests

Drawing on previously published tests of human children on the effects of attachment, Harlow compared the behavior of single-surrogate-reared monkeys with monkeys raised without surrogate experience in a novel open field environment. The open field was a small room filled with unusual objects and toys. The monkey's surrogate was present in the environment on half of the open field exposures. It was found that monkeys raised with single cloth mothers used their surrogate mothers as bases of operation from which they explored the novel environment. Monkeys raised with single wire surrogates were found to be highly emotional and distressed even when their surrogate was present in the field. Due to their highly typical rocking and huddling, Harlow likened their behavior to that of autistic "institutionalized human children."

Harlow also continued to assess the nature and strength of the attachment bond by checking the responsiveness of the various groups to their mother surrogates once they had been permanently separated from them. He found that the monkeys raised with access to the cloth surrogates continued to work to gain visual access to her form for at least the next 15 months. Monkeys raised with wire surrogates alone showed no such maintenance. Similarly, retention tests conducted in the open field showed that monkeys reared with cloth surrogates continued to contact the surrogate when tested over the three-month period following separation and showed reduced emotionality in the novel environment. Wire-reared infants, on the other hand, showed no such preference nor ameliorated levels of emotional distress.

In a variant of the open-field challenge, Harlow placed the monkey's surrogate in a Plexiglas box which blocked direct contact. Harlow reports that following several "violent crashes" cloth-surrogate-reared monkeys adjusted to the condition and continued to show levels of reduced emotionality. These results supported the idea that the infants benefited from the presence of the surrogate even though direct contact was prevented. Little of that kind of benefit was observed for the wire-reared monkeys. In other challenge tests, Harlow found that the monkeys would travel a more "dangerous" route to get to the cloth surrogates.

In summary, there are four core findings from these experiments:

1. Infant monkeys preferred to maintain contact with surrogates with a soft body texture regardless of the feeding arrangements.
2. When exposed to fear-provoking situations, monkeys both sought physical proximity to the cloth surrogates and also appeared to calm in their presence.
3. Infant monkeys raised with cloth surrogates would learn to operate a lever in order to get even a brief visual glimpse of their surrogate.
4. After separation from the surrogates, monkeys raised with cloth surrogates showed retention of these indices of attachment for at least the next year.

An additional finding was that the monkeys raised with wire surrogates and exposed to the fear situations showed a host of bizarre and clearly abnormal behaviors like body-rocking and self-clasping. Harlow again likened these behaviors to those seen in severely disturbed and institutionalized autistic children. This finding was to be experimentally exploited to a great extent later as the animal-model approach to the study of abnormal behavior gained support and attention. It was also discovered later that all the surrogate-reared females showed deficient social and maternal behavior when they became pregnant some years later.

ETHICAL ISSUES

These behavioral observations of monkeys reared with surrogate mothers profoundly influenced the acceptance of psychology as an experimental discipline. No less of an influence has been left by the moral problems surrounding the research. The descriptions and pictures of monkeys clinging tightly to cloth-covered cylinders or writhing in distress in their absence made, and continues to make, an indelible impression on readers and students.

Research Benefits

Although these experiments were conducted nearly forty years ago, virtually all modern-day introductory psychology texts prominently discuss their relevance in sections concerned with explanations of human development. Teachers commonly find that the facts of these experiments consistently elicit a strong response. The reality and meaning of maternal attachment is laid bare and unmistakable by the data and the pictures. The pedagogical force of the experimental demonstrations and their ability to communicate important developmental concepts have been repeatedly demonstrated. Many believe that this work profoundly influenced the way modern psychology is conceived.

As discussed earlier, the central focus of the surrogate work was on the debates concerning theories of attachment. Seriously flawed notions about the development of human attachment would be refuted by this experimental work. We would learn that good mental health itself was essentially dependent upon the child establishing and learning to maintain proper attachment relationships. In one observer's view, the discovery of this conclusion "may be compared to that of the role of vitamins in physical health."[17] Interpreting the attachment process as "derived" from more primary factors had helped maintain a blindness to this fundamental principle, with potentially disastrous consequences for the promotion of proper child-rearing practices and the treatment of mentally ill children.[18]

Harlow's experiments have also revealed a great deal about the cognitive and emotional life of monkeys. The pictures of infant monkeys cuddling and rubbing their bodies on the soft surrogate mothers or crying out in fear and distress during the challenge tests, coupled with the findings from the learning experiments, filled the behaviorist's empty animal with feeling and thought. The meaning of Darwin's concept of mental continuity in the species in nature (see chapter 1) was illustrated in clear relief. Others have argued that advanced appreciation of human-like characteristics and rearing requirements of monkeys provided by these experiments eventually helped to improve the welfare of laboratory animals as the findings informed the evolution of animal husbandry techniques.[19]

Costs and Harms to the Animals

These benefits must be placed in context with the substantial costs and harms to the animals that resulted from a variety of sources. There are, for example, background costs associated with establishing a breeding colony, which required the purchase and importation of monkeys trapped in the forests of Southeast Asia. There is the stress and pain of trapping, separation from group members, injury, disease and death of animals in transport, and the stress of adaptation to a laboratory environment upon arrival. Standard laboratory existence consisted of individual housing in stark metal cages with little or no opportunities to interact socially; adaptation for an animal that had spent its entire life in a social context was quite difficult. Once the breeding females gave birth there was the stress of the separation experienced by both the mother and the infant.[20]

During the first experiments designed to test the preferences for the wire and cloth surrogates, while being provided the fundamental elements of warmth, postural support, and nutrition required for survival, the infants were deprived of the common maternal care responses such as holding, cleaning, and grooming. They were required to live alone in individual cages, a condition completely alien to the evolutionary preparation of the species.

In terms of the challenge experiments, the direct examination of the effects of stress and fear was to a great extent the purpose of the experiments. Attachment, by definition, is a process that is revealed by behavior generated by stressful situations. Therefore the initial and retention challenge tests are described as purposely producing reactions in the infant monkeys such as crouching, rocking, convulsive jerking, self-clutching, and freezing—or as Harlow himself put it, "abject terror."[21] One could ask whether the entire array of tests was necessary to make the point that attachment had been established and maintained to the cloth mothers. The later experiments seem to depict a hunting for an ever more dramatic demonstration of an already demonstrated attachment finding.

As several psychologists have maintained, it is not clear whether Harlow discovered anything new—or at least anything that could not have been discovered without the use of the monkeys involved. Even Bowlby, one of Harlow's staunchest supporters, seems to suggest that the work had primarily a rhetorical effect on debates that were already under way.[22] Is a new "emphasis" in a field a discovery worthy of the suffering of the animals in these experiments? Must we even accept the entrenched belief that a scientific study requires a controlled experiment for acceptance?

We might also ask whether we would approve this work if it were proposed today and came before an institutional animal care and use committee. What modifications would be needed? Is a dramatic demonstration and powerful teaching tool worth the discomfort and suffering of an intelligent and emotionally complex animal?

The Problem of Retrospective Moral Judgment

When reviewing Harlow and his work, we should recall the assumptions of the period in which the work was done. The Animal Welfare Act did not exist until 1966 and did not directly influence experimental designs until 1985. It is today widely believed, as the chairman of the Chemical Manufacturers Association recently put it, "You cannot judge people or a company based on today's standards or knowledge for actions taken 40 to 60 years ago."[23] This thesis suggests that people who use animals cannot be held responsible for catching, transport, and research practices that were deemed professionally appropriate a half century ago. But is this thesis right? Can we not judge Harlow and the institution where he worked at all?

It may help here to introduce a distinction between judging the *rightness or wrongness* of an action and judging the *blameworthiness or praiseworthiness* of the agents who perform those actions. In many circumstances, it is reasonable to say that an action was wrong, but that the agent had no basis for knowing that it was wrong and therefore is not blameworthy. Blame is often mitigated by lack of factual information, cultural beliefs, a person's good character, and perhaps by institutional expectations. But were these mitigating conditions in place in the case of Harry Harlow? On the more fundamental level, is there any basis even for judging that he did anything wrong?

NOTES

1. O. L. & Tinklepaugh and K. G. Hartman, "Behavioral Aspects of Parturition in the Monkey *(Macaca rhesus),*" *Comparative Psychology* 11 (1932): 63–98.

2. R. A. Hinde, T. E. Rowell, and Y. Spencer-Booth, "Behavior of Socially Living Rhesus Monkeys in Their First Six Months," *Proceedings of the Zoological Society of London* 143 (1964): 609–49.

3. R. A. Hinde and Y. Spencer-Booth, "The Behavior of Socially Living Rhesus Monkeys in Their First Two and Half Years," *Animal Behavior* 15 (1967): 169– 96.

4. L. A. Rosenblum, "Harry F. Harlow: Remembrance of a Pioneer in Developmental Psychobiology," *Developmental Psychobiology* 20 (1987): 15–23.

5. See M. Stephens, *Maternal Deprivation Experiments in Psychology: A Critique of Animal Models* (Jenkintown, PA: American Antivivisection Society, 1986).

6. See E. G. Boring, "The Validation of Scientific Belief," *Proceedings of the American Philosophical Society* 96 (1952): 535–39.

7. H. F. Harlow, "The Formation of Learning Sets," *Psychological Review* 56 (1949): 51–65.

8. See K. W. Spence, "Cognitive versus Stimulus-Response Theories of Learning," *Psychological Review* 57 (1950): 159–72.

9. H. F. Harlow, "Mice, Monkeys, Men, and Motives," *Psychological Review* 60 (1953): 23–32.

10. Based upon the previous work of Gertrude van Wagenen; see E. J. Farris, *The Care and Breeding of Laboratory Animals* (New York: Wiley, 1950).

11. A. J. Blomquist and H. F. Harlow, "The Infant Rhesus Monkey Program at the University of Wisconsin Primate Laboratory," *Proceedings of the Animal Care Panel* (April 1961): 57–64.

12. See H. F. Harlow, "The Development of Learning in the Rhesus Monkey," *American Scientist* 47 (1959): 459–79.

13. See H. F. Harlow, "Of Love in Infants," *Natural History* 69 (1960): 18.

14. J. Bowlby, "The Nature of the Child's Tie to Its Mother," *International Journal of Psychoanalysis* 39 (1958): 350–73.

15. H. F. Harlow, M. K. Harlow, and S. J. Suomi, "From Thought to Therapy: Lessons from a Primate Laboratory," *American Scientist* 59 (1971): 539.

16. H. F. Harlow, "Affectional Responses in the Infant Monkey," *Science* 130 (1959): 421–32. We have chosen this paper for three reasons: first, because the paper is a quite complete description of the initial surrogate experiments written for a wide scientific audience and not just for psychologists; second, the paper introduces the use of observational methods and illustrative photography which was to become a keynote of Harlow's work during this period; third, because of the very nature and stature of the journal in which the report appears.

17. J. Bowlby, *Child Care and the Growth of Love* (Harmondsworth, England: Penguin Books, 1953), p. 69.

18. See J. Bowlby, *Maternal Care and Mental Health* (Geneva: World Health Organization, 1951); R. Spitz, "Hospitalism: An Enquiry into the Genesis of Psychiatric Conditions of Early Childhood," *Psychoanalytic Study of the Child* 1 (1945): 53–74.

19. See G. C. Ruppenthal and D. J. Reese, *The Nursery Care of Nonhuman Primates* (New York: Plenum Press, 1979).

20. It is important to note that the establishment of primate laboratories also creates health risks to humans brought about by disease transmission, bite wounds, and such. For example, since 1930 at least 18 laboratory and animal care technicians have died and several have been paralyzed from encephalitis caused by B-virus infections contracted from laboratory housed rhesus monkeys. See A. E. Palmer, "Herpes virus Simae: Historical Perspective," *Journal of Medical Primatology* 16 (1987): 99–130.

21. Harlow, "Affectional Responses," p. 423.

22. J. Bowlby, *A Secure Base* (New York: Basic Books, 1988), p. 26.

23. "Ex-owner of Toxic Site Wins Ruling on Damages," *New York Times,* 18 March 1994, p. 5B.

V

WILDLIFE RESEARCH

10

THE DEATH OF A VAGRANT BIRD

In August 1991 several amateur bird-watchers were encamped in southern New Mexico at a place called Rattle Snake Springs, just inside Carlsbad Caverns National Park. This small oasis in the midst of the parched Chihuahuan desert attracts a large number of bird species and had become a popular observational area. For some time the attention of some members of the group had been drawn to the sight and song of a lone, small olive-and-yellow bird about six inches long who seemed oddly out of place. Descriptions and taped recordings of its song strongly suggested that the bird was a yellow-green vireo.

As far as anyone knew, the established range of the bird was from Central America to Mexico. In an arresting use of language, individual birds sighted out of their established geographical context are referred to as "vagrants." One common usage of *vagrant* is someone who travels "idly . . . without lawful or visible means of support . . . (as a prostitute or drunkard),"[1] but the usage here is a pure derivation from the Latin root *vagari,* meaning to wander. Many circumstances lead vagrants to be out of place, and they are associated with different degrees of scientific importance. For example, the bird simply may have overshot its migration target, been blown off course by a chance encounter with a storm, or hitched an unintended ride on a boat or plane; or it may be in an active search for a new habitat.

While there had been scattered rare sightings of vagrant yellow-green vireos in southern Texas and Arizona in the 1970s, there was no record of the bird having ever been sighted as far north as the latitude of Carlsbad, New Mexico. The status of the yellow-green vireo in South America is somewhat uncertain, since it has a strong resemblance to the closely related red-eyed vireo, and their populations are sometimes confused. Both species have yellow flanks, an olive crown, and head striping.[2]

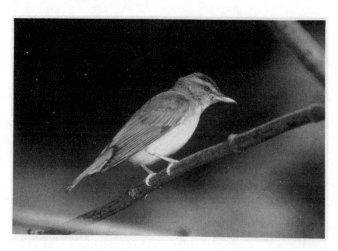

A yellow green vireo is 6–7 inches long, about sparrow-sized. It is identified by its yellow flanks, olive crown, and head striping. These vireos are found in streamside thickets and woodlands. They sing with a series of deliberate musical phrases which they repeat throughout the day. One was sighted in 1991 in southern New Mexico and was reported on the Rare Bird Hotline, a service used by amateur bird watchers. Credit: Vireo, The National Academy of Sciences, Philadelphia, PA.

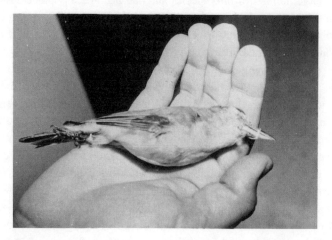

This is the yellow green vireo who was lured out of the Carlsbad Caverns National Park in New Mexico by a student ornithologist and killed. The dead bird now resides as a museum specimen at the University of New Mexico, Albuquerque. Credit: Professor John P. Gluck, University of New Mexico.

The sightings in the Southwest had raised interesting questions. Was the species in the initial stages of a northern expansion, and if so, why? Might it be because of a loss of habitat? It was known that in its home range the bird inhabited canopy, forest borders, and lighter woodland, terrain all under ecological challenge. According to reports, this vagrant bird remained in the vicinity of Rattle Snake Springs until September of 1991, when it precipitously disappeared. It was concluded that the bird had either died or had migrated back to Central America for the winter.

On the first of July the following year, another bird resembling a yellow-green vireo was once again sighted at the spring. Several observers who had made the 1991 sighting believed that this bird was identical to the one observed the previous year. The sighting was reported on the Rare Bird Alert Hot-line, a service managed and used by the amateur bird-watching community, or "birders" as they also known. Shortly after the posting on the hotline, bird-watchers began to arrive from around the United States in hopes of observing the bird.

KILLING AND COLLECTING

On July 8, 1992, John Trochet, a graduate student in ornithology from the University of California at Berkeley who was collecting goldfinches for his dissertation research, traveled to Rattle Snake Springs. Once there he talked with several birders who informed him of the presence of the vireo. He eventually sighted the bird and recorded its distinctive song with his portable tape recorder. At some point soon after the sighting, Trochet made a decision to collect this individual.

The term *collect* refers to the practice of killing a bird with a shotgun or capturing it in a trap or net and then killing it. The bird is then converted into a specimen for deposit and study in an ornithology museum. The tradition in museum ornithology involves the creation of a repository of information by preserving large numbers of specimens of existing groups of birds. The collections are composed of three types of specimens: mounts, skins, and "alcoholics." Mounts are specimens on pedestals in lifelike poses. Skins are specimens where the skeleton (other than the legs and wing bones) and internal organs are removed leaving the skin and feathers, head and beak intact. Alcoholics are the internal soft parts which are preserved in solution. These collections are then used to study morphological differences and similarities between species and between populations within a species.

Trochet's Problem

John Trochet possessed a legal permit to collect any nonendangered bird species in the state of New Mexico for scientific purposes, but by federal law collecting is not permitted in national parks. National parks have the legal status of being sanctuaries for the wildlife contained within their borders, but only as long as they remain there. If Trochet wished to legally collect the vagrant vireo, he was going to have to wait until it was out of the park. This could be a long wait with long odds of success.

Whereas there is a clear prohibition about interfering with animals on parkland, there is no specific wording in the regulations that in fact prevents someone from luring an animal out of the park. Apparently being aware of this distinction and not willing to adopt a more passive and chancy waiting strategy, Trochet used the tape recording he had made of the bird's own song and began to play it aloud at the springs. This technique is frequently used by ornithologists to stimulate a bird whom they can hear but not see clearly to reveal itself. Apparently the bird hears the recording and reacts as though it were coming from another individual and seeks it out in a territorial display. According to Trochet's own account, the procedure worked, and the vagrant vireo flew out of the canopy and began to search for the source of the song. Trochet continued to play the song to the vireo as he walked off the protected property of the national park and toward a private ranch where he had set up a trap of mist nets.[3] On private land the bird was no longer legally protected, and Trochet's collecting permits were in force.

As expected, the vireo followed the replay of its taped song out of the park, flew the quarter of a mile to the ranch site, and was quickly captured in Trochet's nets. Trochet removed the bird from the net and noted that it was indeed a male yellow-green vireo in excellent nesting condition. After the examination, Trochet grasped the body of the vagrant in the palm of his hand, closed his fingers around it, and squeezed tightly. The hand pressure prevented the bird from breathing and it soon died of suffocation. The procedure is called "thoracic compression" and is commonly used to kill birds in the field. Once dead, Trochet prepared the bird as a specimen and sent it back to the University of California ornithology museum.

The Reaction

The reaction of the various interested parties to the collection of this vireo was swift and loud. The ensuing debate between professional ornithologists, birders, and the public at large highlighted the relationship between the legal and the ethical as well as the costs and benefits of the perceived need of some scientists to chronicle an unexpected occurrence contrasted with the wishes and enjoyment of the public. Trochet and other "professionals" asserted the authority and obligation of science to swiftly and accurately describe, record, and explain nature as it exists and changes, even if it means stretching the overall intent of a formal regulation. Birders were outraged that the scientist either failed to consider or undervalued their interests in seeing this unique individual bird alive. Other members of the public who commented seemed to be concerned about the infringement on this bird's life per se. They seemed to take the position that the value of the vireo was independent of the uses to which either the scientists attached to the specimen or the birders to the observation of a living yellow-green vireo. Others expressed surprise that there was furor about the death of a single bird.

Despite the many disagreements between the parties, there was agreement about certain aspects of the vireo incident. All parties eventually agreed that luring a bird off the protected confines of a national park was inappropriate, even though not illegal. Park regulations only speak to animals being killed or disturbed on actual parkland, and therefore no legal action was possible. Nonetheless, the action was seen as a violation of the spirit of the regulations.

In order to consider the more significant ethical conflicts presented by this case, we need first to review briefly the various conceptual and value frameworks of the participants.

THE PURPOSE AND VALUE OF ORNITHOLOGICAL MUSEUM COLLECTIONS

In a recent article, Kevin Winker of the Bell Museum of Natural History at the University of Minnesota reviewed the traditional historical and modern justification for bird collecting.[4] In the most general sense, collecting is the primary way the avian record is preserved. It records and maintains exemplars of what has been seen, where it has been seen, when it has been seen, and under what conditions. Examination of the skins and tissues helps to reveal the variations and similarities that are an expression of the process of evolution.

The discovery of the theory of evolution itself was in part dependent upon the process of comparing the morphological relationships of birds collected by Charles Darwin in the Galapagos Islands. Although painted illustrations and photographs also have served this function, they have always been considered secondary to an actual specimen that can be handled, visualized, measured, and remeasured. Scientists point out that collecting must continue because nature is dynamic and our knowledge of it requires constant updating. Ranges expand and contract, populations become isolated from one another, morphological variations arise or are newly recognized. For example, during the last ten years over six hundred new species of birds have been identified and verified using the process of observation, collection, and comparison.[5]

While North American museums alone house upwards of three million bird specimens that have been collected over the past century,[6] the development of newer genetic analyses has rendered many of the older specimens obsolete.

Additionally, techniques of preservation are now found to interfere with these new biochemical procedures. At the same time, comparison of morphological and genetic information has reinforced the fact that species membership is often obscured by morphological similarity. Therefore, scientists find a need for collections that permit these comparisons.

Specimens provide information beyond that required to detail the variation within the bird world and to specify further the action of evolution in the process of speciation. These data may also offer information important to conservation efforts. The argument is that precise knowledge of the extent of bird diversity is required in order to develop strategies to protect species. Therefore as long as collection does not threaten the well-being of a *population,* the judicious collection of *individual birds* is prudent and in the interest of the overall population. The information potentially provides important insights into our understanding of the processes of evolution, speciation, and biogeographical distribution. In addition, the information may inform conservation and protection plans.

Nonetheless, the practice of ornithological collecting is waning and has been for some time. In 1980, Robert Ricklefs[7] pointed out that specimens were being acquired at a very low level even though many important taxonomic questions remained unanswered. He suggested that the museum tradition in ornithology was dying and being replaced by the study of ecology, ethology, and physiology—something of a paradigm shift in scientific investigation. Yet it is still crucial for students of ornithology to recognize the importance of the collection tradition and the fact that data relevant to the new focus is tied up in the collections. The collections are not merely anachronistic dust collectors.

The Scientific Value of the Collection of a Vagrant

How much valid scientific information was acquired by collecting and examining the specimen of this vagrant individual? The scientist in this case took the expected and requisite attitude of asking whether the individual seen and heard was in reality a yellow-green vireo. Science is about accuracy, and because it is well-known that the yellow-green vireo is hard to distinguish from the red-eyed vireo, photographs and taped song data were not determined to be sufficient for species identification. If it is a yellow-green vireo other questions arise, such as which of the subpopulations has it come from? Answers to such questions required a much closer look than that provided by a photograph or audio tape. In fact, the final determination of species or subpopulation membership may have required biochemical analysis, which requires a significant amount of tissue and, for this purpose, sacrifice of the bird.

Specific identification of the vireo is important for reasons other than mere taxonomic considerations. Collection permitted the acquisition of additional data such as age, sex, fat condition, diet (from stomach contents), general health, pesticide level, parasite load, and existence of injuries and disease. Was this vagrant among an initial wave of pioneering individuals expanding the species range? If so, why the expansion? Are there problems associated with habitat loss in the home range? Is there an overabundance of individuals who cannot find suitable mates or nest sites? The implications of these alternatives might inform further investigation and contribute to conservation and protection activities important to the professional and the public alike.

THE PURPOSE AND VALUE OF BIRDING

Birding exists at many levels of interest and commitment. Fascination with bird life and behavior is widely shared and tends to express respect for the values of conservation and protection. At one end of the continuum, birders are represented by those who simply place feeders on their windowsills to attract members of the local bird community, and they take pleasure in the observations. A classic exemplar of this perspective is presented in the book *Wings at My Window,* by Ada Clapham Govan. In her book she describes that as a housebound invalid she became fascinated with birds when a chickadee visited her window feeder. She eventually became so involved and gained so much pleasure from the pasttime that it helped relieve her chronic incapacitating arthritis. Her book served and continues to serve as encouragement for many to adopt the hobby.

Further along on the continuum are those who plant special trees and shrubbery around their homes in order to attract a larger or more specialized array of species. Yet another level is characterized by "listers." These individuals are strongly motivated to observe and identify as many different species of birds as possible. Lists of sightings are scrupulously kept, personally compared with those of other birders, and turned in to local and national organizations as census devices. In this manner birding contributes to one of the fundamental purposes of museum ornithology, the description of what species have been seen and where. The detractors of the importance of these list data worry that they are often created by individuals not sufficiently familiar with the process of identification.[8]

It would be inaccurate to say that, as a group, birders oppose all specimen collecting. Most acknowledge that a certain amount of collecting is necessary as new species are described. Also, the illustrated field guides on which they depend for accurate identification are constructed by examining trays upon trays of specimen skins in museum collections. But their emphasis is decidedly on the observation and identification of living birds. Frank Chapman, a major shaping force in birding and a longtime editor of the magazine *Bird-Lore,* instituted the traditional creation of "Christmas Lists" in 1900 as a way of distracting people away from shooting birds and toward counting and observing them.

Like scientists, birders are interested in the rare and unique, and the appearance of a vagrant is certainly that. It is easy to see that vagrants are of particular interest to birders. The presence of vagrant birds has the effect of stimulating social and educative interactions among interested people. The situation offers the opportunity not only to observe a member of a species not normally accessible, but it also represents a challenge to the birder's skill as a birder. A single individual must be located, observed, and identified. A needle must be found in an avian haystack. The length of and pride in one's lifetime list is increased by potentially a once-in-a-lifetime observation. Other more tangible benefits also must be recognized. While in search for the prize, birders get moderate levels of exercise and spend money. They buy film, audio tape, meals, gas, and motel rooms. What has become known as "ecotourism" is good for the economy. In short, many lives are enriched by the presence and continued life of the vagrant bird. Once the bird is a tagged specimen skin in a drawer filled with other dead vireos, all this activity ceases.

ETHICAL ISSUES

By the end of the day on July 8, 1992, a scientist was in the possession of a specimen, birders were without a fascinating object of observation, and a single yellow-green vireo was dead. From the positions just reviewed, the foundations of the conflict are clear. How shall these conflicts be viewed? Was either a moral rule or a law broken? Was a covenant with the sanctuary status of the national parks broken? Was the understanding of an important issue in a realm of science advanced? Were the interests of birders unnecessarily blocked? Were the interests of the various parties properly considered and, if necessary, balanced? Was a moral wrong done to a vulnerable individual? Was the bird at least killed humanely?

The Birder-Scientist Conflict

It has been generally acknowledged that Trochet broke what was called an "unwritten" rule by using information acquired from birders actively observing the vagrant to make a scientific collection. More important are some issues raised by an open letter dated September 28, 1992, written by Professor Ned K. Johnson, curator of ornithology at the University of California at Berkeley, and Trochet's dissertation adviser. He wrote, "My personal rule is that the collecting of vagrant individual birds that birders have been observing and enjoying is unwise. Despite the fact that it is often scientifically desirable, and perfectly legal under many permits, too much ill-will is generated by such an act. Obviously, Trochet disregarded this unwritten rule in the incident under discussion."

The choice of the term "unwise" in Professor Johnson's letter is revealing. Its use seems to imply that the matter is one of public relations rather than a consideration of the moral justification of the action. The unwritten rule that Johnson refers to has to do, in his interpretation, with prevention of the creation of ill will and not the weighing and balancing of the interests of scientists and nonscientists or the individual bird. One implication of the statement would seem to be that as long as birders are currently unaware of the existence of a vagrant, and collection by a scientist would therefore not cause a reaction of ill will, their concerns and interests need not be considered.

It could be argued that the collection of a vagrant sets in motion consequences that affect the lives of birders regardless of whether they have seen or know about the collection. Some of the consequences are more tangible than others. For example, some number of vagrants are no longer available to be discovered and enjoyed, and the legitimate interests of birders in seeing living nature are considered irrelevant and are blocked. It may be that the claims of scientists should take precedence in such a situation, but the priority ultimately is justified only by an analysis of the claims of all affected, not merely those aware of a specific situation.

Following the vireo incident, the New Mexico Department of Game and Fish scheduled a meeting where ornithologists and birders could openly discuss their concerns. It was expected that the meeting would result in the development of a set of policies that would be adopted by the department and serve as guidelines for professional and public conduct. On February 19, 1993, a set of regulations made the following points explicit and was officially adopted:[9]

1. The taking of wildlife for scientific and educational purposes is a highly important activity but must not be harmful to wildlife populations and must not abridge the legitimate "rights" of others who use wildlife.
2. The sacrifice of vagrant birds solely for documenting of occurrences is "discouraged."
3. No vagrant birds appearing on the Rare Bird Alert Hot-Line shall be collected. An individual who violates this provision will be assessed one violation point. The accumulation of three points will result in a suspension or revocation of his or her collection permit.[10]
4. All collected specimens are to be considered state property and are to be deposited in an approved institutional museum where they can be inspected by members of the public as well as scientists.
5. Professionals with collecting permits must make their status and purposes known to those with whom they come in contact in the field.

While affirming the importance of scientific and educational collecting, the regulations clearly state that there are others who "use" wildlife and their interests must also be considered. In fact, in the case of vagrant birds, the interests of birders are allowed to take priority over the interests of scientific collectors. While protecting the activities of the amateur naturalist, the provision seems to question whether scientists as a group can be trusted to take the interests of others into account as they conduct their work.

Alternatives to Killing

The birders in this case argued that the vagrant was more important to them and their activities than it was to the scientists, and therefore their interests deserved priority. From this point of view, the scientific benefits of collection must be shown to significantly outweigh these and other related benefits. Whether this point of view is correct, we can ask if the increased certainty of identification that underlies the collecting of the vireo is worth the losses to the birders and others. From the birder perspective, the answer is decidedly no. But is this judgment the most impartial and morally appropriate judgment?

One relevant consideration is that it was widely held by the New Mexico birder community that a reasonably certain identification could have been made without killing the vireo. Field notes, photographs, and audio tapes of the song most likely could have served as an adequate foundation for species identification. If confusion existed about identification, the bird could have been captured, examined, photographed, and then released. If additional biochemical analyses were needed, they could have been done on a retained feather or a small blood sample drawn from a wing vein, procedures quite common in ornithological field research.

As an alternative to killing the bird, the vireo might have been banded, or ringed. In this procedure, the identifying information of a particular bird is registered to an identification number that is embossed on a small aluminum band placed harmlessly on the leg of the bird. In the United States, once the bird is banded, the identifying information is filed with the Fish and Wildlife Service in Washington, DC. The plan is that if the bird is found again, the location and condition of the bird is reported to the service and relayed to the individual who first banded the bird.

Although only about 5% of banded birds are returned and reported, this procedure potentially provides important information regarding migratory movements, longevity, and distribution. If banding had been done in this case, future sightings might have shed light on whether this was the same bird that had been returning for two years to Rattle Snake Springs. If it were, the case for accidental vagrancy would have been weakened in favor of the scientifically significant range expansion hypothesis. A serious consideration of these alternatives would have required planning and a consideration of the interests of other people pursuing the vireo. Do these considerations outweigh the demonstrated scientific interest in collecting and amassing information?

The Significance of a Life

The above considerations are all human-centered. They have to do with conflicting human interests in the bird. But what about the bird's interests? What about the bird's life?

Common assumptions about the significance of a bird's life

Many common arguments in science and beyond downplay the significance of the death of a bird, even when it is killed purposely. These arguments sometimes derive from views about the importance of the death of an individual in relation to the size of the overall population and the number of deaths from other causes. From this perspective, since the estimated North American bird population is between five and twenty billion,[11] the death of one vagrant bird is virtually a nonevent.

Other human-caused bird mortalities account for an enormous number of deaths, dwarfing the losses brought about by scientific collecting. These deaths include an estimated annual loss of 148 million birds due to collisions with windows and motor vehicles and the eighteen million fish-eating birds killed under federal permit in order to protect fish hatcheries.[12] The practice of sport hunting is another source of purposeful bird deaths. For example, it has been estimated that in 1970 and 1971, five million mallard ducks were killed by hunters,[13] and the annual hunt of mourning doves kills somewhere between 11 and 42 million birds.[14]

It is also well known that migrating birds, like the vireo, are often killed in large numbers as they encounter natural disasters such as storms. For example, David and Melissa Wiedenfeld[15] established that a single tropical storm that roared across Grand Isle, Louisiana, in April 1993 killed an estimated forty thousand birds, affecting 45 species of neotropical migrants just as they were about to reach the end of their spring flight across the Gulf of Mexico.

A variant of this argument is that the death or deaths of members of a population or species have significance only if the deaths adversely affect the integrity or existence of a population or species. Therefore, the death of a single individual from a large population is insignificant. By this reasoning, the death of a vagrant is of no real significance. Since the likelihood of the vagrant returning to its native population is low, in a reproductive sense the animal is already worthless. Killing the individual only hastens this already established reality.[16]

Arguments from the Intrinsic Value of a Life

From another perspective, however, the life of a bird has intrinsic value. The heart of the concept of the *intrinsic value* of a life is the claim that the value of an animal is not limited to an analysis of its usefulness to humans. The value of something that is a means to an end is an *extrinsic value*. For example, a bird may have economic value in that its feathers can be sold and made into a form of adornment and its flesh can be sold as a meal. In less material forms of instrumental value, a bird may bring pleasure to one who observes it or hears its song or it may provide data for a scientific investigation. The intrinsic value of a bird, by contrast, is its worth as an end in itself. In his classic book, *A Sand County Almanac,* Aldo Leopold challenged us to look on our ethical relationships with "all things on, over, or in the earth" as a relationship of ends with ends, not merely means and ends.

As we saw in chapter 1, the concept of inherent value has been related by some philosophers directly to questions of the rights and the moral standing of animals. From the utilitarian perspective, philosophers like Bentham, Frey, and Singer view animals as having experiences that are good in themselves—for example, through whatever pleasures they experience. They therefore have a significant stake in how their lives are played out. According to this perspective, we are required to give some moral weight to their experiences. For a nonutilitarian philosopher like Tom Regan (see chapter 1), any animal that is the "subject of a life" has intrinsic value.

Leopold based his justification for the intrinsic value of animals in the nature of the biological world itself. According to this conception, moral sentiments of considering the value and well-being of other beings have evolved from natural selection and the reproductive advantage of social integration. Social living requires some degree of constraint of self-interest. Among social mammals these required constraints have taken the form of other-oriented sentiments such as respect, love, sympathy, and regard. As we have come to understand that all living beings are biologically interdependent, the circle of other-directed concern has broadened. Leopold pushes us to ask whether the idea of the intrinsic value of a living creature as an end in itself may be a philosophical abstraction from these primitive moral sentiments found in many creatures.[17]

Many scientists and birders have incorporated this concept of intrinsic value into the ways that they conduct themselves and speak of animals. To them, the fact that the collection of a vagrant yellow-green vireo might help to demarcate in time and space a population expansion to the southwestern United States or might bring pleasure to group of birders or money to motel owners is not to the point. The bird is an end in itself and not a thing that gains in value by giving pleasure to birders or by satisfying the questions of an ornithologist. Its interests as a living being must also be considered with equal weight along with the interests of others involved.

The Means to Death

A consideration of both the value of the bird and alternatives to killing it suggest the need for an assessment of the means of death. Although published news reports of the vireo incident claimed that the bird died "in a few seconds," implying that the manner of death was insignificant, this claim is debatable.

A panel of the American Veterinary Medical Association (AVMA) has carefully evaluated the appropriateness of euthanasia techniques on a set of dimensions that define the concept of a "good" or relatively pain-free death. The scales include: (1) ability of the procedure to induce loss of consciousness and death without causing pain, distress, anxiety, or apprehension; (2) time required to induce unconsciousness; (3) reliability and irreversibility; (4) compatibility with subsequent examination or use of tissue; (5) issues of safety and emotional impact on human operators and observers.[18] The AVMA panel does not list thoracic compression as a technique that meets these criteria, perhaps because the holding of birds in a tight grasp elicits both resistance and struggle; loss of consciousness is not rapid during suffocation; death may take from one to four minutes; if pressure is not maintained for a sufficiently long time, reversibility can easily occur, requiring that the procedure be reinitiated; and there is a strong chance of a negative emotional impact on observers and operators.

Nonetheless, the panel acknowledges that the requirements of field research may not always be compatible with a pain-free death of experimental subjects. Field researchers use the words "collecting," "killing," or "harvesting" and not "euthanasia" in part to mark this distinction. However, published guidelines for the use of wild birds in research[19] state that thoracic compression is only appropriate to complete the kill of birds already wounded by gunshot. The options recommended for killing birds collected by net or trap include use of various anesthetic agents or physical means such as cervical dislocation or decapitation, all of which either reduce anxiety and fear or rapidly induce unconsciousness.

CONCLUSION

In February 1993, Trochet closed the matter with a letter of apology to the New Mexico Department of Game and Fish in which he said: "Though it probably further reflects badly on me, I must say that I did not realize in advance that the collection of the yellow-green vireo would create such a fire-storm of protest. As in all previous instances when I elected to collect a bird, I made the decision wholly on the basis of the scientific merits. Making such a narrowly focused assessment is not a mistake I will make again."[20]

Despite the passage of time after this case was closed, a mention of the incident still induces quick reactions among scientific collectors, birders, and proponents of the intrinsic value of animals. Despite the new regulations, anger and mistrust prevail. No new yellow-green vireos have been sighted at Rattle Snake Springs, or at least none has been publicly reported. The skin of the vagrant vireo lies flat in a small specimen tray in the Museum of Southwestern Biology at the University of New Mexico in Albuquerque. Records kept on the use of the specimen at the museum show that no one has examined the skin since 1992. A literature search did not uncover any published research about the sighting, and the registrar reports that John Trochet is no longer a graduate student at the University of California at Berkeley.

NOTES

1. *Merriam-Webster's Collegiate Dictionary,* 10th ed.
2. R. S. Ridgely and G. Tudor, *The Birds of South America* (Austin: University of Texas Press, 1989), p. 150.
3. Mist nets are constructed of thin nylon fiber that are virtually invisible to flying birds. Once they strike the net they become entangled in the webbing and are unable to escape.
4. K. Winker, B. Fall, J. Klicka, D. Parmelee, and H. Tardoff, "The Importance of Avian Collecting and the Need for Continued Collecting," *Loon* 63 (1991): 238–46.
5. See C. Sibley and B. Monore, *Distribution and Taxonomy of Birds of the World* (New Haven, CT: Yale University Press, 1990).
6. R. Ricklefs, "Old Specimens and New Directions: The Museum Tradition in Contemporary Ornithology," The *Auk* 97 (1980): 206–7.
7. Ricklefs, "Old Specimens and New Directions," 206–7.
8. J. Remsen, "Use and Misuse of Bird Lists in Community Ecology and Conservation," The *Auk* 111 (1994): 225–27.
9. New Mexico Department of Game and Fish, *Conditions and Provisions for the Taking of Wildlife for Scientific and Educational Purposes* (Santa Fe, NM: *State Records Office,* 1993).
10. While there is no documentation to support the contention, it was widely believed in the birder community that they could personally authorize the collection of a vagrant appearing on the hotline.
11. See The *Auk* 92, no. 3 (1975): supplement 1A–27A.
12. J. Remsen, "Emotionalism Is the Epitaph for Enlightenment," *Birding* (April 1993): 129–32.
13. R. C. Banks, "Human Related Mortality of Birds in the United States," in *US Fish and Wildlife Service, Special Scientific Report, Wildlife* (Washington, DC: US Department of the Interior, 1979) p. 215.
14. Winker et al., "Importance of Avian Collections," pp. 238–46.
15. D. Wiedenfeld and M. Wiedenfeld, "Large Kill of Neotropical Migrants by Tor-

nado and Storm in Louisiana, April 1993," *Journal of Field Ornithology* 66, no. 1 (1994): 70–80.

16. Remsen, "Emotionalism," pp. 129–32.

17. See J. Callicott Baird, "Intrinsic Value, Quantum Theory, and Environmental Ethics," *Environmental Ethics* 7 (1985): 257–75.

18. See "Report of the AVMA Panel on Euthanasia," *Journal of the American Veterinary Medical Association* 202, no. 2 (1993): 229–49.

19. American Ornithologists' Union, "Report of the Committee on Use of Wild Birds in Research," The *Auk* 105, no. 1 (1988): supplement 1A–41A.

20. "Game and Fish OKs Rule on Bird Collecting," *Albuquerque Journal,* 20 February 1993, p. A4.

VI

EDUCATION

11

DISSECTION OF FROGS:
THE JENIFER GRAHAM CASE

In April 1987, Jenifer Graham, a 15-year-old student in Victorville, California, refused to dissect a frog in her biology class. She said it was not squeamishness but moral objections and respect for animal life that led her to refuse. Jenifer offered to do an alternative study in place of dissection that would not involve killing an animal, but this offer was not accepted by the school: if Jenifer failed to perform this requirement, then she would have to suffer the consequences, the principal said. The school lowered Jenifer's grade from an A to a D, but later raised it to a C. As a potentially punitive measure, they added a notation on her official transcript for the purpose of college admission stating, "This student refused to participate in the dissection portion of this class."

Jenifer objected. Two lawyers appointed by the Humane Society of the United States tried to negotiate a settlement for Jenifer. The school argued that there is no substitute for the actual dissection experience: the educational objectives of learning the internal anatomy of a frog cannot be achieved with models, films, and the like. No agreement could be reached.

The case attracted national attention. In the US District Court in Los Angeles, her lawyers argued that Jenifer's ethical beliefs are equivalent to a religion and that the school district had violated her right to freedom of religion under the First Amendment of the Constitution. The *Los Angeles Times*[1] found these arguments weak, because no specific religious teaching speaks out against dissection. Jenifer's moral position was that she wanted no part in the harming and killing of an animal for the sake of her education. Even though she was only 15, she had thought through her moral position on animals to the point that she had become a vegetarian, did not wear leather, and did not use personal care products that had been tested on animals.

Before the case reached resolution, national media attention was further enhanced by Jenifer's participation in a controversial advertisement. In October 1987, Apple Computer released a television commercial featuring Jenifer that distressed some members of the biomedical community. Apple markets a dissection program called "Operation Frog" which is often cited and used as an alternative to actual dissection. The ad, which lasts thirty seconds, was spoken by Jenifer: "Last year in my biology class, I refused to dissect a frog. I didn't want to hurt a living thing. I said I would be happy to do it on an Apple computer. That way, I can learn and the frog lives. But that got me into a lot of trouble, and I got a lower grade. So this year, I'm using my Apple II to study something entirely new—constitutional law."[2] This last was said with a twinkle in her eye, and was an obvious reference to her then ongoing court battle.

This message was criticized by the California Biomedical Research Association, which circulated an "action alert" urging protests to Apple's Chairman, John Sculley.[3] This alert said the ad was "in very poor taste and offensive" to science educators.[4] A spokesperson for the Association of American Universities held that the ad "was a cute marketable commercial for anti-vivisection."[5]

LEGISLATION, COURTS, AND THE PROFESSIONS

In the meantime, humane organizations were busy presenting a bill before the California state legislature that would protect students who objected to dissec-

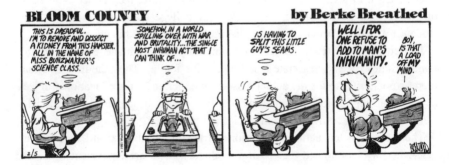

Berke Breathed, who drew this cartoon, has used his syndicated cartoon series many times to present a view sympathetic to the animal protection movement. Credit: Washington Post Writers Group.

tion. Jenifer testified on behalf of the bill and she played an important part in the bill's passage. In March 1988, Governor George Deukmejian signed the Student's Rights Bill into law: beginning in January of 1989, science teachers in kindergarten to twelfth grade would be required to notify students when dissection is part of the curriculum, and to work with them to find humane alternatives if the student objects.[6] This was the first law of its kind to be passed in the United States. Others followed.

Shortly thereafter, in June 1988, the court ruled that the state education system does not require dissection in preparation for admission to California colleges or universities. This ruling undermined one of the high school's major arguments in its refusal to allow Jenifer to receive credit for alternative study. Later, in August 1988, a federal judge dismissed the case and offered a compromise; Jenifer's knowledge of frog anatomy should be tested by using a frog that had died of natural causes. The judge apparently did not know how difficult—if not impossible—it is to find a whole dead frog in the wild.

This unfeasible "solution" does, however, protect Jenifer's right to refuse to dissect a frog, and upholds the school's view that they can insist on testing knowledge of frog anatomy on a real frog, and not on a model, as had been proposed. The notation on her college transcript was ordered removed. But by the time Jenifer graduated from high school in 1989, the school had failed to produce a frog that had died of natural causes. So the matter became moot as Jenifer entered college.

Jenifer's case had wide repercussions. It marked the beginning of a surge of nationwide activity from other students with similar views. Student groups and humane societies initiated campaigns with slogans such as "Say No to Dissection" and "Don't Cut the Frog, Cut the Class." Several animal protection groups established programs to encourage students to opt out of dissection. For instance, a toll-free dissection hotline was established to help students exert their rights to conscientious objection and to be knowledgeable about alternatives. In 1996, the hotline (1-800-922-FROG) was receiving an average of approximately six hundred calls per month (based on a yearly overview since there are seasonal variations). Pat Davis, the director of the hotline and mother of Jenifer, reports that 22% of the calls she receives are about animal dissections in grades kindergarten through six.

As of June 1996, state laws or official policies that allow a student at the grade school level the right to refuse to dissect an animal have been adopted in California, Florida, Pennsylvania, New York, Maine, Massachusetts, and Louisiana. In addition, policies have been adopted in several school districts to remove dissection from the curriculum. Other schools, lacking a formal policy, usually handle the cases in a sympathetic and nonconfrontational manner and find a suitable nonanimal harming alternative.

In the United States, there is no national law that either requires dissection or allows for conscientious objection to it. Animal procedures conducted by precollege students largely fall outside the mandate of the Animal Welfare Act or any other legal requirements.

A 1992 position statement from the National Science Teachers Association (NSTA) endorses dissection at the precollege level. Certain provisions apply— for example, that the activities must be "based on carefully planned objectives . . . appropriate to the maturity level of the student."[7] The position statement further asserts: "Student views or beliefs sensitive to dissection must be considered; the teacher will respond appropriately"[8]—a statement that some administrators have found difficult to interpret. Not everyone agrees with NSTA's endorsement of dissection which, according to one science education specialist, is "contrary to the standards, practices, and possibilities of quality science education for students entering the 21st century."[9]

The most contentious policies are those drawn up by the National Association of Biology Teachers (NABT), a leading organization of over seven thousand biology teachers representing all levels of education.[10] The 1989 official policy, applicable both to grade schools and colleges, supported the use of "alternatives to dissection and vivisection wherever possible,"[11] and the 1990 policy stated, "The lab activity should not cause the loss of an animal's life. Bacteria, fungi, protozoans and invertebrates should be used in activities that may require use of harmful substances or loss of an organism's life."[12] In 1989–90, NABT organized workshops and issued a monograph to help teachers introduce alternatives to dissection.[13]

NABT's actions proved controversial, especially to proponents of animal research.[14] After some political conflict, NABT revised its assessment in a 1994 position statement: "No alternatives can substitute for the actual experience of dissection and [NABT] urges teachers to be aware of the limitations of alternatives. . . . The association encourages teachers to be sensitive to substantive student objections to dissection and to consider providing appropriate alternatives to those students."[15]

A less controversial policy has been formulated by the Institute of Laboratory Animal Resources of the National Academy of Sciences, the policy-making organization for the National Institutes of Heath regarding animal experimentation. Specifically designed for the humane study of animals in precollege education, its 1989 *Principles and Guidelines* do not mention dissection at all. However, they do state, "Observational and natural history studies that are not intrusive (that is, they do not interfere with [a vertebrate] animal's health or well-being or cause it discomfort) are encouraged."[16] One interpretation of this policy could be that if the animal studies are not to be "intrusive" then they should neither harm nor kill the animal.

Policies are still being formulated and it may take many years for a consensus to emerge, if, indeed, one ever does.

HISTORY AND CURRENT PRACTICE OF DISSECTION

Frog dissection first became established as a college-level biology exercise in the 1920s, when there was a heavy emphasis on taxonomy in biology teaching. Over time, dissection gradually moved down to the high school and then the junior high level. In the US the current trend is that dissection of frogs and other species is increasingly being introduced into elementary school education.

In 1988 it was estimated that a total of about four million students took high school biology each year and that approximately 75–80% of these students participated in frog dissection.[17] If each student has one frog, then approximately 3.2 million frogs are used each year for high school use alone, not including those dissections performed in elementary schools and in colleges.

Rana frogs are the most frequently dissected vertebrate species, followed by fetal pigs, perch, and cats.[18] Schools also use invertebrates extensively for dissection—earthworms, grasshoppers, crayfish, and starfish. Reckoned in sheer numbers of dissected organisms, invertebrates only slightly outnumber vertebrates.

It is common that students will participate in repeated frog and other vertebrate animal dissections during their educational career, perhaps one in elementary school, several in high school, more in undergraduate classes, and again in nursing or other professional schools. In some school districts, it is not unusual for students to dissect a frog in eighth grade, a fetal pig in ninth grade, a cat in eleventh grade, and a dog in advanced-placement twelfth grade—and these are in addition to several invertebrate dissections. Students are often required to memorize dozens of names of anatomical parts. Some teachers question the educational value of repeated dissections that are done at the expense of exclusion of other laboratory exercises. Lab exercises have not kept pace with advances in biological knowledge, they claim, and dissection tends to be retained because teachers find it easy to teach. But others argue that the retention of dissection over a seventy-year history proves how valuable this type of lesson is.

Providing millions of frogs and other species for dissection is a profitable business. Biological supply houses purchase animals from various sources and sell them to schools. In the commercial trade, wild live frogs are captured and sold by the barrel. Frogs may be killed and preserved either at the supply house or delivered alive to the schools where either the students or teachers may kill them. Supply houses typically purchase dead cats and dogs from animal shelters[19] and fetal pigs are obtained from slaughterhouses.

In high school biology classrooms, dead materials are common, live organisms rare. Some educators object to the absence of living creatures. How can biology be taught properly, they ask, if the students never study anything living—as happens in all too many high schools? They argue that much better understanding of life processes would come from studying more living things in ways that cause them no harm or destruction.[20]

The National Research Council's Committee on High School Biology Education has strongly criticized the current high school biology curriculum. According to their 1990 report, the high school curriculum is "too inclusive, burdened with vocabulary, and short on concepts. Most students see it as boring and irrelevant . . . the use of laboratories is inadequate."[21] The alarming decline in scientific literacy in the adult American population is often attributed to these failures. A number of people hold that dissection, too, does not teach concepts and is as boring and irrelevant as learning lists of the parts of anything.

According to this committee's report, what the curriculum should include is "an understanding of basic concepts in cell and molecular biology, evolution, energy and metabolism, heredity, development and reproduction, and ecology. Concepts must be mastered through inquiry, not memorization of words."[22] The place of dissection in the accomplishment of these goals is still an openly debated question.

ETHICAL ISSUES

Dissection raises a number of issues about the ethics of using animals for educational purposes, including several of the basic issues discussed in chapter 1 of this volume.

Harms to Animals

For those who believe that dissection is not a very valuable educational pursuit, added weight is given to the basic objection to killing. A number of educators support this view.[23] An opposing view is that the life of a frog is of little significance and is not protected by any form of "right to life." There is, then, a set of substantive issues about whether killing animals is a form of harming and, if so, its significance for dissection.

The degree of human responsibility in causing the death of the animal is also an issue. For instance, the judge in the legal case tried to accommodate Jenifer's objection to killing by requiring that she dissect a frog that had died of natural causes, thus removing human responsibility for the death. Not all animals that are dissected are specifically killed for that purpose. Their deaths may be by-products of another activity. For instance, dead cats and dogs are obtained from shelters where they are killed because of their overpopulation. Fetal pigs sold for dissection are a profitable by-product of the meat industry. If school dissection did not exist, these cats, dogs, and pigs would be killed in any event. Their fate would likely be to serve as fertilizer or in some other product.

These animal carcasses would probably be put to some purpose, not wasted. Also on the benefits side is the learning that occurs for the students in studying the internal anatomy of a frog or other species, as noted previously.

From another perspective, however, there are conspicuous problems of harm. Not only is a life taken, but the method of death can be traumatic. Several controversies have highlighted this problem. For instance, in 1991, a court convicted a leading biological supply house of violating the Animal Welfare Act because it employed cruel methods of killing and injecting cats and other species destined for dissection. In 1994 it was discovered that children in Mexico were being paid to steal pet cats that were then drowned and shipped for dissection in US schools.[24] For many frogs that are delivered live to the classroom, either the teacher or the students do the killing, and their expertise in providing a rapid, painless death is not always assured because not all teachers and students are experienced in these practices.

Harms can also come from the trauma of capture and transport of wild frogs to the biological supply house. The commercial trade sometimes holds the frogs for several days in sacks filled with other frogs. There they may suffer dehydration, contract disease, or die before arriving at the biological supply house. Whether the animal is alive, sick, or dead is not a financial incentive to different treatment, because the economic value of the animal is not affected.

Harm to the Environment

Native populations of frogs, in the United States and worldwide, are now becoming threatened. Scientists first noted the depletion in populations of frogs and toads in the late 1960s. Apprehension has increased as concerns about the environment have mounted. Because species are unique, their loss may have a wider effect, especially by producing adverse repercussions on other living species and disturbing the ecological balance of nature. The food chain may be disturbed, which can harm other animals and plants. While some of these problems are speculative, good evidence supports other concerns. For example, frogs eat insects, including mosquitos and various pests that would almost certainly increase with the disappearance of the frogs that control their populations.

Although many factors contribute to the depopulation of frogs, harvesting frogs for dissection may add to the problem, and some biology teachers now forgo dissection for this reason. The factors that contribute to the depopulation include (in present theory) the state of the earth's ozone layer, the removal of streamside vegetation, deforestation, the use of pesticides, and the continued commercial harvesting of frogs. Thus, dissection is a contributory cause, but not alone *the cause* of the problem.

The deep ethical issue is the global one of how to eliminate threats to the environment without causing even more significant harms (for example, in loss of jobs) in the process.

Harms to Students

Some believe that dissection can desensitize students to animal suffering and reinforce the message that animals are here for humans to exploit, like "things to consume and throw away."[25] The point is generally focused on the moral development of young persons. It is argued that students should be taught to be kind and caring to animals, virtues that are often lacking in the way children are raised today.

In an article entitled "The Psychology of Dissection," Kenneth Shapiro claims that for some students the act of dissection can also be emotionally disturbing.[26] He notes how students often recoil not only at killing, but at the prospect of handling a dead body. A few students and parents view the cutting up of a body as desecration. The desecration aspect is further enhanced if the dissection is poorly done by unskilled persons and if a disrespectful and joking atmosphere intrudes into the classroom, as occasionally happens.

These concerns are of great importance to some students, but the projected risks of harm would only apply to some percentage of the student community. One possible way to handle the problem is to ban required courses involving dissection in the public schools, while permitting instructors to use these techniques in elective courses. But is this the best way to handle the issues? Would such a policy have other negative consequences in the curriculum for those who object to certain teachings and practices? For example, would a school system have to offer biology courses that made no reference to the theory of evolution in order to accommodate students who found such theories offensive to their religious views?

Without some structure of elective courses that allows students the freedom to avoid courses they find offensive, school systems are almost certain to encounter problems with the coercion and possibly the punishment of students. Punitive measures and coercive measures were involved in the Jenifer Graham case, although they may not have been conceived as either punitive or coercive by those who engaged in the actions. Jenifer was exposed to intimidating questioning, given lower grades, and suffered the threat of a potentially punitive comment being placed on her transcript. She was also assigned heavier workloads than those assigned to other students.

Some teachers advocate a "compromise" to escape these problems while maintaining the quality of the science instruction: They would require students to observe a dissection while not requiring them to participate in the cutting of the animal. Margaret Snyder and her colleagues hold that this is the "ideal" solution when a teacher is faced with an objecting student, because they learn the biology without having to take the actions they find offensive.[27] However, requiring observation of dissection is unacceptable to some students, who firmly refuse all forms of participation. Is either party being unreasonable or acting in a morally inappropriate fashion?

Snyder and colleagues also advocate a procedure through which the young student who objects to dissection would have to defend a well-developed moral position on the relationship between humans and animals. In this recommendation, the student is asked to explain the literature or moral or religious foundations on which they base their beliefs. However, these strategies have their own ethical problems. Students, especially those who are young, can easily be intimidated by questions posed by the school authorities, perhaps even emotionally devastated by them. Such treatment is also unfair because other students who willingly dissect are usually not asked to morally justify dissection, nor are their moral views of other matters called into question. If there is to be a moral test of conduct, why not administer the test to everyone equally? One teacher opposed to Snyder's recommendation writes: "The implicit assumption [in Snyder's article] that dissection is a norm and alternative views constitute 'objections,' exposes a bias. . . . The deeper problem here concerns the procedural 'ordeal' that faces a student who does not follow the 'norm.' Why must only those who object to dissection be called upon to explore their motives and reasons? Indeed, we should be concerned about the ethical position of all our students."[28] This comment leads to yet another level of moral problem. Although we should be concerned that students receive a proper moral education, should teachers be in the business of exploring the motives and reasons students have either for participating or not participating? Should there be a burden of proof for any student with any kind of belief?[29]

The Value of Learning

Typically, those in favor of retaining dissection are less concerned about the issues mentioned thus far and more concerned about the value of dissection as a way of learning important lessons in biology. Dissection is not the only way to learn many facts of biology, they argue, but it is the only way to learn some features of the structure, placement, and interrelation of body parts. Without a knowledge of these elements, they believe the student cannot get an adequate grounding in biology. This outcome seems particularly devastating in a period in which study after study has shown a decline in the quality of American science education.

According to those who support dissection, alternatives that avoid using an actual animal (computer simulations, models, X rays, etc.) are inadequate because the experience of dissecting and the comprehension gained through that experience are lost.[30] In particular, the experience of dissection makes a reality of what the internal organs are in a way no other technique quite does. When students learn about the physiological functions of various organs, there is repeated reference to body parts—heart, lung, liver, spleen, kidneys, and so on . For many students these might be just names and pictures in books or on a video screen. Until these organs have been seen and personally handled, students are being confined to a nebulous world of the abstract instead of the more meaningful, memorable world of concrete personal experience.

One high school biology teacher describes her first experience of dissecting as follows:

> I can still remember my first dissection of a mammal. It was a mouse. . . . What ensued was a tremendous explosion of consciousness and understanding. All the things I had been learning were suddenly real. It was a profound experience. But it was something more. By confirming all the things I had been taught, it helped me understand that the world was a rational place, and that knowledge and understanding can come from serious study of real specimens and real data. Every year, I see this same kind of learning occur in my own students.[31]

The declared benefit of such hands-on experience is that the knowledge thereby gained has more impact, is retained longer, and is understood better than if models, charts, or learning from textbooks are substituted. However, this empirical claim is controversial, because little evidence of these claims—or of the counterclaims—is currently available. There is anecdotal evidence on both sides, but very little scientific information.

Alternatives and the Necessity of Dissection

Another way to approach these problems is to ask whether there are any realistic alternatives to dissection that would maintain high-quality science education. Is this possibility well grounded, or is it more fantasy than reality? (On alternatives and their moral basis and importance, see chapter 1.)

Recently, much effort has been given to developing alternatives that specifically substitute for dissection as well as other uses of animals. Many films, videos, models, and computer simulations of dissections are now available from several sources. For instance, a frog dissection package is now available on the World Wide Web (http://tech.virginia.edu/go/frog). Aimed at secondary-school biology students and undergraduates, the package has been highly praised and was voted among the top 500 Web sites by *IWAY* magazine, a computer publication. Also, the UC Center for Alternatives at the University of California, Davis, has developed a sophisticated animal model that is still under test as an alternative to dissection in the high schools. Furthermore, the Humane Society of the United States has established a loan program to provide students and educators with up-to-date alternatives to animal dissection.

Other alternatives to dissection include: various observational anatomical projects of the external anatomy of live animals; student-made models of stomach, livers, and other internal organs; and studies of human anatomy from Xrays, movies of the human gastrointestinal tract after barium meals, pyelograms of the kidney, images of the heart, and computer tomography (CT) scan images. Several organizations, including the National Association of Biology Teachers, have brought out booklets recommending alternatives.[32]

A recent study evaluated "Interactive Frog Dissection," an interactive videodisc developed by the National Association of Biology Teachers as an alternative to dissection.[33] The results showed that this videodisc is as effective as traditional frog dissection in the high school biology laboratory for learning internal frog anatomy. Furthermore, computer simulations are held to be superior to actual dissections for certain purposes, for instance, learning the topography of certain objects from repeatable three-dimensional rotation, and teaching both realistically and diagrammatically the mechanical function and embryonic and postnatal development of various parts of the body.[34]

Proponents for the retention of high school dissection argue that none of these alternatives is adequate for the full range of scientific teaching that needs to be done. Dissection is an essential exercise for learning about internal structures, the interrelationships among tissues, evolutionary relationships, and the physical placement of organs, they say. The remarks of one high school teacher reflect this perspective:

> No model, no video, no diagram and no movie can duplicate the fascination, the sense of discovery, wonder and even awe that students feel when they find real structures in their own specimens. When students know a specimen is real, their attention is heightened, and the information they learn is somehow registered as 'real' . . . I am distressed with the amount of time and energy spent looking for 'alternatives to dissection.' The alternative to dissection is ignorance, and let us never forget that ignorance comes at a terrible price.[35]

Nonetheless, a number of school systems in North America either do not offer or do not require dissection in the high schools. Moreover, school officials in Switzerland, Norway, the Netherlands, and Denmark have prohibited dissection below the university level.[36] In the United Kingdom, the London University Schools Examining Board has removed animal dissection from its syllabus: Instead, its 1990–91 syllabus required pupils to study a computer alternative.[37] There is, as yet, no indication that the scientific literacy of those high school students who do not dissect animals is impaired. On the other hand, as noted previously, careful scientific studies are not available.

Educational Maturity of the Student

The educational value of dissection can vary dramatically with the age and emotional and educational level of the student. The educational goals of including dissection also vary with the group of students being taught. In elementary school, frog dissection has sometimes been used to teach manual dexterity and skill at dissection itself. At the high school level, the objective appears to be mainly to teach basic anatomy of body parts, taxonomy, and labeling of body parts. For college-level students of comparative zoology, the dissection of various species can convey important information about species variations; for veterinary students dissection can be used as a forerunner to doing live surgery just as dissecting the human body is a forerunner for medical students to conducting surgery.

Some people seeking to put forward a compromise for the dissection controversy link the need for animal dissection to the student's chosen career path and specific educational needs. For instance, David Harbster, who has abandoned dissections in his own high school classes, believes that college-level dissection can be valuable because then the students are "closer to their careers."[38] According to this view, dissection can be appropriate for a selected few students, namely, those who have a serious career commitment in the biological sciences and who are at an educational level where such an anatomical study is directly related to their work. In effect, this position would restrict dissection of frogs, cats, and dogs to college-level students or, more likely, to graduate students.

Ethical Significance of Species

Is it necessary to use a particular species for dissection, or could a less sentient species (lower on the phylogenetic scale) by substituted? The recent rise in dissection of cats and even dogs in high schools has caused alarm among opponents of dissection.

On the one hand, some teachers believe that dissecting an animal high in the phylogenetic scale, such as a cat, is both more exciting and will better prepare a student for college biology education. On the other hand, there is generally a descending scale of emotional conflict for students; the higher one goes on the phylogenetic scale, the more the emotional conflict emerges for many students who are familiar with the animals as pets. On the whole, the conflicts (and likely opposition) are greatest if cats and dogs are used, somewhat less if frogs are used, and least if invertebrate animals are dissected.

Just as there is a descending scale of emotional reaction as one goes lower on the phylogenetic scale, so many believe there is rightly a descending scale of ethical concern as one moves lower on this scale. There seems to be a lower ethical cost in destroying invertebrate rather than vertebrate animals, because invertebrates have less well developed nervous systems and are therefore less able to perceive pain. Many policies governing student uses of animals state that invertebrates should be used in preference to vertebrates because they raise fewer ethical concerns and are readily available in large numbers.

The psychological thesis about levels of emotional reaction in students is supported by available evidence; but is the ethical claim correct? Is there any ethical basis to the idea that moral concerns about animals should be connected to the phylogenetic scale, or is this thesis supported more by fantasy than reality?

CONCLUSION

The education of young people has always been a matter of social concern. Over time, styles of education change and curricula change. Some believe that the current resistance to forgoing dissection may be a reflection of the difficulty of changing the status quo. Others see it as a conflict of values pitting valuable education against an undue concern for the protection of animals. As with many other educational changes, the dissection controversy poses ethical concerns that may take years to resolve.

NOTES

1. Editorial, *Los Angeles Times,* 7 August 1988, pt. V.
2. Constance Holden, "Apples, Frogs, and Animal Rights," *Science* 238 (4 December 1987): 1345.
3. Ibid.
4. Ibid.
5. Ibid.
6. California Education Code, secs. 32255–32255.6. Known previous to passage as Student's Rights Bill, Assembly Bill 2507.
7. National Science Teachers Association, "Guidelines for Responsible Use of Animals in the Classroom," *NSTA Reports,* December 1991/January 1992, p. 6.
8. National Science Teachers Association, "Guidelines for Responsible Use," p. 6.
9. David A. Harbster, "Use of Animals in the Classroom," letter, *NSTA Reports,* April 1992, p. 42.
10. National Association of Biology Teachers, policy statements, *1989–94.* The following statements have been issued: "NABT Policy on Dissection and Vivisection," *News and Views* (NABT), March/April 1989; *The Responsible Use of Animals in Biology Classrooms, Including Alternatives to Dissection: A NABT Policy Statement,* approved by NABT Board of Directors, 25 October 1989; *NABT Guidelines for the Use of Live Animals,* January 1990; "The Responsible Use of Animals in the Biology Classroom: A Clarification," approved by NABT Board of Directors, 7 November 1990, published in *American Biology Teacher* 53 (1991): 71; "Position Statements on Animal Use," *News*

and Views (NABT), December 1992/January 1993, pp. 18–19; "Position Statement: The Use of Animals in Biology Education," *News and Views* (NABT), February 1994, p. 14.

11. National Association of Biology Teachers, *NABT Policy on Dissection and Vivisection*, 1989.

12. National Association of Biology Teachers, *NABT Guidelines for the Use of Live Animals*, 1990.

13. Rosalina V. Hairston, ed., *The Responsible Use of Animals in Biology Classrooms: Including Alternatives to Dissection*, monograph 4 (Reston, VA: National Association of Biology Teachers, 1990);

14. One critic called the above-mentioned NABT monograph "an insidiously evil publication—evil because it is a barely disguised tract produced by the animal 'rightists'"; Barbara Bentley, review of *The Responsible Use of Animals in Biology Classrooms*, *Quarterly Review of Biology* 66 (December, 1991): 475–77.

15. National Association of Biology Teachers, "Position Statement," 1994, p. 14.

16. *Principles and Guidelines for the Use of Animals in Precollege Education* (Washington: Institute of Laboratory Animal Resources, National Academy of Sciences, 1989).

17. F. Barbara Orlans, "Debating Dissection: Pros, Cons, and Alternatives," *Science Teacher*, November 1988, p. 38.

18. Orlans, "Debating Dissection," p. 38.

19. See chapter 16, "Where Should Research Scientists Get Their Dogs?" for discussion of laboratory use of cats and dogs from animal shelters.

20. Orlans, "Debating Dissection," p. 40; William V. Mayer, "Biology: Study of the Living or the Dead?" *American Biology Teacher* 35 (January 1973): 27–30; Randy Moore, "Studying Living Organisms," editorial, *American Biology Teacher* 48 (October 1986): 392.

21. Committee on High-School Biology Education, Board on Biology, Commission on Life Sciences, National Research Council, *Fulfilling the Promise: Biology Education in the Nation's Schools* (Washington: National Academy Press, 1990), p. 3.

22. Ibid. p. 21.

23. Carla McClain, "Mexican Cats Killed for U.S. Kids to Dissect," *USA Today*, 2 May 1994, p. 39; Juliana Texley, ed., "Editor's Corner," *Science Teacher*, December 1987, p. 9; David Gilmore, letter to the editor, *American Biology Teacher* 52 (January 1990): 6, 8; F. Barbara Orlans, "Dissection Forum: The Case Against," *Science Teacher*, January 1991, p. 12; David A. Harbster, "Animals in Education," letter to the editor, *American Biology Teacher* 55 (September 1993): 329.

24. McClain, "Mexican Cats Killed."

25. Gilmore, letter to the editor, p. 6.

26. Kenneth J. Shapiro, "The Psychology of Dissection," *Science Teacher*, October 1992, p. 43.

27. Margaret D. Snyder et al., "Dissecting Student Objections: Responding to Student Concerns," *Science Teacher*, October 1992, p. 43.

28. Douglas Allchin, "Dissection: Ethics and Education," letter, *Science Teacher*, January 1993, p. 8.

29. On these issues, see Allchin, "Dissection," p. 8; Sandra Larson, "Dissection: Ethics and Education," letter, *Science Teacher*, February 1993, p. 10.

30. Terry D. Keiser and Roger W. Hamm, "Dissection Forum: The Case For," *Science Teacher*, January 1991, pp. 13, 15; Melissa Stanley, "Member Protests Dissection Policy," letter, *American Biology Teacher* 53 (November/December 1991): 454; Susan Offner, "The Importance of Dissection in Biology Teaching," *American Biology Teacher* 55 (March 1993): 147–48.

31. Offner, "Importance of Dissection," p. 147.

32. Hairston, *Responsible Use of Animals; Objecting to Dissection: A College Students' Handbook* (San Rafael, CA: Animal Legal Defense Fund). Also available are handbooks for high school and elementary students; e.g., Laura Simon, ed., *Beyond Dissection: A Sampling of Innovative Teaching Tools for Biology Education* (Stanford, CT: Ethical Science Education Coalition, 1992).

33. Richard T. Strauss and Mable B. Kinzie, "Student Achievement and Attitudes in a Pilot Study Comparing an Interactive Videodisc Simulation to Conventional Dissection," *American Biology Teacher* (October 1994): 398–402.

34. Alexander S. Davies, "How Computers Can Reduce the Use of Animals in the Teaching of Veterinary Anatomy," *ANZCCART* [Austrailian and New Zealand Council for the Care of Animals in Research and Teaching] *News* 6 (Summer 1993): 1.

35. Offner, "The Importance of Dissection," pp. 147–49.

36. Jason Black, "A City Without Cats," *The Animals' Agenda*, March/April 1994, p. 15.

37. Jane A. Smith and Kenneth M. Boyd, eds., *Lives in the Balance: The Ethics of Using Animals in Biomedical Research* (Oxford: Oxford University Press, 1991), p. 228.

38. Harbster, "Animals in Education," p. 329.

VII

FOOD AND FARMING

12

FORCE-FEEDING OF GEESE

Foie gras (literally, "fat liver") is an expensive food created for French restaurants and the gourmet food market. Foie gras comes from the livers of specific breeds of domesticated geese raised on a carbohydrate-rich diet. Various preparations of fresh foie gras and pâté de foie gras are the most popular and the most profitable items on the menus of many French restaurants, but the way the geese are raised and fed has generated international controversy.

Geese have been fattened in France and a few other countries to produce foie gras since the Roman period. The French cities of Strasbourg and Perigueux have become world famous for the quality of their foie gras. Crossbreeding, particularly in Europe, has improved the hardiness and liver weights in today's domesticated geese. Although France still produces about 60% of the world's foie gras, it is produced and marketed in several countries, including the United States. Some, most noticeably Germany,[1] prohibit the feeding practices required to produce marketable goose livers.

These practices—so-called force-feeding procedures—have raised questions about cruelty to animals that have been at the center of a larger controversy concerning the treatment of farm animals for commercial profit. Some of the issues are distinctly ethical: For example, can these geese be farmed and shipped in an ethically acceptable manner and still produce the desired product? Other issues are both political and ethical. The issue that has generated the most discussion is, should a country condone force-feeding by allowing it on farms or by allowing sales from foreign farms, or should the country prohibit it through legislation?

THE NATURE OF FORCE-FEEDING

Commercial production of fresh foie gras and pâté using force-feeding methods—known as *gavage* (meaning cramming) in France—aims to enlarge an animal's liver through mechanical force-feeding of up to 6½ pounds of salted, cooked maize per day, per animal, for up to one month. The prevailing

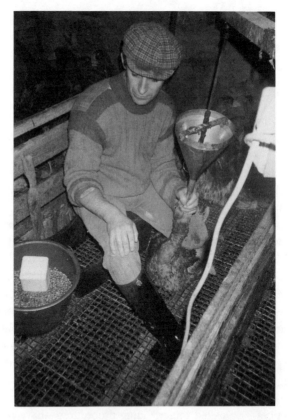

A farmer restrains the goose's body and forces a maize gruel through a funnel-shaped tube that is inserted several inches into the bird's throat, a technique that prevents regurgitation. Each feeding is repeated two to six times a day until the bird's liver enlarges to several times its original size. These livers are then used for production of pâté de foie gras, considered by some to be a luxury food. Credit: Compassion in World Farming, Petersfield, Hampshire, UK.

practice is to restrain the animal's body in a metal or canvas brace and mechanically pump the maize through a funnel-and-tube device that is inserted several inches down the goose's throat using techniques that prevent regurgitation. The feedings take approximately one minute and are repeated two to six times a day until the liver enlarges to several times its original size.

Until four to five months old, geese are usually left to range free on a farm. At approximately five months of age, they are brought indoors and force-fed for 15 to 28 days and closely confined between feedings to prevent them from burning off fat. Shortly thereafter, they are killed. The forced intake is well in excess of normal food consumption. As a result, the liver swells in size. The average weight of the goose roughly doubles; the average liver roughly triples in size. The weight of the liver may increase tenfold in two weeks, and may account for up to 10% of the animal's total weight. A goose that has been force-fed has a liver weighing approximately 800–1000 grams, while a goose that has not been force-fed has a liver that weighs approximately 120 grams. Male livers retain more fat than female livers and are heavier.[2]

Although some geese die from intestinal, liver, or heart malfunctions produced by the force-feeding, most do not. The Landes Experimental Station reported in 1984 that unplanned mortality resulting from force-feeding runs up to 10% of the geese on a farm; autopsies on these geese reveal intestinal lesions, ruptured liver cell membranes, necrosis, and cirrhosis as the causes of death.[3]

A CONTROVERSY AT IROQUOIS BRANDS

Some moral questions about these practices have spread beyond the farm to manufacturing, shipping, importing, and other parts of commerce. Among the best known controversies in the United States occurred at Iroquois Brands, a US corporation located in Greenwich, Connecticut. Although not engaged in the farming and feeding of geese, the corporation had been questioned by one of its shareholders about the company's importation of pâté de fois gras. Peter C. Lovenheim, a shareholder, argued that the force-feeding procedure consisted of inhumane treatment and that shareholders have the right to know and investigate this practice. Iroquois Brands was eventually forced to respond to his inquiry by mailing to its shareholders information explaining the upcoming vote at the company's annual meeting regarding the company's importation of pâté de foie gras from French suppliers. Shareholders were asked whether they wished the corporation to investigate charges made by a minority of shareholders concerning cruelty to geese in France in the process of force-feeding.

Lovenheim, who held two hundred shares of stock, was initially attracted to the company because of its health food orientation and its broad range of specialty products. When he received proxy materials detailing a new product,

Edouard Artzner Pâté de Foie Gras, he was distressed. A proponent of animal welfare, he objected to what he understood as cruelty.

Lovenheim had brought his concerns to a stockholders' meeting and obtained just over the 5% support from other stockholders necessary to introduce the issue to shareholders and management. Lovenheim pushed to have proxy materials mailed to the shareholders, advocating the formation of a committee to investigate the methods used to fatten the geese. However, Lovenheim was met with stern resistance from management. Officers of Iroquois refused to include his proxy materials in the shareholders' report on grounds that the issue lacked economic significance to the company, the only condition management believed to be relevant for shareholder consideration.

Lovenheim replied that ethical and social issues should not be excluded from proxy materials merely because these issues fail to be of economic interest. He and other like-minded shareholders saw the proper treatment of animals as a perennial problem of Western morality that any sensitive person should consider, and therefore as relevant to the operations of a business. They maintained that if undue stress, pain, and suffering are inflicted upon the geese, it is questionable whether further distribution of this product should continue unless a more humane production method could be developed.

In his proposal, Lovenheim requested that a committee be formed to study the methods by which the French supplier produced pâté and report to shareholders its findings, together with an opinion about whether this process caused undue distress, pain, and suffering to animals. Management at Iroquois Brands rejected the need to investigate Lovenheim's allegations. It cited figures that discounted the financial importance of the pâté, claiming the company suffered a net loss on the product. Its figures may be summarized as follows:

Iroquois's annual revenue: $141 million

Iroquois's annual profit: $6 million

Iroquois's sales from pâté: $79,000

Iroquois's net loss on pâté: $3,121

Management acknowledged that moral problems of cruelty to animals were of considerable social importance. The board claimed to "deplore cruelty to animals in any form"[4] and commended the Humane Society of the United States for its work to alleviate problems of animal treatment. However, the company denied that a reseller of the product should be responsible for the means of production. It did not view itself as responsible for the practices of the French over which it had no control. It maintained that upon importation, the product was tested and approved by the federal Food and Drug Administration (FDA). Since this approval indicated an official recognition of the legality of production, executives took the view that all responsibility was thereby lifted from the company.

Iroquois also argued that it was illogical to form a panel to study an issue that the company could not control, especially when the costs of obtaining expert consultation would exceed any reasonably anticipated profit from the product. Management contended that even if a committee were formed to investigate these issues, it would have little if any impact on Iroquois's actual business and even less impact on the world pâté market or the feeding practices in France.

Lovenheim objected to the company's line of argument. He claimed that through importation, advertisement, and sale of the product, Iroquois was indirectly supporting animal mistreatment and must be held responsible. Furthermore, it was precisely the availability of a market for products obtained in this manner that he thought contributes to the continuation of such treatment.

This struggle was eventually presented to a US District Court, which treated the case as a matter of law, avoiding engagement with the ethical questions. Specifically, it considered whether a 1983 rule of the US Securities and Exchange Commission (SEC) should be determinative in this particular case. This rule allows a company to omit proxy materials proposed by shareholders if the relevant operation of the firm—for example, importing pâté—accounts for less than 5% of the firm's total assets and is not "otherwise significantly related to the issuer's business." Iroquois management adopted the view that it was not compelled under this rule to issue the proxy materials.

However, Judge Oliver Gasch sided with Lovenheim on the legal issues, without attempting to rule on the moral issues.[5] Judge Gasch held that the history of the rule in question showed no decision by the SEC that permitted economic considerations to be the sole criterion compelling a given company to issue proxy materials. Judge Gasch ordered that the proxy material be sent to shareholders. Lovenheim claimed that his effort successfully "reasserts the rights of shareholders in all companies to bring moral issues to the attention of management."[6] Thereafter, the unit responsible for the importation of the pâté was sold by Iroquois Brands and management officially pronounced the issue dead.[7]

Despite the withering of the issues at Iroquois, the case has continued to receive public attention in the United States and still is considered in some European countries a major moral and political issue about animal welfare.

STATEMENTS FROM ANIMAL WELFARE GROUPS

Several animal welfare groups have condemned force-feeding and have supported boycotts of the practice and the distribution of the product. The American Society for the Prevention of Cruelty to Animals (ASPCA) has stated that force-feeding "is not just raising animals for food. This is an aberrant and unethical practice."[8] John F. Kullberg, executive director of the organization, explained the ASPCA's position on the force-feeding of geese:

> We consider the force-feeding of geese an act of cruelty and remain committed to having this practice stopped.
>
> Hundreds of thousands of geese are subjected to force-feeding yearly. The pain and stress they endure is very real. The fact that all of this is justified solely on the basis of producing a luxury food item not only promotes the unethical stand that the end justifies the means, but makes the matter even more objectionable because of such a meaningless end.
>
> We are distressed that the results of this inhumane feeding practice are promoted for sale in the United States. It is further the opinion of our legal counsel that force-feeding violates several state anti-cruelty laws.[9]

Compassion in World Farming (CIWF), headquartered in Great Britain, has maintained that, despite its entrenched position in French farming, force-feeding contravenes the European Convention for the Protection of Animals Kept for Farming Purposes. CIWF argues that painful physical abnormalities and diseases of the heart and liver are produced by force-feeding.[10] People for the Ethical Treatment of Animals (PETA) has been sharply critical of foie gras production in the United States. PETA campaigned to shut down Commonwealth Enterprises, a producer in the Hudson Valley in New York. PETA also mounted a campaign to get restaurants, hotels, and airlines to stop serving foie gras.[11]

Critics from several animal welfare groups now argue that the geese deserve increased protection against various methods of research, production, and slaughter. They contend that animal interests and suffering, and not merely their utility to the human species, must be taken into account.

ETHICAL ISSUES

Benefits and Costs

As discussed in chapter 1 of this volume, problems about the use of animals for food are often framed in terms of the relative weight of the costs and benefits involved. "Costs" include all harms, adverse effects on the animals, sacrifices, and resources required to produce a benefit; they are negative effects of pursuing and realizing an objective. "Benefits" are items of positive value such as life, health, and happiness. They are the positive results of incurring costs. To determine whether the force-feeding of geese is justified, one might try to weigh the costs and benefits to see if the suffering of the geese is offset by gains to the animal or to humans.

Benefits

Defenders of foie gras production need not reject the premise that geese are harmed by force-feeding. Their defense may rely entirely on a claim that the benefits to the various parties of the practice simply outweigh the harms. There do appear to be compensating benefits, both to the animals and to the human lovers of their livers—though whether this compensation is adequate for justification is, of course, a prominent issue. One benefit to the animal may be the animal's life itself; the geese are born and raised on the farms, and owe their lives to the farming industry. They would never have become what Tom Regan has called "subjects of a life" were it not for this industry. Whether their lives have, on balance, been worth living under the conditions on the farms is a separate question from that of the value of the lives that have been lived. It is not clearly a benefit to be born into a life lived under inhumane conditions.

However, almost everyone involved in discussion of the ethical issues in this case would agree that the clearest and most relevant compensating benefits are to humans, not animals. The benefits to consumers of a treasured food are obvious, but other benefits are less apparent. For example, roughly twenty thousand French farmers make their livelihood from foie gras production. The income from the farms is a clear benefit, and most of their farms are so small and specialized that a ban on foie gras would produce significant economic costs to these farmers. (However, they sometimes can switch to other farming practices and products.)

Costs

The costs to the geese are premature death and various forms of fear, tension, stress, anxiety, distress, confinement, discomfort, ill health, and pain.[12] But how are we to quantify or otherwise measure these costs? The death of force-fed geese is often not significantly different from the death of many other farm animals sent to slaughter, but some geese often die slowly and in pain over a 24-to-48 hour period. The breadth of the concept of suffering, different evaluations of animal behavior and health complicate these evaluations, and our lack of access to the inner, subjective side of animal behavior complicates the task of assessing the costs incurred by the animals (see chapter 1, pp. 10–12, 19).

Controversy surrounds the interpretation of both the behavior and the physical condition of geese. It has often been reported by those who observe force-feeding that geese strongly resist the feeding machines and find it difficult to breathe after their livers have expanded. There is physical discomfort in the bloated condition of the gastrointestinal tract. However, defenders of force-feeding contend that there is no reason to believe that the geese are caused pain and significant suffering or that any malformation or disease produced by the swelling of the liver causes the animal to suffer in the short period of time prior to being slaughtered. Defenders of force-feeding also argue that if these geese were unconfined and in migration they would, like wild geese, consume much larger amounts of food than they normally do. The argument is that geese are fitted by nature for some expansion of their livers.

Some of these claims are highly controversial when attributed to domesticated animals (which do not migrate), suggesting a need for increased research as to the degree of suffering involved, but it is doubtful that such research will resolve many of the deeper underlying issues. The problems become more complicated as a result of clashing cultural beliefs and attitudes that are sometimes at work in these debates. Presentation of even basic "facts" about animals' positive and negative experiences may be shaped by the observer's position on whether the practice is morally defensible.

Anthropologists have discussed a dazzling variety of attitudinal differences across and within cultures, over the treatment and suffering of animals. What appears in one culture or subculture to be no cost at all will appear a massive cost to another group. For example, in some cultures geese, ducks, and chickens are plucked alive and yanked by the neck for sport, and terrorized in ways persons in other cultures find horrifying examples of abuse and suffering.

Weighing costs and benefits

Even if we could sort out all these problems of benefits, costs, and harms, thinking about the moral issues through cost-benefit comparisons raises its own set of questions: What constitutes a comprehensive list of costs and benefits? How are they to be compared and balanced? Which and whose values should be considered in a calculus of costs and benefits? Can a method of arraying costs and benefits be devised that is comprehensive, while not highly subjective or biased? Each of these questions is difficult to answer not only because various parties have different lists of costs; but also because each has a different priority of values.

These problems have caused some persons to wonder whether the weighing of benefits and costs is possible or, for that matter, desirable. Perhaps the side receiving the benefits will always see the benefits as worth the costs, whereas those who do not receive the benefits will always insist that if the benefit receivers were (in a huge reversal of fortunes) themselves the cost givers, they would never see the practices as justifiable. Could it be that weighing costs and benefits is either not the real issue or an issue that has no resolution?

Moral Issues in Public Policy

Defenders of a political ban on force-feeding argue that the costs to animals are usually ignored in making public policy, so that what is legal is simply that which maximally benefits the human community—without costs to animals playing a role in the balancing. Defenders of animal farms, by contrast, argue that powerful lobbying groups for animals have magnified the suffering involved.

Underlying this political struggle are moral questions of whether, as Stuart Hampshire once put it, "large-scale computations in modern politics and social planning bring with them a coarseness and grossness of moral feeling, a blunting of sensibility, and a suppression of individual discrimination and gentleness."[13] The way geese are raised on a farm may easily desensitize farmers, veterinarians, and all persons connected with the industry. This desensitization in itself constitutes a significant moral problem. From this perspective, trying to decide issues of animal welfare through cost-benefit tradeoffs is not as important as looking directly at the suffering involved—both the quality and the quantity of suffering—to see if it can be made coherent with our overall moral commitments.

Opponents of force-feeding generally find this way of framing the issues more satisfactory than framing the question as one of weighing costs and benefits. They believe that human biases in the political arena are too powerful in circumstances in which one side of the tradeoff benefits humans and the other side harms another species. Farmers, retailers, and others who will be harmed by a political ban can directly represent their interests in the political arena, but animals can only be indirectly represented by surrogates who have taken an interest in their plight.

This problem of potential bias and fair representation raises the question of whether a threshold of suffering should be drawn in public policy for animals, just as we draw such thresholds for humans; beyond the threshold line tradeoffs would be legally impermissible. (See chapter 1 on drawing thresholds) The argument is that just as we do not allow a slave trade in humans or the selling of human babies, irrespective of benefits that might flow from these activities, so we should not allow a high threshold of suffering for farm animals.

In this conception, if force-feeding exceeds an established threshold limit, then force-feeding is prohibited, irrespective of compensating benefits. But is this the right way to determine public policy, and does force-feeding exceed a reasonable threshold?

The Diffusion of Responsibility

Peter Lovenheim argued that Iroquois Brands' importation, advertisement, and sale of a pâté de foie gras made the company indirectly responsible for supporting animal mistreatment and for the continuation of such mistreatment. The company vigorously resisted this charge. It held that it was not even responsible for notifying its shareholders that some public concern exists about the way animals are raised on farms that produce the product it imports.

Assuming that there is a bona fide moral issue about a product that is significantly related to a company's business (or a consumer's purchase), what obligations exist either to object to the practices or to notify those with a potential interest in the information? From this perspective, was it the company's moral responsibility to comply with Lovenheim's request that information be mailed?

Many persons take the view that a corporation's primary and perhaps sole purpose is to maximize profits for stockholders—a view made prominent in the writings of the Nobel prize–winning economist Milton Friedman. Friedman argues that stockholders own the corporation and that profits belong to them as a result. Managers are agents of the stockholders. If the management diverts time and resources to charity or extraneous moral ideals, it is engaged in an illegitimate—indeed immoral—use of the stockholders' assets.[14]

A very different view is that all individuals and social institutions ought to adhere to certain moral standards that bind all persons irrespective of questions of profit. If there are basic moral obligations to which all institutions, including businesses, must adhere, the pursuit of profit in violation of those rules is morally irresponsible. One analysis of this claim is that society cannot legitimately impose affirmative duties on corporations to promote the welfare of other persons and animals, but society can legitimately impose negative injunctions on corporations that require them not to cause harm or to aid others who cause harm in order to promote the business's interests. From this perspective, corporations must take active steps to prevent potentially harmful activities; it is morally acceptable for society to prevent companies from harming animals but not to impose on companies an obligation to donate to charitable causes that promote the interests of animals.

If there are such basic obligations, do they filter down to importers of French foie gras? If so, what about to consumers of these products? Where do we call a halt to our responsibilities?

Mental and Emotional Responses

In addition to costs such as pain and suffering, the cost to the *emotional* lives of the geese merits consideration. As with many other creatures, the *psychological* lives of geese remain largely a mystery. But much is known or can be reasonably hypothesized based on what is known.

As Konrad Lorenz notes in his well known work *The Year of the Greylag Goose,*[15] the emotions of the goose are particularly difficult for the novice student—including many experienced farmers—to discern. Little can be determined by the passive facial expressions on geese, and the meaning of bodily communications are even more difficult to decipher. Yet, Lorenz argues, a close student of geese can read the meanings of both facial expressions and bodily movements. For example, the position of the neck tells a great deal about whether the goose is disheartened, feeling submissive, and the like. In the tradition of Darwin (see chapter 1), Lorenz claims to be able to tell when geese are sad, feel threatened, feel uncertain, feel tense, and so on. He tries to examine the love and affection shown between mates, including the ways in which they fall in love—and the sorrow they experience when a mate is lost.

It has often been recommended that animal behaviorists study the way animals behave—the laws of behavior—without attributing too much to emotion in the explanation of the behavior. A student of behavior needs to be cautious in making claims, because emotions are very difficult to understand. However, this recommendation may be poor advice for those seeking to make a moral assessment. It could be that what little we can learn about the emotions of animals tells us more about appropriate human ethical responses than does a large amount of behavioral information.

According to investigators from Compassion in World Farming, the domesticated farm geese who supply us with our foie gras exhibit some of the telling body signs that Lorenz has noted. CIWF claims that the geese huddle against the farthest wall at a feeding time, turn their backs to the farmers, and will not watch fellow geese during the feeding period. They show signs of pain, discomfort, and emotional distress during the last 15 to 28 days of their lives, when they are closely confined and no longer in contact with the other geese.[16]

Practical Options

One possible practical solution to some of these problems in the farming of geese would be to require more humane provisions of handling, housing, slaughter, and care during the critical periods. Perhaps the isolation could be eliminated, veterinary services increased, and the like. Codes of practice could be introduced to help ensure good welfare standards in farming. In addition, animal welfare requirements could be established that would override agricultural productivity targets so that farmers would be penalized if they violated the standards.

It would also be possible to feed the geese less. The gain in the size of the liver would then be slowed, affecting the quality of the product and the profit margins for the farm. But these human losses might be justified in light of the animal's gains.

Another practical approach would be to stop eating foie gras. However, it is not as clear as it might at first appear how much would be gained, from a moral point of view, depending on which foods one substituted for the foie gras. If vegetables were substituted, for example, then the moral problems would be resolved. However, one of the most likely substitutes is chicken, and as the case of "Fowl Deeds" (chapter 14) indicates, related moral issues about the raising of chicken make it questionable whether the chicken is better off in modern farming than the goose. One might make a case that the goose overall has it better.

The Problem of Drawing Well-Defined Lines

Awareness of the emotional lives and forms of awareness in animals prompts us to ask whether there are relevant similarities between humans and geese that are hidden from view in the way emotions often are. Although we often notice these similarities when interacting with dogs, primates, and other animals whose behavior we think we can readily interpret, do we fail to notice similarities in our encounters with geese? What precisely are the differences between geese and the human species—as well as other human-favored species—that justify the food industry in treating animals in ways they morally cannot treat humans? The challenge presented by this question is to find some bright line that justifies the vastly different ways in which the various species are treated.

Perhaps the premier question is whether we can draw nonarbitrary *moral* lines that have the same precision as *biological* lines between the species. What, ask some defenders of animals, distinguishes the life of a human infant or a child's puppy from the life of a five-month-old goose, so that human infants and puppies are protected in ways that geese are not? What gives the human a moral standing that geese can never gain, and why are dogs offered more protection than geese? If we would not tolerate treating a dog in the way geese are treated, what is the morally relevant difference between them?

It cannot be merely the human capacity to feel pain and suffering that makes the difference, because geese and many other animals share that capacity to a significant degree with humans. Nor can it be, for example, that humans have "reason," the "use of language," or "the capacity to interact with the human community" in ways geese and other animals do not. In these respects, the retarded, the irreversibly comatose, and young infants fall into many relevantly similar categories as geese and other animals that lack these same abilities. (See the chapter 1.)

Nonetheless, the view persists in society as well as in much of the literature of ethics that even if animals have some moral standing, animal life is not valuable in ways parallel to human life. From this perspective, geese do not rank high on any continuum of comparative value that might be constructed across species. Geese share some of the elements of a rich life with humans—food, sex, pleasure—but in other respects humans vastly exceed lower animals—for example, in moral reasoning and intellectual pursuits.

Critics of this view reply that unless we can have the experiences animals have, we cannot appreciate the subtleties of their experiences or the importance to those who have them. To argue that our lives are morally weightier, based on our knowledge of living those lives may only be a way of begging the question that springs from how little we know about other species such as geese.[17]

It is a significant moral problem whether the criteria used to draw the lines between a goose, a dog, and a human will include either too little or too much to provide protection to human persons—especially for what are sometimes called the "marginal cases" of infants, fetuses, the severely demented, the profoundly brain-damaged, and the like. Tradeoffs are as dangerous for these vulnerable humans as they are for vulnerable animals. (See chapter 1)

NOTES

1. FRG, *Protection of Animals Act (Tierschutzgesetz)* 3, sec. 7. This clause is a general prohibition of force feeding animals except when necessary for the sake of their health.

2. Dominique Hermier, "Plasma Lipoproteins and Liver Lipids in Two Breeds of Geese with Different Susceptibility to Hepatic Steatosis: Changes Induced by Development and Force-Feeding," *Lipids* 26 (May 1991): 331–39, esp. 331, 333–34; R. Rouvier et al., "Parmètres génétiques des caractères de croissance, de gavage et de foie gras . . . ," *Génét. sél. Evol.* 24 (1992): 53–69; M. A. I. Salem et al., "Studies on Fatty Liver Production from Aged Geese and Ducks, I: Serum Protein, Glucose and Cholesterol," *Egypt Journal of Animal Production* 23, nos. 1–2 (1983): 109–12; M. A. I. Salem et al., "Studies on Fatty Liver Production from Aged Geese and Ducks, II: Fatty Acid Composition of Liver and Some Chemical Aspects," *Egypt Journal of Animal Production* 23, nos. 1–2 (1983): 113–18.

3. *Agscene* 74 (February 1984).

4. Iroquois Brands, Notice of 1983 Annual Meeting of Shareholders and Proxy Statement, Tuesday, 10 May 1983, Greenwich Public Library, Greenwich, CT.

5. *Peter C. Lovenheim v. Iroquois Brands Ltd.* US District Court, Washington, DC. Civil Case No. 85–0734 (24 May 1985).

6. Quoted by Philip Smith, "Shareholders to Be Given Pâté Question," *Washington Post,* 28 March 1985, p. E3.

7. Personal correspondence from attorney Ralph L. Halpern of Jaeckle, Fleischmann & Mugel (Buffalo), 13 April 1988.

8. American Society for the Prevention of Cruelty to Animals, Supporting Statement to Shareholders' Proposal, in *Peter C. Lovenheim v. Iroquois Brands Ltd,* appendix 3.

9. From a letter written 13 January 1984 by ASPCA Executive Director John F. Kullberg, in *Peter C. Lovenheim v. Iroquois Brands Ltd,* appendix 5.

10. Eileen Lemass and Carol Long, "Pate de Foie Gras: Report on a Visit . . . to an Alsace Farm," CIWF Release, 12 December 1986.

11. "The Foie Gras Factor," *New York Times,* 25 May 1992, op-ed page; Marc Humbert, "Cuomo's Help Sought on Cruelty Allegation," *Daily Gazette* (Schenectady, NY), 30 April 1992; Associated Press, "Group Takes 'Exploding Ducks' Plea to Cuomo," *Watertown Daily Times* (Watertown, NY), 30 April 1992, pp. 1, 7. PETA conducted an undercover investigation of Commonwealth Enterprises that convinced a county district attorney to bring charges against the farm. These events were widely reported in New York newspapers.

12. See Andrew N. Rowan, "Animal Anxiety and Animal Suffering," and A. F. Fraser, "Animal Suffering: The Appraisal and Control of Depression and Distress in Livestock," both in *Applied Animal Behaviour Science* 20 (1988): 127–42; David B. Morton, Gordon Burghardt, and Jane Smith, "Critical Anthropomorphism, Animal Suffering, and the Ecological Context," *Hastings Center Report* 20 (May/June 1990): S13–S19.

13. Stuart Hampshire, "Morality and Pessimism," in *Public and Private Morality,* ed. Stuart Hampshire (Cambridge: Cambridge University Press, 1978), pp. 5–6.

14. Milton Friedman, "The Social Responsibility of Business Is to Increase Its Profits," *New York Times Magazine,* 13 September 1970.

15. Konrad Lorenz, *The Year of the Greylag Goose* (New York: Harcourt Brace, 1978).

16. Lemass and Long, "Pate de Foie Gras," pp. 4–5, and note 12.

17. See Stephen F. Sapontzis, *Morals, Reason, and Animals* (Philadelphia: Temple University Press, 1987), pp. 218–20.

13

VEAL CRATES AND HUMAN PALATES

On 1 February 1995, Coventry Airport in England was alive with animal welfare campaigners protesting the transport of very young calves to Europe to be reared for veal. The animal protesters were persons of all ages and backgrounds, even old-age pensioners. Some watched animal rights protester Jill Phipps try to block the path of a large transport truck by running alongside it and finally cutting in front of the truck and raising her hands. To their horror, she slipped and was crushed to death as the wheels ran over her chest and belly. Just before her death she had given an interview and said, "We will continue even if someone gets hurt. Someone will eventually be hurt."[1] This 31-year old mother became a martyr for her cause. Her funeral some weeks later was attended by representatives of many animal rights and animal welfare organizations. Even the movie star and animal rights campaigner Brigitte Bardot flew from France to attend the ceremony.

The issue of "veal crates" has probably affected more persons directly than any other animal welfare issue in recent times. According to a senior police officer, on the force for more than 37 years, the protests were a new phenomenon. He had never seen so many people, from such diverse backgrounds, unite on an issue. It had brought together vegans [strict vegetarians] and villagers, grandmothers and mothers, animal rights activists and pensioners in a campaign of civil unrest.[2] Why were so many people so concerned about these calves?

Many of the protestors had never been involved in a public protest before. What was the incentive for so many "new" protestors to join the ranks of animal rights campaigners?

THE VEAL TRADE AND METHODS OF PRODUCTION

Veal calves are on the market as a by-product of the dairy industry that supplies consumables such as milk, cheese, cream, butter, ice cream, and yogurt. For cows to produce milk they have to become pregnant. Shortly after birth, calves are removed from cows so that all the milk produced by the cows can be taken and used by the farmer. Typically, calves either feed once from the cow, or are artificially fed so they receive antibody-rich colostrum—the milk produced by the cow for a few days after she gives birth. Calves can absorb antibodies from this milk only for the first 48 hours of life. Colostrum provides important protection for calves against disease.

Not all calves are sold to produce beef or veal, but most are. Some dairy calves are genetically unsuitable for beef or veal production. This is because

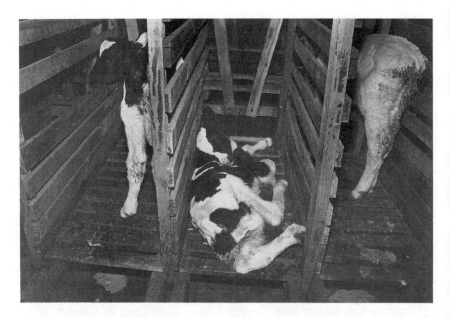

In factory farming production, veal calves spend almost all their lives in crates, as shown. In crates, they cannot lie down in comfort, turn around, or adopt a normal sleeping posture, nor are they able to walk, run, groom, nor make social contact with their neighbors. They are fed exclusively on milk that is low in iron so that the animals become anemic and produce white flesh for the meat trade. Credit: Farm Animal Reform Movement, Bethesda, MD.

dairy calves have been selected genetically for milk yield and milk quality, but not for fast growth rates or lean meat. The genetically unsuitable calves may be killed after a week or two and used to make processed meats such as "veal-and-ham" pies. The majority of dairy calves end up in some form of meat production. Of these calves, most go to traditional forms of beef farming, but there is also a significant trade in the production of veal. It is the methods of producing veal that have raised so much concern about animal welfare.

Because so little veal is consumed in the UK, there is virtually no home market for these animals. There are approximately twenty veal producers in the United Kingdom, killing some five thousand calves a year. As a consequence, calves from the United Kingdom, often less than two weeks of age, are exported to be reared for veal in Europe, notably in France and Holland. The United Kingdom subsequently imports a small amount of "European" veal for gourmet restaurants catering for an elite trade, and some of this veal may have come from UK calves.

The traditional way of keeping these newly born animals for the production of veal has been individually in small wooden crates with slatted floors, in the dark with no bedding,[3] though it is now illegal to keep them in complete darkness in Europe. They are fed twice daily on an exclusively liquid diet of milk replacer for some 16 to 24 weeks, after which they are killed. Keeping calves in crates prevents them from licking and sucking each other and from expending energy on natural activities. Keeping them in the dark and feeding a milk-only diet has been thought essential to produce the coveted pale white meat.

Welfare concerns about this system are that the crates are so small that as the animals grow, they cannot turn round, or lie down naturally with their legs out sideways, or adopt a normal sleeping position. They are unable to carry out natural patterns of behavior such as walking, running, grooming, playing, and cannot make social contact even though they may be able to hear, smell, and sometimes touch their next-door neighbor. The exclusive feeding of milk that is low in iron for such a long time results in the animals developing anemia (perhaps essential to produce the white flesh).

Because the animals are not permitted access to roughage such as straw, grass or hay, the gut (rumen) fails to grow normally. In order to obtain roughage, the calves, if permitted, "overgroom" themselves and eat their coats, which causes hair balls and chronic indigestion. Moreover, fully grown calves may suffer heat stress because of the intensive conditions and poor ventilation. The incidence of infectious disease is often high and has to be controlled by the repeated administration of antibiotics, perhaps as a result of animals not receiving adequate colostrum.

In the first three weeks of life up to 5% of animals in veal units die from infection.[4] In the first six weeks, 10% may develop enteric disease (diarrhea), and over 55% will have a respiratory disease. Also, 21% will have injuries such as abraded and swollen knees and hocks.[5] Animals show stereotypic behaviors such as licking their crates, tongue rolling, and excessive grooming. If they are able to make contact with the animal in the adjacent crate, they often suck each other's mouths and tongues. These sorts of behavior are associated with stressful housing conditions and indicate that animals are not adapting to their environment.

In 1990 the use of veal crates in the United Kingdom was prohibited by government regulations,[6] which require that animals must have room to turn around, must have adequate iron to maintain them in full health and vigor, and after 14 days must have access to roughage to allow their gut to develop normally. In practice, the regulations have led to calves being kept in groups on straw bedding, providing them with room to carry out natural behavior patterns and to have social contact. Similar legislation was subsequently proposed in the US Congress as an amendment to the Animal Welfare Act, but it has not been enacted into law.[7]

THE PROTESTS

The campaign against the export of live animals, mainly sheep and calves from the United Kingdom to Europe, started in February 1994. It was motivated by animals being taken on long journeys, sometimes several days, without breaks for feeding, watering and resting, in violation of European laws and guidelines.[8] Animal "detectives," usually Royal Society for the Prevention of Cruelty to Animals (RSPCA) inspectors, followed the trucks and recorded the suffering of these animals on videotape.[9] The tapes included scenes of animals dying, as well as many suffering from heat stress, dehydration, and food deprivation. Some were also being slaughtered inhumanely, again in breach of European laws. Animal welfare campaigners called for meat animals to be exported "on the hook and not on the hoof." In 1995, British laws were tightened and heavy fines introduced for such illegal journeys—up to 1000 pounds sterling (1500 US dollars) per animal. If several hundred animals were carried at one time, the total fine could be substantial.[10] In addition to transport and slaughter, various aspects of the export trade were denounced as offensive—for example, veal production in crates and the exportation of live lambs from the United Kingdom to be killed in France.

The export trade therefore attracted publicity. Minor demonstrations began at ports. The larger ferry operators stopped taking live exports for fear of losing trade. This resulted in expanded publicity, followed by independent ferry operators trying to pick up the animal trade from the minor ports. Public reports of these events shocked the British public. Protests against the export of animals took place at seaports all over the country. Ferry operators refused to carry farm animals, and, even though exporters subsequently made their own arrangements for sea transport, boarding the ship still required port access, which was successfully blocked by the protesters. As the exporters were unable to use the seaports, they commissioned private companies to fly animals to Europe,[11] but the protesters followed them to the airports.

Some violence has occurred during the protests,[12] but violence has been condemned by the campaigning organizations and the majority of protesters. The protests became well organized picket lines, and it was claimed that the organizers could muster a vigil of around two hundred persons on ordinary days, with up to two thousand on days when an export was likely to take place.

Several countries have condemned the veal crate system,[13] but calf exports continued to increase while lamb exports decreased. Alan Clark, former minister for defense, warned that the government and others involved could not continue to flout public opinion without expecting some form of backlash. William Waldegrave, UK minister of agriculture at the time of the recent protests, warned farmers, "Veal crates and conditions of transport are clearly at the forefront of public and political attention at the moment. But concern and pressure about welfare will continue even when we have dealt with the current problems. Other aspects of modern farming will come under scrutiny."[14]

THE INTERESTED PARTIES

For farmers in the United Kingdom, the live-animal export trade is claimed to be worth 200 million pounds (300 million dollars), and comprises 2.5 million lambs and calves a year. In 1992, approximately 416,000 calves were exported to Europe[15] where around 90% of French and 80% of Dutch veal production is in crates.[16] It is likely, therefore, that the majority of calves exported to these countries will end up in veal crates. Because so little veal is consumed in the United Kingdom and the crating system of producing white flesh has been banned, many purebred dairy calves are worth relatively little and more money can be made if they are sent to market, where they may be bought by foreign buyers or exporters who send them over to Europe. The view of the National Farmers' Union is that so long as the veal trade is legal it should be permitted to continue,[17] and a spokesperson for the Dutch farmers has disputed the claim that veal crates cause problems for the animals.[18]

But some dairy farmers do appear to be changing their breeding system to produce calves more suitable for the British beef market, rather than European veal production.[19] Other farmers have capitalized on the welfare sensitivities of the general public by agreeing to produce veal in a welfare-friendly way. By so doing they have secured contracts with large supermarkets. They have also agreed to restrict transport time to less than one hour to slaughterhouses where the animals are killed immediately.[20]

Exporters and haulers have fought to retain their legal trade despite ferry companies and airlines banning live animals on their boats and airplanes. Exporters (probably less than twenty people in the United Kingdom are involved) have therefore commissioned their own boats and airplanes. As a result, some individuals and their families have been personally attacked and harrassed. There is little doubt that some haulers are guilty of atrocities.[21] Part of the problem stems from a need for better training of haulers and for improvements in the design and standards of their trucks. The port authorities claim that by law they have to take any cargo and have no option but to accept live animals for export.[22]

The veterinary profession finds itself in a dilemma because a government veterinarian has to sign a certificate stating the animals are fit to travel prior to transport. By not signing such certificates, all exports of live animals could be prevented. Veterinarians have been under pressure from within their own ranks, as well as from outside bodies, not to sign certificates.[23] The chief veterinary officer has stated, however, that government veterinarians cannot refuse to sign an export certificate on grounds of conscience if the conditions for the certificate are in order—that is, if the animals are fit for travel and comply with disease control regulations.[24] The professional Hippocratic oath commits veterinarians "to ensure the welfare of animals committed to their care"; as a consequence veterinarians are caught in a position of being able to prevent the cruelties of long-distance transport and veal production, but would likely have to resign their position as government employees.

Governments in Europe and the United Kingdom have responded in a variety of ways. For example, the United Kingdom has banned practices in veal production that promote poor welfare[25] and has tightened up on national standards of animal transport. Possibly as a result of the demonstrations, the UK government has also commissioned a research project (at a cost of 30,000 pounds sterling, 45,000 US dollars) to demonstrate that high-quality veal can be produced profitably and humanely.[26] The UK government has been under considerable pressure to ban the export of calves, but insists that it cannot do so because of the single-market trade agreement within the European Union (EU). The UK government considers that the way forward is to raise standards throughout member states in the EU. Major concerns are how to implement national legislation and how to monitor standards fairly and effectively.[27]

The transport of live animals has caused considerable furor with little agreement between member states on journey times or on rest, feed, and watering intervals. There has been some progress with European agriculture ministers, who reached a "significant agreement" on journey times and the like. However, welfare groups are not satisfied. They argue that animals will still continue to suffer long and stressful journeys (for example, of up to 31 hours) and that the new law will be difficult to enforce.[28]

Animal welfare organizations, notably the RSPCA, the International Federation for Animal Welfare (IFAW), and Compassion in World Farming (CIWF) have joined together to obtain an independent legal opinion on whether the United Kingdom could impose a unilateral ban on the export of live animals to Europe.[29] On the basis of this opinion, they have taken the UK government to court, claiming that it would be lawful for the government to ban the export of calves for veal production.

Farmers claim that many of these calves are worth very little because of their conformation and genetic makeup. If they did not send them to market, their only other option would be to kill them at birth. CIWF disputes that the poor conformation of some dairy calves prevents them from being raised for beef, because 40% of the beef sold in the United Kingdom is sold as minced meat used in meat pies, making quality of conformation irrelevant. They argue that farmers simply want to make "a few pennies more" and are choosing to sell to the highest bidder, likely to be the heavily subsidized continental veal producer.[30] CIWF goes even further and argues that UK dairy farmers are disadvantaging their beef counterparts, as well as slaughterhouse owners, by obtaining such high prices for their calves. They claim that this strategy prevents beef farmers from buying and rearing homegrown calves. Another consequence is that there will be reduced work for UK slaughterhouse workers.

The public in the United Kingdom consumes little veal, both because veal is expensive and because many consider it unethical to eat veal. Veal consumption in France averages 5.6 kg per capita, Italy 4.0 kg, the United States 0.68 kg—compared with 0.1 kg in Britain.[31] The increase in public concern has been heightened by the media coverage and the sight of the large, baleful eyes of calves poking their heads out between the bars of the trucks held up at the ports. These emotive scenes have engendered empathic public responses and have encouraged some people to protest against the live-animal export and veal trades.

The protesters range from those who have never been on a demonstration before and who have been shocked by what they have recently learned about the veal and export trades, to those who are frequently involved in peaceful protest against various misuses and abuses of animals. The protests have also attracted those who are committed to violence and who use any demonstration or crowd-gathering event for their own violent or anarchistic ends.[32]

The police are in a difficult position, because they are legally bound to enforce what is lawful, despite the public protests. At one port, the police introduced a restriction that exports could take place only on two consecutive days of the week in order to reduce the costs of police protection. In a recent court action by a livestock transport company, the judge ruled that this restriction was unlawful.[33] The police are now likely to be sued for compensation for the loss of trade.

The retailers, including many supermarkets, now claim to sell only British veal, which accounts for one-third of that consumed, the rest coming from Europe and sold through other outlets, presumably to the restaurant trade. Some supermarkets have contracted with farms to produce veal in a welfare-friendly way; but these changes, together with relabeling the veal as "baby beef" or "lightweight rose beef" still do not seem to have changed the public's views.[34]

Several professions have been affected by these developments. Gourmet restaurants frequently serve veal, which is described in the *Larousse Gastronomique* as "pale meat, smelling of milk, with satiny white fat."[35] Julia Child has similar tastes: "Pick veal by its color—pale creamy pink about the shade of raw chicken thigh. Some cuts of the dark pink or reddish so-called free-range veal may be tender, but in my opinion, it neither looks nor tastes like veal. It should be called calf."[36]

Milk-substitute manufacturers have also been affected, and one manufacturer (Volac) has withdrawn from supplying the veal farmers with milk powder: "British people don't like it and it will never lose its reputation for cruelty whatever the welfare standards are."[37] Finally, some members of the clergy have become involved and have occasionally blessed truckloads of calves before they were transported to Europe.[38]

ETHICAL ISSUES

Animal-Rearing Systems: Cruel or Welfare Friendly?

Many methods of farm animal husbandry, particularly those that involve confinement or intensive systems, raise concerns over the welfare of animals. One analytical approach by which to assess welfare was first put forward by the Brambell Committee in 1965 and is termed the "Five Freedoms."[39] They proposed that animals should have the freedom to stand up, lie down, turn around, groom themselves, and stretch their limbs. These five freedoms were subsequently modified by the UK Farm Animal Welfare Council as follows.[40]

1. Freedom from thirst, hunger and malnutrition
2. Freedom from discomfort
3. Freedom from pain, injury and disease
4. Freedom to express normal behavior
5. Freedom from fear and distress

The New Zealand National Animal Welfare Advisory Committee[41] has adapted them as five basic requirements for animals to meet their needs:

1. freedom from thirst, hunger and malnutrition
2. the provision of appropriate comfort and shelter
3. the prevention, or rapid diagnosis and treatment, of injury, disease or infestation with parasites
4. freedom from distress
5. ability to display normal patterns of behavior

The veal crate system fails to meet these requirements, particularly those relating to being able to carry out natural behaviors, the provision of comfort, and freedom from malnutrition. If loading, transport, and unloading of calves is also taken into account, then fear and distress will also be incurred.

Many participants in these discussions have pointed out that there are alternative, more welfare-friendly, husbandry systems. For example, it is possible to rear animals in groups to provide the social contact and the space for them to display many of the natural behaviors that they would display in fields. The provision of higher levels of iron keeps the animals from becoming anemic, but the flesh will be pink, not white. No evidence suggests that keeping these animals in the dark causes their meat to be white; natural daylight therefore could be provided. The provision of straw provides for normal physiological development of the rumen without affecting meat quality other than its color. The provision of dry food, rather than an exclusively liquid diet, helps meet the physiological needs of the animals but does make the system slightly less profitable.

One question that arises for veal, dairy, and beef farmers, and others associated with the trade is, under what conditions, if any, should farmers be permitted to sacrifice animal welfare for personal gain? Farmers receive substantial agricultural subsidies from the public purse, without which they would not be able to survive. Does this support oblige them to be responsive to public opinion about animal welfare?

Many modern farming systems leave much to be desired from an animal welfare viewpoint. Do farmers therefore have a moral responsibility to use only welfare-friendly alternatives? If the public will not buy the welfare-friendly product and will buy cheaper, less welfare-friendly alternatives, then welfare-friendly farmers will not survive (or perhaps will survive less well). What responsibilities, if any, does the general public have in making purchases?

Another question is whether farmers have a stronger obligation to protect animals than do other members of society. It could be suggested that farmers are society's stewards of animals. If they fail to meet society's (reasonable) expectations of animal welfare, they not only undermine their guardian status, but set in place a resistance to eating meat and other animal products. The rise in vegetarianism from 2–3% in 1983 to 7%[42] in 1993 is due to a mixture of financial, health, and animal-welfare implications of meat eating. This trend away from meat eating,[43] in the long term, may endanger the future of some types of farming.

Do Veterinarians Have Special Responsibilities?

Veterinarians commonly subscribe to an oath to protect animals. As a result of their commitments and training, society accords veterinarians special privileges and assigns them certain responsibilities, though any wording that states those responsibilities is very general and in need of specification. What are veterinarians entrusted to do in caring for and protecting animals in the present case? By not signing the certificates of fitness for animals to travel, veterinarians would not be committing an illegal act, but would they be living up to their social responsibilities? Or is it not *social* responsibilities that are at stake, but *personal* responsibilities that derive from the moral ideals of veterinarians?

It would be an act of omission based on their conscience, and conscientious objection has had an honorable tradition in Western moral and political thinking. Moral conflicts of conscience sometimes emerge because people regard as unethical some role obligation or official order that descends from a hierarchical structure of authority. In many cases, such as the refusal to sign a certificate, the individual does not rebuke others or obstruct them from performing an act but only says, "Not through me." Occasionally this situation arises when a veterinarian refuses a procedure requested by an owner, customer, or institution.

If a veterinarian wishes not to comply with a request for a normal responsibility, these conscientious convictions should be respected, and he or she should be free to withdraw from the circumstance. In some situations, however, the question is not whether the veterinarian has a right to refuse involvement, but a duty to refuse involvement. Which, if either, is it in the present case?

Moral Coherence and Social Solidarity

Veal crates were banned in the United Kingdom in 1990. The method was considered unacceptable on grounds that it caused avoidable animal suffering. Questions of moral coherence arise when a country bans a product for ethical reasons yet still permits its importation from another country. (Veal importation was permitted even before the single market agreement in the European Union was signed.) Furthermore, retailers and restaurant owners in the United Kingdom are permitted to sell veal, the public to consume it, farmers and exporters to provide animals for its production, and haulers to transport it long distances. They are all part of a society that has deemed veal crates to be cruel and unacceptable, and yet they are supporting the trade in the full knowledge of what happens to those animals.[44]

If animals are deemed worthy of protection from this method of farming, can ethical principles of avoiding harm be justifiably used to reach the conclusion that veal produced by this method ought not to be produced or sold?

Another problem of moral coherence and a related problem of conflict of interest arise in the case of the UK minister of agriculture and his wife, Caroline Waldegrave. Is it morally permissible for her to support the veal trade by recommending its use in recipes, when her husband is the minister of state responsible for ensuring veal crates are not used in the United Kingdom? How far are people bound by the public responsibilities and position of their spouses, and can they opt out of being involved? How far should Minister Waldegrave go to ensure that calves from his own farm do not end up in veal crates in Europe? Does the minister have an untenable conflict of interest?[45]

The Ethics of Gourmet Writers and Chefs

Finally, do gourmet recipe writers and chefs have a responsibility not to encourage people to eat animal products that are produced inhumanely? In Southeast Asia, dogs are strung up off the ground and beaten and bruised in order to tenderize the flesh before they are killed and consumed, snakes are skinned alive, and cats are immersed in cauldrons of boiling water to kill them, rather like lobsters. Would it be acceptable for gourmet writers to produce recipes specifying these ingredients? Are these even comparable events? If not, how do we delineate the boundary between an unacceptable and an acceptable use of farm animals?

In a dialogue between top chefs Julia Child and Paul Prudhomme,[46] Child recalls that male calves "in the old days" were disposed of by being left in a ditch to die, but now can be raised as veal. She suggests that today's practices in raising veal are acceptable because they upgrade a worse bygone practice. Is this a valid line of argument? Could it be said that it is all right to kill farm animals (e.g. bulls and horses) using low standards of humaneness but without first rendering them insensible, because at one time we used to bait these animals with dogs?

Prudhomme and Child go on to discuss the "Bambi syndrome," whereby animals are elevated to the same value as human beings. No doubt cartoons and Disney movies depict animals unrealistically, but does the fact of fantasy in this realm provide any basis for saying that animals have no value—or if some value, much less value? Finally, Prudhomme states, "I would love that person to be really hungry and put in the same place as [location with] that animal and still think of it as something they can't touch. They'd take out a knife, cut its throat, and eat it very quickly." Hungry people have been known to eat other humans at such time! Is this a valid test of value or yet another challenge to moral coherence?

Do Some Animals Have Higher Moral Standing Than Calves?

In order to prevent the export of unwanted horses to Europe to be killed for meat, the UK government permits horses only over a certain value to be exported. The value is high enough to make the trade uneconomic. This special treatment of horses raises the question of whether, and why, horses are morally different from other species, such as cattle and sheep? Many members of the public appear to hold horses in high esteem and attribute higher moral standing to them than to beef cattle. Is it because of our closer relationships with some animals that we award them higher standing? Since ancient literature, horses have been seen as noble creatures, and we interact with them more closely than with other farm animals such as cattle. Does this general outlook justify making them a special case given increased protection? Is this the same kind of problem we have in conferring higher standing on primates (see chapter 1) or a different problem?

How Far Should Protesters Go?

Protesters who feel that a lawful activity is wrong have several options beyond becoming vegetarians. They can make their views known and try to change practices. For example, they can communicate their concerns to the public, to governments, and to producers. However, when these actions fail or protesters feel ignored, they often feel helpless in the face of what they consider a deep moral wrong. They may consider their only recourse to protest more forcefully. What has been so exceptional in the case of the export of veal calves has been the strength of feeling by so many people who had no particular calling or axe to grind, and who came from such diverse backgrounds.

Although there was some violence by a small number of persons (damaging trucks and harassing police), the picket lines were generally peaceful, though noisy. Civil disobedience can be nonviolent and has been used by many social movements to achieve change after other efforts have failed. However, lying down in front of trucks to try to prevent them moving forward had a tragic consequence in the veal protests and may, like many tactics, be questioned as a morally justified form of protest. But how does one draw the line between a justified and an unjustified strategy?

Although public awareness and sensitivities have been heightened in the United Kingdom, in Europe, and further afield, the export of calves goes on. These exports may not endure for much longer, because the European Union is scrutinizing many agricultural practices, including veal production.

NOTES

1. "Calf Protest Victim Was Sacrificed to a Vile Trade," *Daily Telegraph,* 16 August 1995, p. 5.

2. See, for example, *The Guardian,* 5 January 1995, *The Independent,* 5 January 1995 and "Thirty were arrested as veal loader reaches port" in the *Daily Telegraph,* 11 February, 1995, 19 February, 1995. (At Brightlingsea, out of the 30 who were arrested for

willful obstruction of the highway, one was a 78 year-woman.) and *Today* radio broadcast of 22 August 1995.

3. J. Webster, C. Saville, and D. Welchman, *Improved Husbandry Systems for Veal Calves* (Bristol, England: Department of Animal Husbandry, University of Bristol School of Veterinary Science, 1986).

4. *Veal Production,* RSPCA Farm Animals Information leaflet (Horsham, West Sussex, UK 1995).

5. A. J. F. Webster et al., "Some Effects of Different Rearing Systems on Health, Cleanliness and Injury in Calves," *British Veterinary Journal* 141 (1985): 472.

6. Welfare of Calves Regulations 1987 (SI 2021) came into force 1 January 1990, now embodied in Schedule 2 to the Welfare of Livestock Regulations of 1994.

7. HR 263: To amend the Animal Welfare Act to require humane living conditions for calves raised for the production of veal. Introduced 4 January 1996 by Andrew Jacobs (D-IN) in the 104th Congress.

8. The RSPCA has archival evidence in house, according to a Compassion in World Farming briefing on "The Export of Live Animals," 4 February 1994.

9. Compassion in World Farming video tape, "For a Few Pennies More."

10. The Welfare of Animals during Transport Order (1995), made under the Animal Health Act of 1981.

11. Phoenix Aviation tried to open an "air-bridge" for live exports to Europe from Bournemouth, but the local authority refused them a license. One of their planes crashed 21 December 1994, killing five crew. *Independent,* 5 January 1995; *Daily Telegraph,* 9 February 1995.

12. Truck windshields have been smashed, and haulers have had themselves and their homes and families threatened with attack. *Daily Telegraph,* 3 February 1995; 9 February 1995; 21 February 1995. *Guardian,* 16 January 1995, reported that the minister of agriculture had received razors in the mail.

13. *Daily Telegraph,* 24 January 1995.

14. *Daily Telegraph,* 9 February 1995.

15. *Veal Production.* RSPCA. Of the over 400,000 calves, 192,000 went to France, 177,000 to Holland and 46,000 to Belgium/Luxembourg.

16. *Welfare of Calves: Lawfulness of Export Restrictions,* opinion of Judge G. C. Barling, Queen's Counsel (London: S. J. Berwin & Co., 1995) p. 4, para. 6.

17. *Daily Telegraph,* 8 February 1995, reporting speech of Sir David Naish, President of the NFU.

18. A spokeswoman for Dutch Landbouwschap Farmers organization said there was no evidence that rearing the calves in crates harmed the animals' welfare. *Reuters,* 10 January 1995.

19. *Daily Telegraph,* 11 February 1995, reporting that pedigree beef bulls were fetching record prices.

20. Katy Brown, "Veal: The Facts You Should Know," *Country Living,* April 1995, pp. 45–46.

21. The RSPCA found nine out of ten trucks exceed maximum journey times, one consignment supposedly destined for Holland ended up in Greece two and a half days later with four hundred of six hundred animals dead. *Independent,* 5 January 1995.

22. The Harbors, Docks and Piers Act (1847) on one interpretation compels a port to accept any lawful cargo.

23. *Veterinary Record,* 8 April 1995, p. 371.

24. *Veterinary Record,* 25 March 1995, p. 282; *Veterinary Record,* 3 June 1995, p. 571.

25. Welfare of Calves Regulations 1987 (Statutory Instrument 2021).

26. Demonstration unit at ADAS Research Center, Rosemaund, Hereford, England. Ten to twelve animals will be kept in large pens and reared on milk, water, and barley straw. *Daily Telegraph,* 24 May 1995; 21 July 1995.

27. There have been a string of cases "uncovered" by the RSPCA normally following UK haulers. For example, on January 6, 1995, three British firms that export live calves were found guilty of animal cruelty. The prosecution claimed calves were packed into trucks for 37 hours without food, water, or rest for a journey of 1,100 miles to southwest France. *Reuters.* For Compassion in World Farming videos and cases, see *Agscene* 118 (Summer 1995): 3–8.

28. "European Ministers Reach Agreement on Animal Transport," *Veterinary Record,* 1 July 1995, pp. 2–3.

29. *Welfare of Calves,* p. 4. Barling claims that article 36 of the Treaty of Rome would permit the ban if animals were being caused to suffer or if public morality was being offended.

30. *Agscene* reported on a Meat and Livestock Commission conference in April 1995. *Agscene* 118 (Summer 1995): 14.

31. *Independent,* 13 January 1995, quoting NFU figures.

32. "Rent-a-Mob Fear Drives Away Farm Campaigners," *Guardian,* 5 January 1995; "Protests Continue as Live Exports Resume," *Veterinary Record,* 29 April 1995, p. 427.

33. *Daily Telegraph,* 27 July 1995.

34. Brown, "Veal," pp. 45–46.

35. Emily Green, *Independent,* 13 January 1995.

36. Julia Child, *The Way to Cook* (New York: Alfred A. Knopf, 1995), p. 207.

37. Brown, "Veal," p. 46.

38. The bishop of Dover made the blessing. *Daily Telegraph,* 11 June 1995.

39. F. W. R. Brambell, *Report of Technical Committee to Enquire into the Welfare of Animals Kept under Intensive Husbandry Systems* (Cmnd. 2836) (London: HM Stationery Office, 1965).

40. Farm Animal Welfare Council, *Second Report on Priorities for Research and Development in Farm Animal Welfare* (London: Ministry of Agriculture Fisheries & Food, Tolworth, 1993).

41. "New Zealand Code of Recommendations and Minimum Standards for the Welfare of Bobby Calves," (1993) *Code of Animal Welfare,* no. 8 (Ministry of Agriculture and Fisheries, Wellington, New Zealand).

42. Figures vary between 4.3% and 11.4% for a "mainly" vegetarian diet. Mintel & Gallup (1993).

43. Figures indicate that red meat consumption is down but poultry meat consumption is up.

44. D. B. Morton, "Ethics of Farm Animal Exports," *Veterinary Record,* 11 March 1995, p. 252.

45. The *Daily Telegraph,* 9 February 1995, reports that William Waldegrave admits that some of his calves were sold for export from his Somerset farm.

46. *Modern Maturity* (Winter 1994). Quoted in *The Animals' Agenda* 15, no. 4, p. 13, 1995.

14

FOWL DEEDS

If someone said, "This must constitute, in both magnitude and severity, the single most severe, systematic example of man's inhumanity to another sentient animal,"[1] what would you think he or she was talking about? The person who made this claim went on to reveal that in the United Kingdom alone, one-quarter of the heavy strains of these animals are in chronic pain for one third of their short, six-week lives, only 10% are able to walk normally, up to 6% die during rearing, 4% have chronic arthritis, 3% break their bones, and 2 million of them die during transport each year. In 1994 some 7 billion of these animals were eaten in the United States, 4 billion in Europe, and 719 million in the United Kingdom. We are, in fact, discussing broiler chickens, and the person who made these statements is John Webster, professor of animal husbandry at the University of Bristol's School of Veterinary Science.

THE BROILER CHICKEN INDUSTRY

In less than fifty years, broiler chicken, so called because of the way it is cooked, has become one of the commonest animals consumed in many people's diets.[2] The poultry meat sector is a significant employer (40,000 to 50,000 jobs in the United Kingdom alone) and a major consumer of cereals, soya, and meat and bone and fish meal. These birds are reared intensively, in large numbers and at relatively low cost, thus providing a ready source of palatable tender meat for many people. The time taken to grow from chick to table is less than seven weeks, and farming methods have become heavily engineered and automated to satisfy the birds' physiological requirements, as well as to facilitate their catching, transport, and slaughter.

Some 10,000 to 50,000 (sometimes as high as 100,000) day-old chicks are reared as a single batch on a bed of wood shavings, chopped straw, or shredded newspapers in windowless sheds. A farmer (sometimes called producer or grower) might have responsibility for several sheds.[3] The birds are maintained under nearly continuous low-level lighting[4] for 23, even 24 hours a day in order to discourage the birds from becoming overactive, which would lead to aggression and divert energy consumed in the diet away from desired forms of growth.[5] Little cannibalism or feather pecking takes place, unlike chickens kept in battery cages for egg production. The litter is gradually "replaced" by feces and the original shed floor is difficult to see after two to three weeks. In areas of

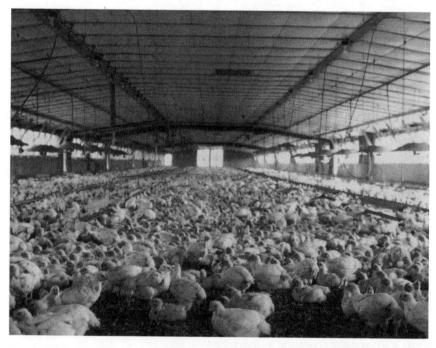

Factory farmed hens are maintained throughout their lives in overcrowded sheds that typically house from 10,000 to 50,000 chicks. The birds are maintained in near-continuous low-level lighting in order to reduce aggression. These animals have been intensively bred for rapid growth, high appetites, and breast muscle volume. Credit: Farm Animal Reform Movement, Bethesda, MD.

water spillage, or if the ventilation is inadequate, it can become damp and smelly and lead to skin lesions.[6] Moreover, the surface of the litter can become hard and cause breast blisters.

Ventilation is provided by means of louvers and automated fans in the roof and sides of the building. The ventilation controls ambient temperature and humidity by way of regulating air flow, which also helps avoid the build-up of irritant and toxic gases such as carbon dioxide and ammonia from the litter. In cold weather the ventilation rate is reduced, which can lead to a build-up of these gases (particularly ammonia), and cause damp litter. High outside temperatures are very important, because the ventilation system has to cope with the hot weather and also with the heat the birds themselves produce.

The heat produced by the birds increases substantially as they get heavier and so towards the end of their commercial growth period, a spell of hot weather can be critical.[7] In hot weather, surplus heat has to be removed or the birds will grow slower or, at worst, die of heat stress and high humidity.[8] If the ventilation fails through a power failure then literally tens of thousands of birds can die overnight.[9] In hot, dry climates, such as parts of the Middle East, the provision of adequate humidity to prevent the birds' dying of dehydration is a problem.

The birds have been intensively bred and almost exclusively selected for rapid growth, food conversion rate, high appetite, and breast muscle volume. They are provided with a nutritionally balanced, high-protein, high-energy diet, which accounts for about 70% of the cost of production. Water and food are always available throughout the shed in specific feeding areas. Various dietary formulations are given to the birds depending on their age. Initially, they are fed a high-protein "starter" diet and then a lower-protein "grower" diet. Both diets contain growth promoters, as well as antibiotics and antiparasite drugs to prevent clinical infections. Over the last five days or so they are given a "finisher" diet free from chemical additives.

In Europe there is a space allowance of 0.5 square feet (450 cm^2) per bird at the outset of stocking, but toward the end of the production time, when the birds have significantly increased in size and weight by some 25 fold, this appears less adequate and the floor becomes "carpeted" with birds. In the United States and the United Kingdom the maximum recommended stocking density is around 7 pounds of bird mass for every square foot, which is approximately equivalent to a single sheet of legal-size paper for each bird.[10]

The birds are put through the system on an all-in/all-out policy. That is, the birds are all started at the same time and, at the end of the growing period, are all killed at the same time. Sheds are thoroughly cleaned and disinfected between batches in order to minimize the risk of cross-infection. As a rule, disease due to infection is low, with animals routinely being given vaccines and other therapeutic measures. When a predetermined date has been reached, or when sufficient numbers of birds have reached the finishing weight, the batch is ready to go to slaughter.

The food is removed overnight to reduce the risk of intestinal perforation during evisceration, and therefore fecal contamination of the plant, before teams of catchers come in and load the birds into crates, which are then packed onto open trucks. The birds are unloaded at the processing factory and shackled by their legs onto a moving conveyer belt. From there they are stunned instantaneously by an electric current passing between the rail and shackles to their heads, which have been dipped into a water bath to complete the electric circuit. They then pass to a mechanical neck cutter where their throats are cut. They bleed to death before passing into a tank of scalding water to make plucking easier. The carcass is then eviscerated, inspected for reasons relating to public health, dressed, cooled, and packed according to the retailer's requirements.

PROBLEMS OF HEALTH AND WELFARE

There are inherent practical difficulties in the production methods used with these chickens that make normal good farming practices, such as daily inspection and killing birds that are irretrievably sick, difficult to ensure. This problem is exacerbated because of the large number of birds per stockperson, the low lighting levels, and the high density of stocking, all of which make adequate inspection difficult, if not impossible.[11]

Problems of Leg Weakness

Daily inspection of all animals to cull sick and moribund birds becomes important because many develop a lameness called "leg weakness," which is sometimes severe enough for them to die from not being able to reach food and water. It is thought that the leg weakness is partly due to the disparity in growth between the muscle tissue and the skeletal frame needed to support the weight of the body and muscular activity, particularly in the last two weeks of their lives.

S. C. Kestin and co-workers[12] carried out a survey of leg weakness in four flocks of broilers comprising 1127 birds at slaughter weight, reared under normal commercial conditions. They scored the birds for lameness and found that only one-tenth of the birds walked normally. The rest (90%) had detectable gait abnormalities. Gait was scored on a scale from 0 to 5: A score of 0 represented no detectable abnormality, the bird being dextrous and agile. At the other end of the scale, a bird with a score of 5 was incapable of sustained walking, though it might be able to stand. Locomotion in score 5 birds could only be achieved with the assistance of wings or by crawling on the shanks. Between normal and severely abnormal gaits, a score of 3 was given when a bird had an obvious gait defect, which might comprise a limp, a jerky or unsteady strut, or severe splaying of one leg as it moved. The bird often preferred to squat when not made to move, and its maneuverability, acceleration, and speed were adversely affected. Overall, in the studies of Kestin and co-workers, some 26% of birds had gait scores of 3 or above.

When the behavioral patterns of these birds were examined, it was found that broilers without any leg weakness spent 80% of their time lying down. This figure increased to 88% in moderately lame birds, and they spent some 40% less time in walking. Further studies have shown that unaffected normal-gait birds made 70 visits to the feeders for a total of 67 minutes a day, whereas gait-score-3 birds only made 32 visits but for the same length of time. Other work has shown that analgesic drugs can reverse some of these observations and increase the number of visits, indicating that the birds may well be in pain.[13]

Lameness is important not only because of the pain involved, but because the birds may not be able to feed properly, which stunts growth. One study showed that when the birds were kept longer, to 85 days of age, 20% of males and 16% of females died.[14] Studies of the causes and pathology of leg weakness indicate that it is a complex disease with three main causes. The cartilage from which the drumstick bone (tibia) grows and develops can be malformed (tibial dyschondroplasia), there may be a septic arthritis, or the tendon of the main muscle in the drumstick can become displaced from the hock or ankle bone. In humans and other animals, all these conditions are directly, or indirectly, likely to cause pain, which suggests that many of these animals are constantly in some sort of pain. Millions of birds in the United Kingdom and United States would fit this description.

The genetic makeup of these birds has inevitably exacerbated the leg problems through selection for appetite and fast muscle growth, coupled with a highly nutritious and energy-rich diet. The lack of space for exercise during the latter part of their rearing could also contribute to leg weakness, as exercise is likely to promote strength and proper bone development. Alternatively, even if there were sufficient space the birds might not be able to use it because of their leg and respiratory problems (see below). Many birds with severe leg weakness might die of dehydration or be trampled on by others as they become exhausted trying to reach the food and water stations (which are raised off the ground); that is why good-practice recommendations require twice-daily inspections.

Lung, Heart, Blister, and Burn Problems

Leg weakness is not the only problem for these birds. They also suffer from lung infections, and heart disease (1%), leading to congestive heart failure and an accumulation of fluids in the abdomen (ascites).[15] Other birds develop blisters over the breast as well as hock "burns" or "scalds" due to the close contact with the damp litter when they squat, which is more likely with leg weakness:[16] One survey showed that 29% of birds had hock burns.[17] Such superficial skin lesions are likely to be uncomfortable or even painful and may be likened to grazes or wet eczema on ourselves. The mortality of birds in the sheds before they are taken to the slaughterhouse increases with age, but typically may be 6%.

Problems in Catching, Transport, and Slaughter[18]

The catchers of the chickens are faced with "depopulating" sheds that contain tens of thousands of animals. The litter, dust, darkness, and high levels of ammonia make it an arduous and unpleasant task for both humans and birds. The birds are "harvested" early in the morning, as fast as possible, because it appears less stressful for the birds, and also so that the processing plants can be kept busy during the day. They process birds at five to ten thousand per hour. Usually four birds are held in each hand by the feet (and sometimes wings but this method is illegal in some countries),[19] creating several disadvantages for the animals. The birds may be frightened by being handled roughly and carried upside down,[20] and by the noise of others trying to escape and vocalizing due to fright or pain.[21] If the animals are already in pain from the leg disorders described above, then this handling will compound any suffering.

The birds are packed into crates, then removed from the transport crates at the processing factory. There is risk of injury during both procedures, through inept handling. Such procedures lead to bruising and even to fractured bones, and studies have shown that 3% of birds have broken bones before they are stunned.[22] Between 0.19% to 0.42% of birds arrive dead at the processing factory: the deaths being due to preexisting pathology (25%), catching and transportation injuries (35%), or stress and suffocation (40%), with the proportions varying throughout the year. Some birds had more than one injury, 51% had died from congestive or acute heart failure, and 35% showed evidence of trauma such as dislocated hips (which the reader might have seen as hemorrhage around these joints when carving cooked chickens), dislocated necks, ruptured livers, crushed heads, and intraperitoneal hemorrhage.

Catching can be made more humane, and there can be significant differences in mortality rates between different teams of catchers.[23] If birds are removed from the crates one at a time, holding two legs instead of one, fractures are less common (4.6% versus 13.8%).[24] Mechanical harvesters, driven through the broiler house, have been designed to catch the birds using a sweeping system. The harvester has a retractable boom and sweeper arms fitted with rotating foam-rubber paddles that move the birds onto an inclined conveyor and transfer them into a crate behind the harvester.[25] These machines appear to frighten the birds less than human contact[26] and have lower injury rates.[27]

During transport, the control of ventilation and temperature inside the carrying crates on the trucks is minimal, and birds are often exposed to all weathers. The animals may suffer not only thermal stress but noise, vibration, and motion stress, depending on the design of the truck, the route and the driver.[28] It is difficult to attain acceptable transport conditions at all times in a journey, because temperatures and ventilation rates while standing still (for example, while loading and during traffic delays), are inevitably different from when the vehicle is in motion.[29]

Finally, slaughter is an area of concern. Death is achieved by an electrically induced stoppage of the heart followed by bleeding to death. If insufficiently high currents are passed when the birds are being electrically stunned, then they may recover consciousness before they are bled out. There is a tendency in the industry to use too low a current because a high electric current may cause carcass downgrading due to hemorrhages in the breast muscles. Surveys have shown that the currents necessary to achieve cardiac arrest are not always reached, and that if the automatic neck cutters operate ineffectively,[30] then a small proportion of animals may still be conscious when they enter the scalding-water tank on the automated line. Processing plants sometimes employ people specifically to ensure effective stunning and neck cutting, so that the animals are dead before entering the scalding water.

Problems in the Production of Breeding Birds

Birds kept for breeding have to be reared to sexual maturity to produce eggs for future generations of broilers.[31] This involves about 1% of those eaten. Genetic selection of the breeding stock is for lines that grow fast, convert food into muscle efficiently, and develop muscle in the right places (breast, thigh). However, the lifespan of these broiler birds, given unrestricted feed, would rarely be long enough for them to reach sexual maturity due to the leg weaknesses and the other diseases mentioned earlier.

In order to keep these breeders alive and fertile, they are fed only from a quarter to a half of their normal intake for their sixty-week production life.[32] This restriction appears to cause them to carry out abnormal behaviors such as abnormal preening and pecking at inanimate objects, presumably in an effort to satisfy their hunger drive. It has been suggested that these birds are in a constant state of hunger because of their restricted rations. Male breeding birds may have their toes removed and both sexes may have their beaks trimmed which has been shown to cause acute and chronic pain. It is now being advocated that birds be caged in order to overcome poor breeding and fertility rates, which would then restrict their ability to carry out natural behaviors such as dust bathing and wing flapping.[33]

These problems could be compared to systems of production thirty years ago, when chickens such as these grew at half the rate and relatively few were lost.

The birds took 86 days to reach five pounds, compared with 42 today. The average flock size then was nearer 1500 birds, compared with 20,000 today. Husbandry and killing were not so mechanized, and poultry production was part of family farming. Moreover, chicken meat 25 years ago cost $3.75/lb., whereas now it costs $1.30/lb. The "improvements" that have occurred over the past thirty years have led to increased production, so that chicken is now widely regarded as a cheap, highly palatable, and healthful meat. These improvements have also led to high animal death rates with evidence for animal suffering exceeding that of the past.

ETHICAL ISSUES

Several ethical questions arise from these practices. Obvious questions are, if animals are to be used as sources of protein, can it be done at a lower cost to the animals and, if so, are we morally obliged to reduce the suffering to the minimum level, even though it may mean paying more? These are not the only questions, however.

Death Rates, Disease Levels, and Pain and Suffering

First, the death rates and disease levels found in the broiler chicken industry are not tolerated in any other area of farming, raising questions about the justification for such an uncommon practice. In other parts of the food industry, the farmer would likely take remedial action, such as calling for a veterinarian when a dairy cow is lame. Similarly, the owner of a lame pet dog, cat, or racehorse would call the veterinarian. Is our current legal tolerance of the situation to do with ignorance of what is happening on farms, or size of animal, or margin of profit, or has it to do with the nature or moral standing of the animal concerned?

One essential question to ask is, do these birds feel pain, and can they suffer? There is no evidence that chickens are not able to experience pain, and a considerable amount of physiological and behavioral evidence that they do and are also able to experience other unpleasant mental states such as fear, anxiety, hunger, thirst, discomfort, and distress, as do many other birds and mammals.[34]

Clearly we need to *justify* any treatment of animals that causes suffering on a basis that takes account of their interests—utility from the animal's perspective—and not merely their utility as food. We also have a moral obligation to prevent avoidable and unnecessary suffering in animals,[35] even if the fulfillment of that obligation has the consequence of losing benefits for humans. (See chapter 1.) These obligations need not be interpreted as requiring that animals not be used as food sources, but they do suggest that practices in the chicken industry may need considerable rethinking.

Intelligence and Moral Standing

Current evidence also suggests that some birds display signs of intelligence, which may increase their suffering. It is generally acknowledged that animals with highly developed nervous systems are more likely to suffer as a consequence of their advanced mental abilities. For example, higher mental abilities may enable some animals to predict what may happen to them in the light of their earlier experiences, or they may have their desires frustrated. Such anticipation or mental frustration may make suffering worse than for animals lacking these abilities.

The intelligence of some birds is connected to questions about their moral standing. Moral claims on behalf of animals do not have anything to do with their intelligence if pain, suffering, and overall welfare are taken to present the only moral issues. Nonetheless, intelligence may play a significant role in the moral standing assigned to an animal and may deeply affect how we view the animal.

Consider, for example, the work of Irene Pepperberg with Alex, an African gray parrot.[36] Alex has demonstrated that he has the ability to count, identify shapes, colors and objects, and even use words to get what he wants. He is able to identify objects that are presented in different shapes (for example, paper), link novel shapes and colors, and even identify shades of color correctly. In this way the bird shows he is able to make new, previously unlearned connections, confirming that he is not simply learning by rote. More remarkably, he apparently uses words like "no" to express feelings of annoyance, displeasure, and noncooperation, rather than his "native language" of a squawk or a screech. Experiments on other species of birds have shown that various birds are capable of various forms of intelligence.

If chickens are able to experience pain, fear, and distress and have limited intelligence, are we justified in treating them differently from other farm animals, such as sheep and cattle, which to date have not shown such advanced developments (which is not to say they are not able to do so!)? In particular, if chickens are able to suffer, ought we to be farming them in the ways currently practiced?

Desensitization and Lack of Social Connection

Perhaps it is the vast scale on which the birds are reared that desensitizes producers, veterinarians, in fact all those connected with the trade. Such desensitization presents its own ethical issues. The care of one animal is different from the care of tens or hundreds of thousands kept in this way. The same desensitization may occur in the treatment of some humans in prisoner-of-war camps, or in schools or universities, or in the lives of busy physicians, veterinarians, and politicians. But can the prevalent lack of care be justified? A duty of care should extend to all as much as to one, but this is plainly impossible with broiler chickens as they are reared today. Does this fact suggest that a compromise may be in order? For example, perhaps we could and should allow industrial farming techniques, but require more-humane provisions of handling, slaughter, and care during the critical periods of growth.

Perhaps the current lack of concern for broiler chickens also has to do with the size of the animal: the bigger an animal, the more we take notice of it. This may be because large animals show more obvious signs of pain, such as louder noises (pigs) and cause more damage to the surroundings when trying to escape the pain (horses with colic) than do small animals. Humans may find it easier to relate and recognize signs of pain in the larger animals, especially if those animals live in close proximity to humans.

We may also forget that small things feel pain, because we ignore the ways in which they are limited in their abilities to respond to painful situations. These animals may struggle, but be relatively powerless in our restraining grasp. They may cry out in ultrasound frequencies that we are unable to hear, or they may remain immobile as a response that we interpret as "not feeling any fear or pain." We may simply not recognize when small animals are afraid, distressed, or in some form of pain. Finally, small animals may find things painful that we cannot conceive as being so, for example, high-frequency sounds, odors, and low or high temperatures. Can we even recognize in many cases what causes suffering in animals *from the animal's point of view?*[37]

Is it a factor that these animals appear so different from ourselves and other mammals that we cannot identify (empathize) with their suffering easily? If so, we would more likely be able to identify signs of pain in animals that look like ourselves (for example, the great apes—gorillas, orangutans, chimpanzees) or to whom we are closely connected socially. In the law of some countries, primates, dogs, and cats are given special protection whereas other animals are not deemed worthy of consideration at all, even though they might be remarkably similar to dogs and cats.[38]

Practical Questions and Alternatives

What might actually be done to eliminate or alleviate some of the problems mentioned above? Here are some possibilities that bear discussion.[39] Many of these possible courses bear on questions about alternatives and the obligation to seek alternatives that are found elsewhere in this volume (see chapter 1).

1. We could stop eating chicken. Undoubtedly, in a short time this would

decrease animal suffering. Not eating chicken raises the issue of whether people should become vegetarians or simply eat more welfare-friendly meat products. Most of us eat meat because of tradition and because it adds to our pleasures in life. But is the human benefit outweighed by the cost to the animals? Believers in animal rights could accept only vegetarianism as a way forward because they believe that animals have a right to a life and should not be caused to suffer in any way, independent of considerations of utility for humans. Animal welfarists, on the other hand, tend to be utilitarians who acknowledge that humans have a duty not to cause animals avoidable harm, but are prepared to use animals for human benefit. They accept that some minimal level of suffering may be inherently necessary to produce their food, and certainly do not see animal life as sacrosanct. But, from either perspective, one might be able to justify not eating chicken: The animal rights advocate believes chickens should never be killed and the animal welfarist believes the harms done to the chickens are not outweighed by the benefit of eating chicken.

2. Codes of practice could be introduced (as has happened in some countries, including Canada and Sweden) to help ensure welfare-friendly farming standards and practices in farming. This would help ensure practices such as a backup power supply, minimum ventilation rates, maximum stocking densities, training of stockpersons, minimum inspection regimens, proper stunning currents, and so on. In addition, animal welfare, as opposed to agricultural productivity targets, could be set (for example, acceptable levels of mortality, lameness, fractures, ineffective killings) so that breeders, farmers, catchers, and processors would be penalized if the established limits of suffering were exceeded. Self-auditing could also be encouraged so that producers are encouraged to assess their own performance based on score ratings for relevant criteria.[40]

On a practical basis it is possible to feed the chickens less. The weight gain would then not be so rapid, and the disparity between body weight and skeletal growth not so great. This strategy may reduce leg problems by as much as 50%, but the financial profit per bird would also be reduced. In addition, as the birds have been bred for appetite, such a restriction would probably make the birds chronically hungry. Perches could be provided for the birds that would increase exercise and strengthen their legs for as long as they were motivated to get on and off the perches, but this maneuver might also increase breast blisters from perching. In addition, periods of darkness could be provided, which has been shown to improve skeletal strength. Perhaps most importantly, breeders could select for birds that have strong legs and incorporate other health and welfare criteria into their selection programs, as is now starting to happen in some breeding locations.[41]

Crates could be improved with larger openings, so that it would be easier to pack and unpack the birds, and the birds could be killed in the crates by exposure to lethal concentrations of natural gases (such as carbon dioxide or argon), rather than electrocution and bleeding. This strategy would eliminate the stresses and pain associated with unpacking and shackling. Teams of catchers could be paid a "welfare bonus" based on fracture and bruising rates.

3. The public could pay more for chicken so that broilers could be reared more humanely and profitably. The public could be educated about production methods and the suffering and the "losses"; chicken products could be labeled to indicate the system of production, giving consumers a choice. If consumers were not prepared to pay more, or not that much more, then other avenues might have to be explored, such as lower profits for producers, processors, or retailers.

Animal welfare is itself currently becoming a factor in the market, and more retailers are advertising products as animal friendly (for example, dolphin-friendly tuna and free-range eggs and chicken). But will these advertisements just become a war of words, misrepresentation, and mislabeling by advertisers and marketing managers? The RSPCA has recently launched a Freedom Food campaign with which farmers can register, using the RSPCA label if their methods of production meet certain criteria.[42] Many animal welfare organizations have initiated programs to reduce the plight of these birds.

4. National laws could be changed. In the United States, poultry are sometimes exempt under state laws regarding animal cruelty, because they are not considered "animals," or perhaps were never considered at all. In Europe, under article 36 of the Treaty of Rome, which regulates trade in a free market, all farmed animals are classified along with insentient commodities such as vegetables and fruit. A significant moral difference seems to exist between sentient animals and objects that do not have the ability to experience pain and pleasure. If the status of animals were changed so that their ability to feel pain and to suffer were legally recognized and differentiated from other traded goods, that change might help strengthen and increase welfare legislation.

5. International agreements and laws could be changed. We live increasingly in a world market, and the General Agreement on Tariffs and Trade (GATT) promotes world trade. A country that banned the importation of goods from another country on the basis of the method of producing those goods would be acting illegally and would be penalized in some way. The implication is that if stricter laws are introduced within a country to protect the well-being of animals, then cheaper, poor-welfare imports may undercut welfare-friendly, home-produced products such as chicken meat. But how far is the World Trade Organization (the controller of GATT) prepared to take the argument that methods of production are morally neutral and irrelevant? More important to ethical debate, how far should such organizations exert controls?

Finally, it seems appropriate to finish, as well as start, with a quote from Professor John Webster:

Personally, I almost never eat broiler chicken unless it is of a light, slow growing strain, free range and usually corn fed. By so doing, I can eat smaller portions of a better tasting bird, the heavier strain of broiler being, in my opinion, little more than an edible plate, all flavour to be added retrospectively. By such means I satisfy the needs of my conscience, my health (by eating relatively less meat and more vegetables) and my palate. To this consumer, this chicken has real added value.[43]

NOTES

1. John Webster, "A Cool Eye Towards Eden," in *Animal Welfare* (Oxford, England, and Cambridge, MA: Blackwell Science, 1995), p. 156.

2. In the United Kingdom in 1992, broilers comprised 84% by weight of the poultry meat market, with 1,013,000 tons of chicken being consumed, which represented some 27% of the total meat supply. See *The Agriculture Committee Second Report on the UK Poultry Industry* (London, UK: HMSO) p. 10.

3. See A. Elson, for a general reference on systems, "Housing Systems for Broilers," in *Proceedings of the 4th European Symposium on Poultry Welfare,* ed. C. J. Savory & B. O. Hughes (Universities Federation for Animal Welfare, 1993), pp. 171–84.

4. The lighting is around 2 to 20 lux. An office would normally be between 300 to 500 lux.

5. F. J. Jensen, "Stocking Density, Lighting Programmes and Food Intake," in *Proceedings of the 4th European Symposium on Poultry Welfare,* pp. 185–94.

6. "Report of the Farm Animal Welfare Council UK (1992) on the Welfare of Broiler Chickens." Available from MAFF/FAWC, Tolworth Tower, Surbiton, Surrey, KT6 7DX, UK, p. 9.

7. In addition, feed intake falls by about 1.5% for every degree centigrade rise above normal temperatures (around 21 degrees Celsius, or 70 degrees Fahrenheit): the higher the temperature, the greater the depression of food intake.

8. Each bird produces 8 w; if the shed has 40,000 birds then 320 kw has to be removed at ambient temperatures such as 32 degrees Celsius, or 90 degrees Fahrenheit.

9. In some countries there is a legal requirement for there to be standby generators.

10. Report of the Farm Animal Welfare Council UK (1992) on the Welfare of Broiler Chickens gives 34 kg/sq. meter, which is about 750 sq. cm. per 2.5 kg bird (0.8 square feet per 5.5 lb. bird).

11. One man in charge of four sheds (each with 40,000 birds) spending 4 hours-day on inspection would need to check 11 birds/second and no blinks! It is recommended that birds are inspected at least twice a day and sometimes they are inspected more frequently. Scanning of birds achieves a minimum level of inspection but not sufficient to pick up all sick animals.

12. S. C. Kestin, T. G. Knowles, A. E. Tinch, and N. G. Gregory, "Prevalence of Leg Weakness in Broiler Chickens and Its Relationship with Genotype," *Veterinary Record* 131 (1992): 190–94. Kestin has extended his work into leg weakness to some 21 flocks and basically similar results are being obtained.

13. S. C. Kestin, personal communication, 1996.

14. P. Hunton, "The Broiler Industry: 34 Years of Progress," *Poultry International,* July 1995.

15. B. H. Thorp and M. H. Maxwell, "Health Problems in Broiler Production," in *Proceedings of the 4th European Symposium on Poultry Welfare,* pp. 208–18.

16. See Report of the Farm Animal Welfare Council (1992) on the Welfare of Broiler Chickens, p. 9.

17. N. G. Gregory, and S. D. Austin, "Causes of Trauma in Broilers Arriving Dead at Poultry Processing Plants," *Veterinary Record* 131 (1992): 501–3.

18. M. A. Mitchell and P. J. Kettlewell, "Catching and Transport of Broiler Chickens," in *Proceedings of the 4th European Symposium on Poultry Welfare,* pp. 219–29.

19. P. A. Bayliss and M. H. Hinton, "Transportation of Broilers with Specific Reference to Mortality Rates," *Applied Animal Behavioral Science* 28 (1990): 93–118.

20. G. Kannan and J. A. Mench have found that carrying birds upright stresses them less. Influence of different handling methods and crating periods on plasma corticosterone concentrations in broilers. *British Poultry Science* 37 (1996): 21–31.

21. P. J. Cashman, C. J. Nicol, and R. B. Jones, "Effects of Transportation on the Tonic Immobility Fear Reactions of Broilers," *British Poultry Science* 30 (1989): 211–21.

22. N. G. Gregory and L. J. Wilkins, "Broken Bones in Chickens: Effect of Stunning and Processing in Broilers," *British Poultry Science* 31 (1990): 53–58.

23. Bayliss and Hinton, "Transportation of Broilers," pp. 93–118.

24. N. G. Gregory, L. J. Wilkins, D. M. Alvey, and S. A. Tucker, "Effects of catching method and lighting density on the prevalence of broken bones and on the ease of handling of end-of-day hens," *Veterinary Record* 132 (1993): 127–29.

25. P. A. Bayliss and M. H. Hinton, "Transportation of Broilers," pp. 93–118.

26. I. J. H. Duncan, G. S. Slee, P. Kettlewell, P. Berry, and A. J. Carlisle, "Comparison of the Stressfulness of Harvesting Broiler Chickens by Machine and By Hand," *British Poultry Science* 27 (1985): 109–14.

27. J. F. Gracey, *Meat Hygiene,* 8th ed. (London: Balliere Tindall, 1986), pp. 455–57.

28. C. J. Nicol, A. Blakeborough, and G. B. Scott, "Aversiveness of Motion and Noise to Broiler Chickens," *British Poultry Science* 32 (1991): 249–60.

29. P. D. Warriss, E. A. Bevis, S. N. Brown, and J. E. Edwards, "Longer Journeys to Processing Plants Are Associated with Higher Mortality in Broiler Chickens," *British Poultry Science* 33 (1992): 201–6.

30. For example, if only one common carotid artery is cut instead of two, it takes 2 minutes for a bird to die as opposed to 1.5 minutes.

31. Hunton, "Broiler Industry."

32. *Chickens' Lib Fact Sheet* 32 (May 1992). Available from Farm Animal Welfare Network, P.O. Box 2, Holmfirth, Huddersfield, HD7 IQT, U.K.

33. J. A. Mench, "Animal Welfare and Management Issues Associated with the Use of Artificial Insemination for Broiler Breeders," in *Proceedings of the 1st International Symposium on the Artificial Insemination of Poultry,* ed. M. R. Bakst and G. J. Wishart (Savoy, IL: Poultry Science Association, 1995).

34. P. N. Grigor, B. O. Hughes, and M. C. Appleby, "Effects of Regular Handling and Exposure to an Outside Area on Subsequent Fearfulness and Dispersal in Domestic Hens," *Applied Animal Behaviour Science* 44 (1995): 47– 55; J. H. Duncan and J. A. Mench, "Behavior as an Indicator of Welfare in Various Systems," in *Proceedings of the 4th European Symposium on Poultry Welfare,* pp. 69–80.

35. D. B. Morton, "Is Unnecessary Suffering Avoidable?" *Veterinary Record* 133 (1993): 304.

36. See review of Pepperberg's work with Alex and other evidence in Marion Stamp Dawkins, *Through Our Eyes Only? The Search for Animal Consciousness* (Oxford and New York: W. H. Freeman; Heidelberg: Spektrum), pp. 119–27

37. This has been the subject of other investigations. D. B. Morton and P. H. M. Griffiths, "Guidelines on the Recognition of Pain, Distress and Discomfort in Experimental Animals and an Hypothesis for Assessment," *Veterinary Record* 116 (1985): 431–36.

38. In the United Kingdom the Animals (Scientific Procedures) Act, 1986 London, HMSO 182, requires special justification for experiments involving dogs, cats, primates and horses. In the United States, the Animal Welfare Act (1966, 1990) governing research does not cover experiments on rats, mice, or birds. See also F. B. Orlans, *In the Name of Science* (New York: Oxford University Press, 1993), pp. 58–60.

39. See *Practical Approaches to Broiler Welfare,* eds. M. Baxter, D. B. Morton, and Anna Clemence Mews, report of a seminar, 14–15 September 1995, Ammerdown, Bath (*Alastair Mews Memorial Trust,* 1995).

40. Foundation for Animal Care. Saskatchewan Inc. produces such a leaflet. *Broiler Management Review.* Available from FACS, 502 45th Street West, Saskatoon, S7L 6H2, Canada.

41. Joy Mench, personal communication, 1995.

42. Farm Animal Welfare Council, *Second Report on Priorities for Research and Development in Farm Animal Welfare* (London: Ministry of Agriculture, Fisheries and Food, 1993).

43. John Webster, "Cool Eye," p. 163.

VIII

COMPANION ANIMALS

15

SHOULD THE TAIL WAG THE DOG?

Paul Plonka bred a litter of 11 boxer puppies in March 1994, and telephoned his local veterinarian to arrange for them to be docked, as he had done with his last litter some years previously. Imagine his surprise when the veterinarian declined to do so. What was he to do? If he didn't have their tails removed he might not be able to sell the puppies, and, anyway, who had ever heard of a boxer with a long tail? He must do it himself—but how? He reasoned that cutting off the tails with a knife or scissors might cause excessive bleeding and also make a mess, so instead he tied each tail at its base with cord to cut off the blood supply, anticipating that the tails would drop off in time. This did occur, and Plonka felt he had done a good job.

A few weeks later, an inspector from the Royal Society for the Prevention of Cruelty to Animals (RSPCA) called and asked him who had docked the puppies, at what age, and how they had been docked? Plonka subsequently found himself in court, emerging with a fine of 350 pounds (550 dollars) and having to pay legal costs of 50 pounds.[1] He was found guilty of contravening the UK Veterinary Surgeons Act, 1966 (amended 1991), by carrying out an act of veterinary surgery without being appropriately qualified.

On the surface, the docking of puppies seems a trivial issue. Docking appears only to cause a few seconds of minor pain shortly after birth and all is soon forgotten—almost as innocent as circumcision in male human newborns. However, docking has become a matter of some controversy in a number of countries. The debate has focused around a number of questions, each of which will be considered below.

1. Why are the tails removed, and why in some breeds, but not others?
2. Does docking have adverse effects on the animals?
3. If docking is to be performed, what is the best procedure? Who should dock, how should it be done, and at what age?
4. Finally, ought docking to be performed at all?

HISTORICAL, MEDICAL, AND LEGAL ASPECTS OF DOCKING

Historical Aspects

Docking has been practiced for centuries.[2] Until the eighteenth century it was thought that undocked dogs were more likely to develop rabies. Many dogs were docked, and the owners of undocked dogs were liable to a tax. In addition,

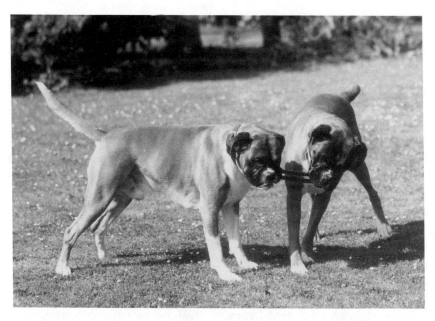

These boxer dogs—one with a docked tail (on the right) and one without (on the left)— are among the 50 or so breeds of dogs that are customarily docked. Docking is sometimes a required standard set by national kennel clubs for many breeds of show dogs. The British and Australian veterinary associations oppose tail docking in the belief that it is an archaic and pointless practice. Credit: Animal Photography, London, UK.

dogs were used for hunting and shooting, and some of these dogs damaged their tails in this work. It was thought that docking reduced the chance of injury in some breeds. Spaniels, for example, flush game by going into the hedgerows and other cover, and are thereby more likely to damage their tails than retriever-type dogs, which work in the open and bring back game after it has broken cover and been shot. Consequently, spaniels, but not retrievers, were docked. Other reasons put forward for docking were strengthening the back, increasing speed, and impeding some breeds from chasing game.

Today, docking is carried out for a variety of reasons. These include: not wishing to break with tradition, improving appearance, preventing dogs from injuring themselves while involved in shooting and hunting, better hygiene, and providing for more harmonious cohabitation with humans in confined living conditions. At present, some fifty breeds are customarily docked.

Medical Aspects

The tail in a dog is formed from a line of 15 to 20 vertebrae with flexible joints, strengthened by ligaments, and covered by muscles that extend, flex, and bend the tail in all directions. A tail serves as an organ of balance, and for communication with other dogs, animals, and humans. Its position and actions, together with body stance, can signal pleasure, friendliness, dominance, playfulness, unhappiness, lack of well-being, defensiveness, inquisitiveness, aggression, nervousness, and submissiveness, as well as other characteristic breed stances (for example, pointing toward hidden game). The tail also carries a scent gland used to mark out territory. Although animals appear to adapt well to docking, under certain circumstances the lack of a tail will adversely affect balance and communication.

"Docking" is the surgical process by which a varying length of tail (depending on the breed)[3] is removed by means of scissors, scalpel, razor, knife, or rubber rings. It is normally carried out without anesthetic in the first few days of life. After cutting off the tail the stump may be stitched or treated with an antiseptic powder. Rarely is an analgesic (pain reliever) given before or afterwards.

Pain is a characteristic property of higher vertebrates, including mammals, birds, reptiles, amphibia, and fish. Pain perception is essential to alert an animal to potential or actual injury, helping prevent further damage. Pain sensors are located in the skin, which would be the first part of the body to be exposed to an external threat, and respond to excessive pressure, heat or chemical stimuli. Impulses from these sensors travel to the brain (at speeds of 50 m/sec.—that is, at more than 100 mph) and the individual can then consciously locate the source and intensity of the stimulus and take appropriate action.

One fundamental and largely unresolved question is whether a puppy in the first week or so of life is capable of feeling pain or whether its nervous system is too immature. Their ability to feel pain is indicated by their behavior during docking, as the puppy often squeaks or squeals. Some argue that such squeaking is a reflex response and does not necessarily indicate pain. However, because pups whimper for some time afterwards, and seek comforting behavior from their mother,[4] it is unlikely to be a simple reflex, which would occur within fractions of a second and then cease. Although immaturity of the nervous system has been advanced as a reason why puppies do not feel pain when their tails are docked, others have argued the reverse, that is puppies feel more pain because of the immaturity. Those that say the animal does not feel pain admit that the immaturity would simply slow down the speed of reaction, not that pain would be absent.[5] Those that argue for the young feeling more pain extrapolate from work in rats that shows that the pain-inhibiting fibers in adults are not present at birth and take some weeks to develop.[6] Therefore, until they have fully developed, neonatal animals are likely to feel more pain than adults for a given stimulus.

Docking by means of rubber rings rather than by surgical methods has been advocated as not being painful, particularly by the Council of Docked Breeds. But evidence of pain has been found in lambs, calves, and goat kids for at least two hours after ringing, and extending in some animals to abnormal behaviors for two days or so.[7]

Legal Aspects

The Council of Europe, with its 34 member states, recently opened its Multilateral Convention for the Protection of Pet Animals,[8] and this has revived the debate over docking in the United Kingdom. Article 10.1.a. of the convention specifically prohibits the docking of dogs' tails. Other sections ban ear cropping, devocalization, defanging (removal of canine teeth) and declawing (with exceptions allowed for therapeutic purposes). A partial repeal for *docking only* is permitted under the convention; that is, countries can sign the convention but not implement the ban on docking. To date it has been signed by 13 countries,[9] including Belgium, Denmark, Finland, Germany, Greece, Italy, Luxembourg, the Netherlands, Norway, Portugal, Sweden, and Switzerland. Some countries have retained an option on docking. The convention prohibits surgical interventions primarily carried out for aesthetic reasons or for the personal convenience of the owner or the breeder.

In countries outside Europe there appear to be no specific laws relating to docking dogs, although it is being actively discussed in the United States, Canada, Australia, and New Zealand. In fact, in many countries it is legal for dog breeders to dock their own litters but the conditions under which the procedure is carried out are often far from ideal.

INTERESTED PARTIES AND THE POLITICAL LANDSCAPE

A number of parties have an interest in how the controversy over docking is resolved. Pet ownership continues to increase, and pet animals are supplied by commercial puppy farmers and traditional dog breeders. Veterinarians are involved in the care of pets, and, of course, are the persons usually most directly involved in docking.

Traditional breeders fear it will be difficult to sell undocked puppies of breeds that are customarily docked because of the altered appearance. They fear some unsold animals would have to be killed.[10] Every year in the United Kingdom, around a quarter of a million dogs have had their tails docked and the total annual turnover from docked dogs, including export, is estimated to be around 50 million pounds (75 million dollars). If docking were to cease, potential buyers might turn their attentions to other breeds, and so the traditional breeders of docked breeds, some of whom have spent considerable time and effort in "improving" their breed, will lose out.[11]

Some breeders feel so strongly about this issue that they have threatened to boycott veterinary surgeons who adhere to the guidelines of their professional associations, which obligate them not to dock.[12] Some breeders insist that a veterinary surgeon ought to do what the breeder wants, because they are paying for the service and it is not a matter of professional judgment. A black market–underground movement has now been created with "red" vets who will not dock and "green" vets who will, as well as some breeders who are breaking UK law by docking puppies.[13]

The kennel clubs regulate the registration and showing of pedigree dogs through their councils (made up from breeders). Docking is not required to conform to any breed standard according to the UK Kennel Club (KC), but as the KC has failed to give guidance on what sort of tail judges should be looking for, breeders play safe and try to have their puppies docked. Some breeders are also afraid to speak out against docking because the KC appoints judges at dog shows and judges determine which breeders win or lose; this is a powerful incentive for many breeders to continue to support docking. In Norway, the KC has gone along with the docking ban and is not prepared to accept imported docked dogs for registration, unless the docking has been carried out by a veterinary surgeon authenticated by certification.[14]

The Council of Docked Breeds (CDB) was set up to counter the docking opponents in the United Kingdom, and to defend the breeder's "right" to continue to dock tails (this right was based on legal ownership rather than any moral consideration). The CDB has been accused of scaremongering, because it puts forward the view that docking is the thin end of the wedge to greater controls over breeders, so breeders of undocked breeds should also join.[15]

The veterinary profession has opposed docking for many years, not only on the grounds that it causes unnecessary suffering, but particularly because of the methods used to carry out the operation.[16] In William Youatt's book (1839), entitled *The Obligation and Extent of Humanity to Brutes,* the following passage was written for the Society for the Prevention of Cruelty to Animals.

> If the sharp, strong scissors, with a ligature, were used, the operation, although still indefensible, would not be a very cruel one, for the tail may be removed almost in a moment, and the wound soon heals; but for the beastly knawing off [sic] of the part—and the act of drawing out the tendons and the nerves—these are the acts of a cannibal; and he who perpetrates a barbarity so nearly approaching cannibalism deserves to be scouted from all society.

Some veterinarians carry out docking because, they argue, it would be worse for the animals if they, as trained surgeons, did not. Despite the financial inducement to carry out docking, the profession on the whole is against the procedure. A 1989 survey by the Australian Veterinary Association found that 86% of respondents opposed nontherapeutic docking and described it as "archaic," 'barbaric," and "pointless." A similar survey conducted in 1992 by the British Small Animal Veterinary Association showed 92% of UK veterinarians agreed with the ban and 56% stated that they refused to dock at the present time. It is notable that two veterinarians in favor of docking stood for election to the Council of the RCVS in 1994 (which was a political route to reverse the ban) but failed to be elected. In North America, the American and Canadian veterinary medical associations do not have position statements on docking.

Animal welfare organizations worldwide have not been particularly active in this area, except in the United States, where the Association of Veterinarians for Animal Rights has labeled docking and cropping as "cruel and needless rituals."[17] Other organizations have position statements but do not appear to have mounted significant campaigns. The UK RSPCA has a list of breeders willing to supply undocked puppies.

The public's views have not been clearly determined. In the light of an ever increasing public concern for animal welfare, there is likely to be opposition to docking. A small survey indicated that more than 90% of clients of a veterinary hospital in Plymouth, England, were against docking.[18] The length of a tail will not directly affect most people's choice of pet, as other factors such as temperament, cleanliness, and cost of upkeep will weigh more heavily.

REASONS FOR AND AGAINST DOCKING

Several reasons for and against docking are found in the literature on the subject. These reasons are not clearly *moral* reasons, but they often have ethical implications.

Reasons for Docking

Prevention of injury is one of the main arguments for docking puppies, particularly in breeds used in hunting and shooting, such as spaniels and pointers. The injuries occur because when the dogs go into dense cover, briars may become entangled in the fur (feather) and damage the tail. It is believed that these dogs will injure their tails more if left undocked, but no one can be certain because these breeds have not been left undocked for centuries. If shortening the tail prevents the likelihood of injury, one might predict that within a breed, those animals that had not been docked would incur fewer tail injuries than those that had.

Over the past few years docking has been prohibited in some countries, and so relevant evidence might soon be available by comparing older (docked) with younger (undocked) dogs. For example in Sweden, where docking has been banned since 1989, a 1991 survey in veterinary clinics showed that 73% of tail injuries were in undocked animals.[19] However, these figures were not related to the proportion of undocked versus docked dogs attending the clinic. Until we can establish accurate figures for tail injuries in docked and undocked dogs, together with the circumstances surrounding the injury, that is, whether the injury occurred at home or during fieldwork, we are unlikely to have the sort of data that would substantiate further commentary.

Improved appearance is a second reason that breeders give to justify removing or shortening the tail, believing it makes an animal look more attractive (thus the term "cosmetic" docking). Traditional breeders determine the standards laid down for a breed, in conjunction with the national kennel club, and so when breed standards are revised, they tend to perpetuate the traditional view of what an animal of that breed should look like.

Some find it surprising that docking is acceptable because KC rules state that any dog that has been changed in appearance by artificial means *except as specified in the breed standard* may not compete at any show or obedience trial and will be disqualified.[20] In other areas of a dog's anatomy, corrective surgical interventions are not accepted for show purposes, for example, teeth malalignment, eyelid deformation, altering the set of the ears or tail, removal of excessive skin wrinkle or unwanted color. However, ear trimming or cropping (the same procedure differing in degree) to obtain the desired appearance is approved by some national kennel clubs.[21]

Improving hygiene is the third reason advanced to support docking in the Old English sheepdog, Yorkshire terrier, and Australian silky terriers. Fouling and retention of feces in perineal hairs may lead to maggot infestation, as well as an unwelcome smell in the house. It can be argued that owners of breeds with this potential problem can, by thorough and regular grooming, prevent this problem from occurring, but owners have not proved to be reliable in attending to their animals in these ways. The hygiene argument, like the prevention argument, has attracted suspicion because there are various breeds with the same potential hygiene problem that are not docked (for example, Pekingese, bearded collies, and border collies).

Reasons Against Docking

The pain initially inflicted at the time of docking is likely to be significant, and it may persist as discomfort for a day or more, particularly if rubber rings are used. Animals also may suckle or sleep less. Breeders generally have inadequate training in surgical technique and are often unaware of the potential adverse consequences of docking and how to avoid them. Tails docked improperly can become infected, although infection is not a common problem. In extreme cases infection can ascend the spinal cord or spread elsewhere in the body, and the animal may have to be humanely killed. This is more likely to happen in breeds where the tail is cut very short, for example, the Old English sheepdog or Rottweiler.

Fatal hemorrhaging has been recorded in genetic lines that carry a blood clotting defect, and chronic pain and self-mutilation have also been reported.[22] Some dog psychologists believe a dog with no tail, such as an Old English sheepdog or Rottweiler, can miscue other dogs; as a result severely docked animals may appear to show unwarranted aggression by not being seen to wag their tails, and so become the victim of attack.[23]

Docking is ineffective as a means of preventing harm. In a survey it was found that 78% of all dogs attending the authors' clinic were undocked and that 83% of all dogs with tail injuries were undocked.[24] This clinic's records, extracted between 1965 and 1985, showed that 0.41% of undocked dogs and 0.31% of docked dogs sustained injuries of the tail or stump and the authors concluded that docking could not be recommended as a prophylactic measure. Furthermore, if docking is truly a preventive measure then complete removal of the tail should be even more successful because it would eliminate all risk of injury, and this would hold true for all breeds. In practice, however, breeders and international breed standards vary considerably (even within a breed) and between one-third and three-quarters of the tail is removed according to the breed.[25]

ETHICAL ISSUES

The arguments for and against docking have now been discussed, but we have yet to consider applicable ethical principles and the types of moral problems involved in docking dogs.

Acceptable Criteria for Nontherapeutic Surgery

Many kinds of surgical procedures are carried out in animals. Those defending the docking of puppies often compare it to the docking of other species, such as lambs, piglets, horses, and cattle. In addition, the docking of puppies is compared with neutering, as well as with trimming the beaks of intensively kept poultry. Is the justification for the surgical intervention the same in each of these cases? If not, what are the key differences?

The following criteria have been suggested[26] as appropriate ways of addressing the moral justifiability of docking. The assumption is that if all of the criteria are satisfied in a particular case by answering yes to questions 1–5 and no to questions 6–8, then docking would likely be justified.

1. Is there compelling evidence that leaving the animals intact (for example, leaving the tail on) predisposes those individuals to harmful consequences?
2. Is there compelling evidence that leaving the animals intact predisposes other animals in a group to harmful consequences?
3. Is there evidence that the proposed intervention is in the best interests of the animal? That is, does the intervention confer a benefit for the animal that outweighs the removal of harms?
4. Would the harmful consequences or the benefit occur in a significant proportion of the population?
5. Is the increase in "value" to the animal owner as a result of carrying out the proposed intervention (for example, increased economic value) sufficient to offset the harm done to the animals?
6. Does the proposed interference cause a greater harm than the damage one is trying to prevent?
7. Is there an alternative means with no adverse effects (for example, clipping tail fur) that would achieve the same end (for example, reduce the risk of perineal infection)?
8. Is there a less harmful way of carrying out the proposed intervention that would achieve the same end (that is, would a local anesthetic or sedative make the procedure less painful)?

In effect, these criteria attempt to ensure that a proposed benefit is real, valuable, and attainable—and that some overall good from the surgical intervention can be anticipated. But are these criteria adequate? Do they even address the right issues? Is this just a form of utilitarian balancing of benefits and harms, when it should involve principled reasoning that does not rely on a utilitarian framework? (See chapter 1.)

The Principle of Protecting Structural and Functional Integrity

One possible principle that seems to have little or nothing to do with balancing harms and benefits is the following: *It is important, in principle, not to destroy or unnecessarily disturb the structural or functional integrity of an animal.* This is clearly a strong principle. Is it acceptable? What are its implications?

Many reasons might be offered in support of this principle. A major reason might be derived from the reasoning outlined in chapter 1 of this volume pertaining to the inherent value of animals: removing parts of animals would not seem respectful of the inherent value of animals, if they possess such value. A practice of significant structural or functional alteration seems to suggest that the animal was imperfect in some way beforehand, and that it is necessary to alter it to meet human purposes. There are also limits to what it would be morally permissible to do in the interests of preventive medicine: removal of limbs to avoid fracturing them or removing teeth to avoid the possibility of decay would not be considered acceptable veterinary practices.

What are the implications of this reasoning? Is the above principle to be construed so that no manner of shaping appearance is permissible? Can the hair of poodles not be trimmed to an owner's tastes—or even hair cut away to unblock the eyes of Old English sheepdogs and bearded collies? Perhaps these are not matters of structural integrity. If not, then what about cropping dogs' ears to "improve" their appearance, which many people now judge unacceptable? What are we to say about the removal of claws from indoor pets, or the removal of poisonous mechanisms from pet snakes? What is the scope of the principle, and does it have equally principled limits?

On the other side of this line of questions is this: ought breeders to be able to alter or even mutilate a dog merely because it is their property under law? Does the above principle have no standing or defense whatever? If no pain or suffering is involved in making functional or structural changes, would that fact make it morally acceptable?

It is likely that some surgical mutilations will require more justification than others. Those who believe in animal rights will maintain that it is always wrong to interfere and likely will defend some strong version of the above principle (see chapter 1) on grounds that animals have an inherent right not to be caused to suffer or to be surgically altered unless the surgical intervention is ultimately in their best interests, as is the case with a therapeutic intervention. But would this be the right interpretation of the principle? Should the principle be specified in a different way, or should it be abandoned?

Alternative Possibilities and Slippery Slopes

There may be alternative ways to avoid the very harms that docking is thought to minimize. For example, sportsmen could be encouraged to trim the hair from the tail and to examine their dogs more frequently to remove briars, and so minimize tail damage. They could also avoid using their dogs in close cover or choose a more appropriate breed or strain with different coat characteristics. Pet owners could be taught to groom and trim their animals effectively so that fecal material did not become trapped. Breeders could breed for sensible tail shape, tail feather, and tail length (for example, shorter tails as in the Pembrokeshire corgi). If effective, would these alternatives be preferable to docking, and should they become the standard practices?

Another question about alternatives arises from the thesis that some forms of surgical intervention are *necessary*. A strong thesis is that a surgical harm can be judged necessary only if it is in balance with any gain *for the animal*. A far weaker principle is that a surgical harm can be judged necessary only if it is in balance with any gain for the *animal and/or the human owner*. From either perspective, the claimed benefit and the animal suffering have to be carefully evaluated and balanced, one against the other. But there are additional problems, too. At what level of probability of injury would it be agreed that docking is a justifiable preventive measure: 10, 20, 50, or 80%? Studies on sheep suggest a test case: Can the docking of lambs be justified if, as now appears to be the case, more than 40% of undocked lambs are affected with larvae (maggots) eating the animals' flesh, compared with less than 12% in docked controls?[27] Can preventive docking in dogs be justified if similar proportions apply?

One problem with this test case is that few dogs will ever be used for shooting or hunting, probably less than 1%. Moreover, of those dogs that go hunting, only a small proportion will damage their tails or require a therapeutic intervention at a later date. However, the results of surveys carried out by the Swedish KC and the Veterinary School at Uppsala between 1990 and 1994 have been submitted to the Swedish Department of Agriculture for their consideration to lift the docking ban for the German pointers.[28] The surveys found in a total of 368 hunting dogs some 28.3% of animals sustained tail damage, although the circumstances, extent, and nature of that damage was not specified, and in the 1990–94 survey up to 70% had tail injuries that involved more than superficial damage. In such cases, if the activities involving dogs are themselves justified, the test case of necessity for lamb docking might apply to some subset of dogs in a population that would be affected. However, there would still seem to be no point in docking those dogs that were never going to go hunting.

On a utilitarian basis, this conclusion might seem to receive additional support: the total amount of suffering (pain and discomfort) caused by docking every puppy in a "susceptible" breed is likely to be greater than the suffering of the few adults needing this operation therapeutically. The pain caused by therapeutic docking also could be justified as in the animal's best interests, and also the pain could be mitigated through the use of anesthetics and postoperative analgesics to a point where it should be relatively insignificant. Using a similar utilitarian logic, it could be argued that the benefit gained from having a tail by the majority of intact dogs would outweigh the disadvantage to those small number of dogs that would have to be docked therapeutically.

Of course, a larger utilitarian picture includes human interests. Docking for cosmetic purposes involves balancing human aesthetic sensibilities against animal suffering in a "cost-benefit analysis." Such preferences could be regarded as trivial or important, depending on the individual view taken. But accepting any human pleasure or aesthetic preference at the expense of an animal would also seem to open the door to a justification for many uses of animals widely considered unacceptable and often legally prohibited, such as dog fighting or baiting animals. How does one draw a line at the limits of human benefits in the balance of interests? Here we will soon return again to question whether the consequences of accepting docking as an ethical procedure lead down a slippery slope that would involve accepting other surgical interventions such as ear cropping or trimming and carrying out similar procedures in other breeds of dogs or in other animal species such as horses, cattle, and cats.

A final question about possible alternatives is whether decreasing the harms associated with docking would make docking any more justifiable. If we could refine the operation by relieving the pain associated with docking, and by training those carrying out the procedure, thereby reducing the incidence of faulty technique and painful side effects, would this make docking any more justifiable?

Do Veterinarians Have a Special Moral Responsibility?

Many veterinarians take an oath at the time of qualifying that they will do their best to protect the welfare of animals in their care. "Welfare" can be interpreted in several ways, but most would take it to include not inflicting unnecessary or avoidable suffering. Does society look to the veterinary profession for informed opinion over whether animals suffer during a particular procedure? In the event of any doubt, should the veterinarian give the benefit of that doubt to the animal or to the owner? Should veterinarians simply carry out what they are asked to do by the legal owner—such as tail docking and breeding—or does society entrust them to do more by virtue of being a professional person with special status and, therefore, special responsibilities? For example, are they entrusted with the care and protection of animals, much as guardians are entrusted to protect many vulnerable and incompetent persons? If not, what role do veterinarians have, and does anyone have special responsibilities assigned by society for the protection of animals?

Other arguments have been advanced which are relevant to the issue of docking dogs, in particular, claims about 'rights'. Rights language gives rise to much rhetoric, as proponents of rights must provide an account that "grounds" the existence of rights. Often equal and opposite claims are made in the name of rights, leaving the right of a breeder to dock in opposition to an animal's right not to be harmed by the breeder. Some may claim human rights trump animal rights. Even human rights are played off against each other in the debate: the right of a breeder to insist a veterinary surgeon do what the breeder wants is balanced by the right of the veterinary surgeon to do what he or she wants or feels is right to do.

CONCLUSION

Most would agree that humans have an obligation to protect animals, not to misuse or abuse them, and not to inflict on animals unnecessary or avoidable suffering. It follows that any surgical interference on an animal stands in need of justification. Paul Plonka obviously knew that puppies were born with tails, but perhaps he did not know that docking them would cause them pain, or even that docking requires moral justification. Plonka was found guilty of causing unnecessary suffering to the puppies. It is likely that his justification was simply that he thought it was the "right and natural thing to do." Further reflection might have persuaded him that the matter is more complicated.

NOTES

1. *Daily Telegraph*, 31 March 1994; "Fined £350 for Docking," *Our Dogs*, 10 June 1994.
2. *Dalziel's British Dogs*, 2nd ed., pp. 44–45, in Drury's version of 1905; W. Youatt, *The Obligation and Extent of Humanity to Brutes*, written for the Society for the Prevention of Cruelty to Animals, 1839.
3. "Editorial: Guidelines for Tail-Docking," *Journal of the American Veterinary Medical Association* 152, no. 1 (1968): 60–61; "Standards for Docking Tails of Pups," *Australian Veterinary Journal* 46 (August 1970): 403.
4. Jean Irwin, John Irwin, and Ceri Irwin, "Puppy Behavior at Docking Time," *Dog World*, 22 May 1987.
5. R. Fritsch, (1984, 1992) various letters to the German Kennel Club on docking which apparently were influential in forming the German government's views before signing the convention (and entering a derogation on docking).
6. M. Fitzgerald, "Neurobiology of Fetal and Neonatal Pain," in *Textbook of Pain*, 3rd edition, ed. P. Wall and R. Melzack (London: Churchill Livingstone 1994), pp. 153–63.

7. J. E. Kent, V. Molony, and I. S. Robertson, "Changes in Plasma Cortisol Concentration in Lambs of Three Ages after Three Methods of Castration and Tail Docking," *Research in Veterinary Science* 55 (1993): 246–51.

8. Ad Hoc Committee of experts for the protection of animals (CAHPA), *Convention for the Protection of Pet Animals* (Strasbourg, France: Council of Europe, Publications and Documents Division 1988).

9. "European Scene," *Veterinary Record,* May 20, 1995, p. 505.

10. This figure might be compared with the estimated 50,000 dogs killed a year by the humane societies, and a dog population calculated to be around seven million (both UK figures).

11. P. Shaw, "The Case for Docking," *Dog World,* 29 April 1994; idem, "The Ethics of Docking Tails," *Dog World,* 6 May 1994.

12. In the United Kingdom, the Royal College of Veterinary Surgeons, which licenses all veterinarians in the country, has issued guidance on docking which emphasizes that docking can only be carried out for therapeutic reasons. The sole exception is when the veterinarian can be sure that *the individual puppy* is going to be used for hunting or other endangering activity. Furthermore, records of each individual animal must be kept. "RCVS Public Statement on Docking" (12 November 1992). These guidelines are now incorporated into the *1993 Guide for Professional Conduct for Veterinary Surgeons.*

13. James Erlichman, "Dog Breeders and Vets Admit Tail Docking Law Is Flouted," *Guardian,* 27 June 1994.

14. Anne Moore and Ginnette Elliot, "CDB Update: RCVS Review of Docking," *Dog World,* 10 March 1995.

15. A membership of six thousand has been claimed. See "One Year On: Council of Docked Breeds Update," *Dog World,* 1 July 1994.

16. F. B. Edwards, "The Practice of Docking," *Veterinary Record* 57, no. 17 (28 April 1945): 208.

17. Association of Veterinarians for Animal Rights, "AVAR Launches Campaign to Stop Docks and Crops on Dogs," *AVAR Directions* 32 (Spring 1993): 1–3.

18. "RCVS Docking Working Party," personal correspondence (1995) between J. S. M. Bower and the Royal College of Veterinary Surgeons.

19. Swedish Docking Survey, "Swedish Tail Injuries in Undocked German Pointers," *Dog World,* 8 November 1991, pp. 4, 61.

20. American Kennel Club, "Surgical Procedures May Affect the Eligibility of Dogs to Compete in Shows," *Journal of the American Veterinary Medical Association* 152 (1968): 62–64.

21. For example, dogs with cropped ears are not permitted to be shown in the United Kingdom, Holland, or Scandinavia but are in other parts of Europe, and in the United States. See *Our Dogs,* 29 October 1993, pp. 10–11.

22. T. L. Gross, and S. H. Carr, "Amputation Neuroma of Docked Tails in Dogs," *Veterinary Pathology* 27 (1990): 61–62.

23. R. A. Mugford, personal communication to Mr. J. Bower, 21 February 1989; W. J. Netto, J. A. M. van der Bourg, and D. J. U. Planta, "The Establishment of Dominance Relationships in a Dog Pack and Its Relevance for the Man-Dog Relationship," *Proceedings of the Royal Netherlands Veterinary Association and the Netherlands Association for Companion Animal Medicine* 117 (1992): 51S–52S.

24. P. G. G. Darke, M. V. Thrusfield, and C. G. G. Aitken, "Association Between Tail Injuries and Docking in Dogs," *Veterinary Record* 116 (13 April 1985): 409.

25. The English pointer, unlike the German pointer, is not docked. The *show* springer

spaniel has a tail docked by two-thirds whereas the *working* springer is docked only by one-third. Great Danes, greyhounds, wolfhounds, and labradors are not infrequently docked as adults for therapeutic reasons, but never as puppies.

26. D. B. Morton "Docking of Dogs: Practical and Ethical Aspects," *Veterinary Record* 131 (1992): 301–6.

27. See Al Vizard, "Tail Docking of Lambs in the Control of Flystrike," *Veterinary Record,* 28 May 1994, p. 583. Also see N. P. French, R. Wall, and K. L. Morgan, "Tail Docking of Lambs in the Control of Flystrike," *Veterinary Record,* 29 July 1994, p. 47.

28. Swedish Kennel Club Pointer Docking Survey, *Dog World,* 8 November 1991, pp. 4, 61; See also Nick Mays, "Sweden Is Set to Lift Docking Ban," *Our Dogs,* 4 August 1995.

16

WHERE SHOULD RESEARCH
SCIENTISTS GET THEIR DOGS?

On 3 July 1965, Fay Brisk, a dedicated humanitarian who had worked for reform of the Pennsylvania dog dealers, called the Animal Welfare Institute for help.[1] A Dalmatian dog, named Pepper, had been stolen from his owners, the Lakavage family, and they were seeking his return. Mr. Lakavage had seen Pepper in a photograph taken of the temporary unloading of animals from a Pennsylvania dog dealer's overcrowded truck. The family, which included three children, set off to find their pet. Pepper allegedly had been taken to a big New York dog dealer, named Nersesian. When the exhausted family arrived at Nersesian, they were refused admission.

The politically active Animal Welfare Institute sought help from Pennsylvania's Senator Joseph Clark, a known friend of animal protection and chief sponsor of then pending legislation to set humane standards for laboratory animal care. Congressman Joseph Y. Resnick was also contacted because his office was in the district where Nersesian's dog farm was located. But intercession from these political forces failed to secure entry for the Lakavage family to the Nersesian farm. Congressman Resnick was so outraged at this that shortly thereafter he introduced a bill into Congress to prevent such practices.

The Animal Welfare Institute tells the story: "Meantime, pressure by State Police brought an admission from the Pennsylvania dog dealer that he had taken his load not to Nersesian, as he had first said, but directly to Montefiore

Hospital in New York. . . . Fay Brisk telephoned the hospital . . . [and learned] the dog had died on the operating table the day before and already had been incinerated. The dog dealer insisted that the dog was not Pepper—the evidence had been incinerated."[2] Congressman Resnick introduced a bill on July 9, 1965, that required licensing of dealers in dogs and cats for laboratories and of the laboratories that purchased them. The bill also required that dealers' premises be federally inspected to ensure adherence to humane standards.

Dognapping, as the theft of pet dogs was called, became a national issue when, some months later, *Life* magazine ran the story "Concentration Camps for Dogs," which recounted stories of pet thefts and which carried horrifying pictures of filthy, inhumane conditions at dog dealers' farms.[3] Recounted also were the personal stories of pet owners whose dogs had been safely retrieved from the laboratories of the National Institutes of Health and Harvard Medical School.

After the *Life* exposé, the Resnick bill won rapid passage and played an important role in motivating the 1966 Laboratory Animal Welfare Act, the first US legislation to govern humane standards for laboratory animals and their acquisition. Pepper's name has gone down in animal legislative history: At the 1996 celebration hosted by the US Department of Agriculture (USDA) of thirty

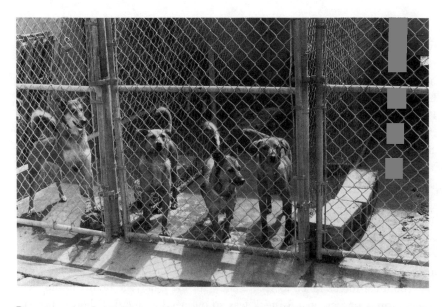

Dogs are group-housed in runs that allow both outdoor and indoor shelter at this facility run by the American Humane Association in Englewood, Colorado. The dogs remain only on a temporary basis and may eventually be either adopted or killed. Credit: American Humane Association, Englewood, CO.

years' enforcement of the Animal Welfare Act which was the subsequent name of the 1996 Act, guests were invited to wear a lapel button bearing his picture.

LEGAL USE OF PET ANIMALS IN LABORATORIES

Under the new law, laboratories became far more determined to avoid the embarrassment of pet owners finding their still-wanted pets on the operating table; in the future, the acquisition of dogs would have to be made in a scrupulously legal manner. There was one avenue of acquisition that was already widely practiced—namely, the use of dogs from city animal shelters. Shelter animals (also variously called pound or random-source animals) include dogs no longer wanted by their owners, strays, and lost animals. Because suitable homes cannot be found for many of these animals, they have to be killed. But instead of killing them, some shelters have developed a lucrative trade of selling these animals to laboratories, either directly, or through an animal dealer.

When the owners of dogs found in shelters no longer want their pets, researchers believe that they are justified in using these animals for experimental purposes. Humane organizations, however, are opposed to the practice of using shelter animals in labs: they claim that shelters should be sanctuaries for pet animals, not a means whereby dogs are placed in potentially painful experiments in alien environments. This bitter controversy between researchers and humane societies goes back several decades and is still politically unstable.

HISTORICAL BACKGROUND

In 1945 the biomedical research and education community became serious about obtaining shelter animals. It established an organization, the National Society for Medical Research (NSMR), whose primary purpose was to work for passage of laws that would make it mandatory for shelters to hand over dogs and cats for research and teaching. The demand for research dogs had risen dramatically with the vastly increased federal funding for biomedical research immediately after World War II. The country was enjoying increased affluence and the household pet population rose dramatically. Along with this came irresponsible pet ownership and consequent pet overpopulation. More animals ended up in shelters than homes could accommodate, and these animals provided a convenient, cheap source of laboratory animals.

Despite the resistance of shelters to giving up their animals for research, NSMR was generally successful. Several states enacted laws to legalize the use of shelter dogs in labs. But over time, resistance mounted. In the early 1950s some community leaders formed new humane organizations, still active today, to counter the efforts of the biomedical community. These organizations included the Animal Welfare Institute, The Humane Society of the United States, and the American Humane Association.

The new humane societies tried to control the vast overpopulation of dogs and cats by launching public-education programs about responsible pet ownership, establishing low-cost spay and neuter clinics, and pressing for mandatory neutering of dogs and cats. However, the problem was out of hand; shelters found that one of their major tasks was to destroy animals because enough adoptive homes could not be found.

Pet overpopulation peaked in the 1980s, when it was estimated that as many as 8 to 10 million dogs and cats were destroyed in shelters annually.[4] By 1996, this figure had fallen to an estimated 6 to 8 million, due at least to some extent to persistent efforts to promote sterilization of pets.

Struggles continued in the state legislatures, and by early 1996 the tally was the following: 14 states had enacted laws that forbade use of shelter animals; 6 states specifically affirmed use of shelter animals; 6 states had laws that permit use of shelter animals. In the other states without specific laws, the use of shelter animals sometimes occurs. Political conflicts occur at the city level also, and with similarly mixed results.

Along with this trade, pet theft continues to be a problem. "Help Stop the Scandalous Trade in Stolen Pets" was the headline of a "Dear Colleague" letter dated 16 September 1993, from Congressman George E. Brown Jr., an influential politician on laboratory animal legislation.[5] In this letter, Brown comments on a CBS report about recently documented cases of theft of pets to be sold for use in medical research, and he cites a recent book by Judith Reitman entitled *Stolen for Profit.* Brown argues that the USDA has not acted to end these abuses.

Aware of these problems, the USDA announced amendments to the Animal Welfare Act regulations to help prevent the use of lost and stolen pets.[6] Under these regulations, which took effect 23 August 1993, shelters must hold dogs and cats for at least five days, including a Saturday, before releasing them to dealers. Prior to this regulation, USDA officials estimated that most shelters held their animals for about three days before releasing them to dealers, insufficient time for a number of owners to reclaim their animals. Congressional interest in pet theft is still active. In the 104th Congress in 1996, two new bills (HR 3393 and HR 3398) were introduced to help ensure that all dogs and cats used by research facilities are obtained legally.

Over the years, new groups have been established to fight this issue. For the biomedical community, the most politically active group is the National Association for Biomedical Research (NABR), an organization that assimilated the older NSMR. Influential groups such as the American Medical Association, the American Physiological Society, and the American Veterinary Medical Association defend positions similar to those of NABR. This constituency supports the continuance of animal experimentation and use of shelter animals for this purpose.

In 1985 the opposition to these groups sought to strengthen its base by forming a coalition: eleven humane societies and antivivisection organizations established ProPets specifically to oppose NABR on the shelter dog issue.[7] But the coalition lasted only four years; the organizations could not reach agreement on whether or not to foster the use of purpose-bred animals (animals bred specifically for laboratory use). But since the breakup of ProPets, the individual organizations have continued their efforts independently.

Patterns in laboratory dog use have changed over the years. Numerically, use has declined in the last twelve years from 202,000 in 1984 to 82,454 in 1996.[8]

Anecdotal evidence suggests that researchers now prefer to use pigs, ferrets, and other species that are less in the public eye. Thus, a decrease in the use of dogs does not mean a decrease in the use of other animals for the same purposes.

There has also been a trend toward greater use of purpose-bred dogs, as opposed to shelter dogs. In the 1950s and 1960s, the use of shelter dogs was at an all-time high in some facilities, representing 100% of all dogs used; by 1989, shelter dogs represented about 60% of all dogs used; the other 40% were purpose-bred and came from commercial breeders.[9] This proportion has remained about the same to 1996. Hoffmann–La Roche, the pharmaceutical company, has used only purpose-bred animals since 1979.[10]

In response to the growing demands for purpose-bred dogs, commercial breeders have stepped up their production efforts. In 1984 for instance, Hazelton Laboratories started a purpose-bred dog colony in Cumberland, Virginia and within five years was producing approximately 13,000 animals per year for research. Here, beagles are kept from birth to the time of sale. Once a day, for 10 to 15 minutes, human handlers pet the animals to socialize and prepare them for their later life in a laboratory. This petting is critical to socialization, especially during the three-to-seven-weeks stage of development, and socialized animals bring a higher price to the breeder.

In some countries there has been a long tradition of using only purpose-bred dogs for research—for example, in England, Sweden, Holland, and Denmark. The Council of Europe in 1985 began a cooperative endeavor involving several European countries; they pronounced that dogs and cats "shall originate from registered breeding establishments. . . . Straying animals of a domesticated species shall not be used in [experimental] procedures."[11]

CONTEMPORARY USES OF LABORATORY DOGS

Dogs are used as subjects for a wide variety of scientific experiments for research on cardiovascular disease, bone injuries, hearing loss, blindness, lung disorders, and infectious diseases. They are also used for testing that involves either development of new drugs or the safety testing of drugs for problems such as adverse side effects. Among the procedures used in the research are induced heart attack in a conscious animal, exposure to infectious diseases or lethally toxic agents, and multiple surgeries. Some projects can continue for months, even years. Dogs are also used for educational purposes to demonstrate basic physiological and pharmacological principles and for practice surgery—the so-called dog labs in medical schools. Some of these procedures are painful in that the animals are permitted to recover consciousness from (sometimes unskilled) surgery; other procedures may be pain-free if the animal is killed without being allowed to recover consciousness. All involve eventual death.

By law, experiments involving dogs (and certain other species) have to be approved by an Institutional Animal Care and Use Committee, an oversight committee for compliance with nationally accepted humane standards including minimization of pain. (See chapter 1, pp. 38–41.) But the operative humane standards do not address the choice between shelter and purpose-bred animals. They require only that the animal is legally acquired, either purchased from a dealer or directly from a shelter or commercial breeder. Dominated by scientist members, no oversight committee is known to have banned the use of shelter animals. The mainstream view among scientists is expressed in an official statement of the American Physiological Society: "[T]he denial of the availability of random source animals would be a catastrophic setback and the Society strongly endorses the continued use of unclaimed pound animals for basic and clinical research and teaching."[12]

Are suitable alternatives available for shelter animals that would constitute a lesser ethical problem? One answer would be, yes, don't use dogs at all; another would be, yes, use purpose-bred animals. However, there are difficulties with substituting purpose-bred animals with shelter animals. One is the financial burden. According to NABR, "The high cost of acquiring purpose-bred animals to replace random-source dogs and cats may price many research projects out of existence."[13] According to officials of the American Medical Association, stopping the use of shelter animals for research "would dismantle medical research . . . medical advances would be compromised."[14] A representative of the Society for Neuroscience asserts that not using shelter animals would be "a major loss for the future of health and society."[15] That these claims are exaggerated is borne out by experience both in some American states and several other countries where shelter animals are not available.

The *New York Times* reported that in 1996 dealers typically purchased dogs from shelters for $15 and resold them to laboratories for $250.[16] According to NABR, purpose-bred animals can cost from $260 to $995, according to breed and status.[17] Michael DeBakey, the heart surgeon and then president of the NABR, estimated in 1987 that a total ban on shelter animals would add $70 million per year to research costs, reducing the amount of money available for research each year.[18] Others thought these figures were exaggerated and misleading.[19]

The reasoning is that the cost of using research animals is the acquisition cost plus the utilization cost. The longer the animal lives, the higher the utilization cost and the less significant proportionally becomes the purchase price. For any animals kept for any length of time, the initial purchase price becomes less important in relation to the overwhelmingly larger utilization costs. So, for long-term experiments of weeks, months, or years, it is misleading to assess financial costs only in terms of acquisition costs.

Buying cheap animals also may not be an economy. Geneticist Michael Festing argues that the use of shelter animals may compromise the validity of the research results because of the uncertain and often inferior health status of these animals.[20] Also, additional costs might be incurred because greater numbers of animals have to be used to compensate for the many sicknesses and deaths among these dogs. According to Festing, upgrading the quality of biomedical research requires upgrading the quality of the animals used.

Neither of the two federal agencies responsible for the oversight of safety testing involving animal use has specific policies that prohibit the use of shelter animals; nevertheless, in practice, shelter animals are not used by all those whom they oversee. A spokesperson for the Food and Drug Administration states, "Pharmaceutical researchers generally do not use shelter animals (random source animals) for drug testing" because of concern that some random source animals may "actually be pets that have been illegally acquired" and also because the health status and age of shelter animals is ill defined; hence "it may be difficult to reproduce research results."[21] Similarly, the Environmental Protection Agency "require[s] certification that any animals [they] receive are free of various microbes, for example, viruses and parasites."[22] In effect, this means that shelter animals are not used.

As is recognized by these federal agencies, selecting a uniform subject sample is often desirable or essential to an experimental design. Sound methodology involves eliminating variables to the point where there is only one variable to be tested. This would eliminate the use of shelter animals where there are many variables in the subject animal—breed, age, pathological history, upbringing, experience—all of which could affect the scientific results. Also, spurious scientific results could occur because shelter animals can be stressed animals, lacking physiological normality. They may even exhibit long-term pathological damage (for example heartworm, which would make them less than ideal for cardiac research). Random-source dogs that carry infectious diseases can be a source of risk for their human handlers.

Some scientists argue that, for selected experimental purposes, the use of shelter animals represents sound judgment. Indeed, the lack of uniformity among random-source dogs is viewed as a plus, because the subjects better mimic the population of human beings that come to be treated in hospitals; the human population comprises different races, ages, and genetic composition, and each individual has a different medical history.

ETHICAL ISSUES

Assessing the Benefits and the Harms

One approach to the justification and criticism of contemporary practices involving shelter dogs is to make a cost-benefit assessment (see chapter 1). This method of analysis attempts to weigh the total harms against the total benefits to determine the highest net benefit for all affected parties.

On the benefits side, several claims have been made. One view is that biomedical research is generally a worthy activity that leads to the improvement in quality of human life and the reduction of suffering. Furthermore, when shelter animals are suitable for certain experiments, their use can be justified if the benefits are relatively high. Some of these animals are doomed to die if not claimed as pets, so is it not better that they die for a good cause? Any pain and suffering is justified if the human benefit outweighs the cost to the dogs. Proponents of this view argue that restrictions on the use of shelter animals hampers a socially important activity.

On the harms side it is argued that a dog is likely to experience considerable pain and suffering as a laboratory subject. The degree of likely pain or suffering has to be considered case by case: it can vary according to the nature of the research procedure (minor for a nonrecovery procedure under anesthesia but major if used in a long-term experiment involving, say, induction of a heart attack). It can also vary according to the animal's previous history and other factors.

Comparison of Purpose-Bred and Shelter Animals

The life history of an animal prior to entering a laboratory is relevant in assessing harms. According to one view, animals specifically bred for laboratory use are a preferred refinement to using shelter dogs because they are likely to suffer less. Purpose-bred animals have endured lifelong restrictions in living space at both the breeders' and research facilities and a permanently restricted way of life regarding diet, reproduction, and so on. They have no choice in cage mates, if cage mates even exist, and have few opportunities to make choices in general. Since they have a more impoverished life to begin with, the argument can be made that they appear to suffer less from deprivation, confined quarters, and the like when used for many research purposes.

Shelter animals, on the other hand, have led more varied lives. Initially, almost all of them, at some time, will have lived as companions to human beings and will have enjoyed certain freedoms and choices not usually available to the purpose-bred animal. They have probably never lived in a cage alone, which is a common fate in a laboratory. Their lives have been relatively rich in stimuli; they have known affection from humans and social relations with other animals; they are used to variety in their environment and food. From the dog's point of view, might it not be better to be painlessly killed at the shelter (when a home cannot be found) than to have a longer life but one that involves assured predictive harms in a laboratory?

For animals, as with humans, new situations can bring additional stresses, including severe new restrictions. For instance, it is natural for pet dogs to mark their territory by frequent urination to leave scents, but when held in a laboratory cage, this behavior has to be suppressed because of space confinement. Some cages have not even allowed room for a dog to lift its leg to urinate. When there is little or no opportunity to express their previously learned behavioral repertoire, dogs suffer. Do these facts constitute a sufficient justification for using purpose-bred dogs rather than shelter dogs?

Harms from Transportation and Handling

For many shelter animals, the trip to the laboratory door can be traumatic. The accompanying diagram illustrates the routes by which animals reach the laboratory. Most commonly, shelter animals are sold to a dealer who often acts as a middleman. Sometimes they are traded repeatedly among dealers. Typically they will spend from five to thirty days in any one facility and they are subjected to potentially traumatic changes and possible contact with sick animals throughout this waiting period.

By comparison, purpose-bred animals are taken from the commercial facility directly to the laboratory. As a result, the potential for neglect and mistreatment is much less. Judging from the number of convictions for violation of Animal Welfare Act standards, dealers who trade in shelter dogs are much more likely to treat animals poorly than are commercial breeders.

**SOURCE AND TRADING ROUTES OF
LABORATORY DOGS AND CATS**

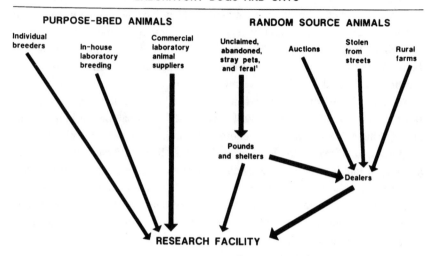

In this schematic representation, routes by which dogs and cats arrive at the laboratory door are shown. The two major routes are from commercial animal dealers or shelters and animal control agencies; several minor routes are also shown. An additional source, not shown here, is of retired and injured greyhounds from the race track. The dealers depicted, so-called class B dealers, who do not breed animals, have to be licensed under the Animal Welfare Act to trade in random source animals. Credit: Dr. F. Barbara Orlans, Georgetown University, Washington, D.C.

The Issue of Pet Overpopulation

Animal advocates claim that the pet overpopulation problem is being exploited as a rationale for using shelter animals. Their view is that the overpopulation of pet animals should be dealt with as a serious problem in itself; the pet trade should not overlap with the research animal trade. The problems inherent in overbreeding should not be confounded by establishing a profitable market for "surplus" animals. The fear is that if such a market is developed, then it will be even harder to try to control unwanted breeding.

Handing over animals for research may adversely affect community efforts to stem pet overpopulation. Evidence for this thesis is provided by S. Shurman, who surveyed 28 city and county shelters in Michigan and found that those shelters that released animals for research were "the least developed in terms of efforts to prevent pet overpopulation."[23]

The presence of a market for former pets increases the possibility of a black market in stolen pets. Despite formal regulations to discourage it, the unscrupulous theft of pets is not likely to be halted. The profits from selling dogs are too compelling. In some measure, pet-napping would be reduced if only purpose-bred animals were used in research.

Are Two Lives Lost Instead of One?

It has been argued that if researchers are denied shelter animals then "more dogs and cats will die," thereby imposing a heavier ethical burden on society.[24] The Foundation for Biomedical Research and its sister organization NABR argue that if a shelter animal is not used, then two animals would die instead of one—a shelter animal in addition to a purpose-bred animal.[25] The implication is that the use of a shelter animal, which will die anyway, saves another animal from being born and killed for human use and helps justify the use of shelter animals. Similarly, WARDS (Working for Animals used in Research, Drugs, and Surgery) argues its case for pound seizure (mandatory release of shelter animals for research) by stating: "When [shelter] animals are not turned over for research, the number that suffer and die are increased needlessly because scientists turn to another avenue for supply."[26]

This argument is a form of utilitarian justification, but is there a fallacy at work? Critics have countered that taking two lives instead of one is an oversimplification because it is not true that if a shelter animal is not available then a purpose-bred animal will be used. There are other possibilities: The investigator may decide to use a different species of animal, or to pursue a different research approach that does not use animals at all, or to abandon that line of research altogether.

Furthermore, the "two deaths are worse than one death" argument suggests that one dog death is morally equal to another dog death and that one dog life equals another dog life. If all dog deaths were judged morally equal, then the death of a wild dog, a laboratory dog, or a pet dog would all be of equal moral significance. Yet human beings typically make keen distinctions among dogs in different circumstances and have a different sense of obligation toward them. With a wild dog, a person feels no obligation to treat the animal when sick or to intervene to prevent a painful death. With a purpose-bred laboratory animal held in human captivity, a researcher is obliged to treat untoward sickness and to provide a painless death, but no obligation not to induce lethal diseases or to shorten that animal's life at will. The owner of a companion dog has an obligation to treat the animals' sickness, provide a painless death where possible, and not to cause the animal pain or suffering purposefully.

Thus, an argument can be made that wild, laboratory, and pet dogs are not "equal" and do not normally carry the same types or levels of human obligation. Such reasoning leads to the conclusion that we have different obligations and likely a lower level of obligations to purpose-bred dogs.

The Special Relationship of Humans
with Domesticated Animals

In *The Little Prince,* Antoine de Saint-Exupéry explains what it is that makes a pet a pet. The prince asks, "What does that mean—'tame'?" and the fox replies: "It means to establish ties. . . . To you, I am [now] nothing more than a fox like a hundred thousand other foxes. But if you tame me, then we shall need each other. To me, you will be unique in all the world. To you, I shall be unique in all the world. . . . But you must not forget it. You become responsible, forever, for what you have tamed."[27]

Similarly, those who want to protect shelter animals from ending up in laboratories believe that pet animals have a specially protected status that should not be violated. By having companion animals, humans, as a group, have obligated themselves to protect pets, as a group, from certain harms—such as being used as subjects in experiments. Humans incur an enhanced obligation to pet animals that is lacking in their relations with dogs bred specifically for experimentation. Can one population of dogs (not merely an individual dog), permissibly be treated differently than another population of dogs?

For example, should a shelter animal continue to enjoy the status of a pet? Opinions range from the view that shelter animals are "commodities" to the view that shelter animals are primarily pets and "once a pet, always a pet," which does introduce a morally relevant difference among different dog populations.

From the total population of shelter animals, it is the well-treated companion animal that is most likely to end up in a laboratory. Typically the shelter population comprises approximately 50% strays and 50% relinquished pets, according to a 1985 survey by the American Humane Association.[28] Unless a new home is found for them, they will either be sold to dealers and may end up in research labs, or they are euthanized. The shelter animals likely to be selected by dealers are those that show unmistakable signs of close association with humans in their friendliness and obedience to human commands. Since many more shelter animals are available than are needed for research, the most friendly, obedient, and easily handled animals tend to be chosen first. Approximately 40,000 dogs per year purchased by dealers end up in laboratories.

But according to a long-held view of NABR, "the small number of abandoned shelter dogs and cats used for research and education are not people's pets. Rather, they are unwanted animals, often abandoned, whose owners have not claimed them or for which adoptive homes cannot be found."[29] That is, once "abandoned," a dog loses its status as a pet. Another interest group, WARDS, with similar views of advocating the use of shelter animals for research, refers to a pet animal as a "prime commodity,"[30] which suggests that a pet is primarily an article of commerce or economic good.

John McArdle, formerly of The Humane Society of the United States, has a different view: "We define a pet from the perspective of the cat or dog and its socialization history with and expectations of humans. It is irrelevant to that definition whether or not the owner remains with the animal."[31] Phil Arkow, a representative from another humane society, shares that perspective: "Inasmuch as most, if not all, strays were once someone's pet," none of them should be used for "questionable purposes."[32]

Are Shelters Sanctuaries?

Another argument against the use of shelter animals is that it violates the central purpose of shelters—to be sanctuaries for lost and abandoned animals. Giannelli, the ProPets former director, wrote that use of shelter animals for research is "a direct invasion of the heart of the animal protection movement, a breach in the wall of what were intended to be places of last refuge and protective sanctuary for animals."[33] Taking shelter animals for research "interferes with everything humane societies represent and attempt to accomplish," said McArdle.[34]

Humane societies argue that they have a hard enough job, as is, in persuading the public to bring in unwanted pets to local shelters rather than abandoning them to the streets. The difficulty increases if the animals coming in through the front door are seen shipped out the back door for sale to laboratories. Shelters that release animals for research could also suffer financially because some people would not support such practices.

A counterargument is that city run animal control agencies (as opposed to privately funded humane shelters) do not have to operate as sanctuaries and have often never been conceived in this role by the municipalities that fund them. From this perspective, shelters have only a responsibility to the public to remove unwanted animals that may be a public nuisance. If not used by laboratories, these "surplus" animals are going to be killed at the shelter, so why not make some human use of the live animal? Under this conception of a shelter, which course is preferable for the animal: a quick and painless death or a longer life as a research subject? This question may not be answerable in the abstract, because so much depends on the particular laboratory and particular use of the dog in research. Yet the formulation of policy often cannot await such contingencies.

Human Uses of Dead Animals

Not only live, but also dead animals can serve human ends. Shelters face an ethical problem in disposing of 6 to 8 million dog and cat carcasses produced each year. There are several options: use them as landfill, incinerate the bodies, or pay to have them carted away to "protein plants" that render down the bodies to make animal food, fertilizer, glue, and ingredients for some cosmetics. The use as landfill has diminished because of environmental laws and currently accounts for about 30% of the carcasses: another 30% are incinerated, and 40% are rendered in "protein plants."

The generally preferred route of incineration is not feasible for a number of shelters because it is too costly to purchase and run the equipment. So shelter managers have little choice other than to provide material for the "protein plants." This choice is often made with reluctance because of the perceived desecration of the animals' bodies; but when budgets are tight, is there any realistic alternative?

An Ethical Compromise?

A compromise solution—one that has not been substantially tried in the United States—is to limit the use of shelter animals to certain purposes. For example, they could be retained in the laboratory only for short-term, nonsurvival experiments in which the animal is dead within 24 hours of leaving the shelter. The rationale is that, from the animal's perspective, there is little difference in terms of pain or suffering. The animal is going to die soon anyhow, and providing that high standards of humaneness are maintained after leaving the shelter for transportation and overnight housing, then death in the laboratory is really only a slightly delayed euthanasia.

For such a policy to work, certain restrictions would have to apply: (1) the animal must be used within 24 hours of leaving the shelter and only used for nonsurvival experiments in which the animal is either killed immediately or fully anesthetized and never allowed to recover consciousness until death; (2) the animals should be obtained directly by the USDA-registered research facility from the shelter, not through a dealer; and (3) this policy should not apply to shelters that fund animal control programs with *private* funds, but only to facilities such as shelters that receive *public* funds to operate animal control programs. The rationale of the latter provision is that shelters receiving only private funds should be free to operate as they choose, but those that receive public funds incur obligations.

The advantages of this "acute-study" proposal is that the animals' measure of suffering is not appreciably increased. Also, an inexpensive source of dogs and cats is provided that is suitable for some scientific purposes.

CONCLUSION

Increasingly in recent years, public opinion has affected the way that animal experimentation is conducted, and reasonable limits have been set on a number of previously unregulated practices. If limits were set on the use of shelter animals for short-term nonsurvival research projects that would ensure the death of the animal within 24 hours of arrival at a laboratory, some of the heat of this debate over use of shelter animals would likely subside. Also, if the source of laboratory dogs were limited to commercial breeders, then the possibility of pet theft would likely be reduced, and some shelter animals would be given a painless death rather than becoming subjects of research. At present, no one seems to have a comprehensive answer to the several questions raised by our current uses of either shelter dogs or purpose-bred dogs.

NOTES

1. Christine Stevens, "Laboratory Animal Welfare," in *Animals and Their Legal Rights: A Survey of American Laws from 1641 to 1990,* 4th ed. (Washington: Animal Welfare Institute, 1990), pp. 73–75.

2. Ibid., p. 74.

3. Stan Wayman, "Concentration Camps for Dogs," *Life,* 4 February 1966, pp. 22–29. See also chapter 1 of the present volume for the historical importance of this article.

4. Andrew Rowan and Alexandra Wilson, eds., *Animal Management and Population Control: What Progress Have We Made?* (Boston: Tufts University School of Veterinary Medicine Center for Animals, 1985).

5. George E. Brown, Jr. (U.S. House of Representatives), "Help Stop the Scandalous Trade in Stolen Pets," letter to colleagues, 16 September 1993.

6. "USDA Announces Amendment to the Animal Welfare Act," *AWIC Newsletter* 4 (July/September 1993): 13.

7. Michael A. Giannelli, "Dogs and Cats by the Pound," *Humane Society News,* Summer 1985, p. 22.

8. United States Department of Agriculture, *Animal Welfare Enforcement* (Beltsville, MD: United States Department of Agriculture, annual reports, 1984 and 1996).

9. Thomas L. Wolfle, director, Institute of Laboratory Animal Resources, National Academy of Sciences, personal communication, 11 July 1989.

10. Martin Hirsch, director, Public Relations, Hoffmann–La Roche Inc., Nutley, NJ, personal communication, July 8, 1994.

11. Council of Europe, article 21, *European Convention for the Protection of Vertebrate Animals Used for Experimental and Other Scientific Purposes,* memorandum prepared by the Directorate of Legal Affairs, 4 June 1985, Strasbourg, France.

12. American Physiological Society, *Statements on Animal Usage: Pound Animals* (American Physiological Society, Washington: 1986).

13. NABR [National Association for Biomedical Research], *NABR Issue Update: The Use of Dogs and Cats in Research and Education* (Washington, DC: NABR, 1994).

14. Steven Smith and William Hendee, "Animals in Research," *Journal of the American Medical Association* 259 (1 April 1988): 2007–8.

15. Robert E. Burke, "The Role of Scientific Organizations in Humane Animal Research," in *National Symposium on Imperatives in Research Animal Use: Scientific Need and Animal Welfare* (Bethesda, MD: US Department of Health and Human Services, PHS, NIH, 1984), p. 318.

16. Evelyn Nieves, "Agency Fails to Protect Pets, Critics Say," *New York Times,* 5 February 1996, p. B7.

17. NABR, *NABR Issue Update: The Use of Dogs and Cats in Research and Education.* NABR 1994.

18. Michael E. DeBakey, "So Where Will Researchers Get Their Dogs?" *Washington Post,* 25 July 1987, p. A13.

19. Michael A. Giannelli, "The Decline and Fall of Pound Seizure," *Animals' Agenda* (July/August 1986): 36; Robert J. Mrazek, "The Least We Owe to Animals That Are Sent to Shelters," *Washington Post,* 25 June 1987, p. A17.

20. Michael Festing, "Bad Animals Mean Bad Science," *New Scientist* 3 (20 January 1977): 130–31.

21. May-Alice Miller, chief, Communication and Education Branch, Center for Veterinary Medicine, Food and Drug Administration, Public Health Service, Rockville, Maryland, personal communication, 14 September 1994.

22. Richard Hill, science advisor, United States Environmental Protection Agency, personal communication, 9 August 1994.

23. S. Shurman, "The Case Against Pound Release," *Shelter Life,* Summer 1985, p. 5.

24. NABR, *NABR Issue Update: The Use of Dogs and Cats in Research and Education.*

25. Foundation for Biomedical Research, *The Use of Pound/Shelter Animals in Biomedical Research and Education* (Washington: 1990), p. 8; NABR, *NABR Issue Update,* 1994.

26. WARDS [Working for Animals used in Research, Drugs, and Surgery], *The WARDS Credo: A Different Way to Care for Forty Years* (Washington: WARDS, Summer 1993).

27. Antoine de Saint-Exupéry, *The Little Prince* (New York: Harcourt, Brace & World, 1943), pp. 66, 71.

28. American Humane Association, "The American Humane Animal Shelter Reporting Study: Some Preliminary Results," *Advocate* 3 (Winter 1985): 14.

29. NABR, *NABR Issue Update: The Use of Dogs and Cats in Research and Education.*

30. WARDS, *WARDS Credo.*

31. John McArdle, "People You Should Know," *Physiologist* 28 (1985): 70.

32. Phil Arkow, "Animal Control, Animal Welfare, and the Veterinarian," *Journal of the American Veterinary Medical Association* 191 (15 October 1987): 940.

33. Giannelli, "Decline and Fall," p. 35.

34. McArdle, "People You Should Know," p. 71.

IX

RELIGIOUS RIGHTS

17

ANIMAL SACRIFICE
AS RELIGIOUS RITUAL:
THE SANTERIA CASE

In the spring of 1987, a controversy arose in the city of Hialeah, Florida. It began when Ernesto Pichardo, the president and priest of the Church of the Lukumi Babalu Aye, issued a public statement on the church's plan to build a worship and education center on city land that the church previously had leased. The announcement triggered discussion and debate among residents of Hialeah, some of whom were opposed to the church's plan.[1] Before the controversy subsided, the US Supreme Court had become involved. The case raises issues about balancing the interests of nonhuman animals against the interests of humans, in particular, the human interests incorporated in First Amendment protection of the free exercise of religion.

The opposition originated in concerns about the sacrifice of animals, a practice associated with the Church of the Lukumi Babalu Aye. Members of the church practice a religion called Santeria. This religion began in the sixteenth century, among Cuban slaves who had been removed from their East African homes. The slaves belonged to the Yoruba people, who practiced a traditional religion in Africa. In Cuba, the Yoruba were not permitted to practice their religion openly. They were often baptized as Christians without their consent before being forced onto the Spanish ships that took them to Cuba.

In response, many Yoruba practitioners incorporated their traditional faith into the Roman Catholic religion. In this merging of the two religions, traditional spirits and symbols among the Yoruba became identified with various Christian saints and symbols. The assimilated references to Christian doctrine enabled Santeria believers to practice their religion more openly, reducing the possibility of persecution and stigma.[2]

The exact number of Santeria believers in the United States is unknown. According to one recent estimate, there are about fifty to sixty thousand practitioners in the southern part of Florida. Other areas with high concentrations of believers are New York City, northern New Jersey, and Los Angeles.[3] Santeria also has adherents in Cuba, Puerto Rico, and Venezuela.[4]

THE RITUAL SACRIFICE IN SANTERIA

A traditional activity that remains important to Santeria believers is the ritual sacrifice of animals. According to Santeria, God has a destiny for each person. To fulfill their destinies, people rely on the help of certain spirits, called *orishas*. Animal sacrifice is viewed as an important way to express one's devotion to the orishas. Indeed, because the orishas are seen as living beings, their very

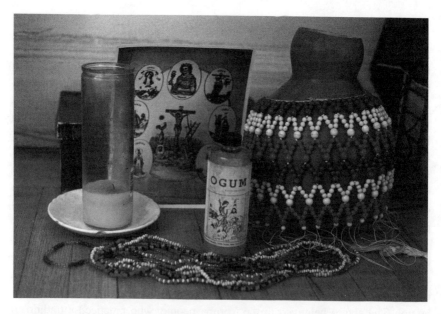

This assemblage of Santeria-related objects includes a votive candle; a picture of Seven African Powers representing deities, saints, and Christ; a canister of a bath mixture thought to confer the influence of the African deity Ogum on the bather; a set of necklaces worn by devotees; and a Shekere, a musical instrument used to accompany ritual chants. Credit: Professor George Brandon, CUNY Medical School, New York.

survival is dependent on receiving food from their devotees.[5] Ceremonies involving animal sacrifice are conducted when new members enter the church; to mark births, deaths, and marriages among members; to heal the sick; and as part of a yearly holiday observance. Based on figures provided by Pichardo, an estimated 12,000 to 15,000 animals are sacrificed each year as part of church initiation ceremonies conducted in the Hialeah area.[6]

Partially due to the stigma and persecution experienced by Santeria practitioners, the church does not have a central authority, a training system for its priests, or written documents setting forth its principles, rituals, and ceremonies. At present much Santeria worship is conducted in private, in groups whose members and priests often have little contact with other Santeria practitioners. As a result, there is some variation among different groups in how animal sacrifice is performed.

According to the statements of Pichardo, as well as other documents admitted as evidence in legal proceedings on the church's building proposal, chickens, pigeons, goats, doves, guinea pigs, ducks, sheep, and turtles are sacrificed in Santeria rituals. Priests are taught the method of sacrifice as apprentices, through observing and assisting more-experienced priests. For the sacrifice, the animal is held on its side while the priest raises the animal's head with one hand and with the other hand inserts a knife about four inches long into the right side of the animal's neck and then pushes the knife through the entire neck. The knife is not inserted into the animals' throat, but into an area behind the throat and in front of the vertebra. The goal is to puncture the animal's two main neck arteries with one movement, producing death rapidly.

A veterinarian and scientist from The Humane Society of the United States participating in the legal proceedings testified that "this method of killing is not humane because there is no guarantee that a person performing a sacrifice in the manner described can cut through both carotid arteries at the same time."[7] In addition, certain physiological events may occur in the animal, particularly in young goats and sheep, to prolong the experience of pain and distress prior to death. Moreover, chickens have four carotid arteries, which makes it more difficult to achieve success with one cut.

Other aspects of the Santeria ritual also raise animal welfare concerns. Because numerous animals may be sacrificed as part of a single ceremony, various species of animals are at times gathered in one room prior to sacrifice, and exposed to the noise and bodily secretions produced by the nearby animal being killed. As a result, they may detect that animal's pain and fear, and may themselves experience fear and distress prior to their own sacrifice. Many of the animals killed in Santeria ceremonies are raised specifically for sacrifice, and may receive inadequate food, water, and housing during the course of their lives.

RESPONSES IN THE HIALEAH COMMUNITY

Some Hialeah residents were disturbed by the impact of animal sacrifice on people in the community. In the usual Santeria procedure, the sacrificed animal's blood is collected in clay pots, which are then offered to the orishas. The animal's head is cut off, and the blood and body remain for a longer period. In some ceremonies, flesh from the animal is cooked and eaten; in others it is discarded. According to court testimony, animals' remains are often found in public places in Hialeah, creating a possible health hazard. Concern was also expressed by Hialeah citizens about the possible psychological effects the sacrifice procedures could have on children observing the ritual.

Their concern that members of the Church of the Lukumi Babalu Aye would engage in animal sacrifice led members of the Hialeah City Council to take a series of formal actions designed to discourage the practice. Two resolutions and four ordinances were enacted, by unanimous vote. The resolutions expressed the city's desire to prohibit and oppose "public ritualistic animal sacrifices" and "all acts of any and all religious groups which are inconsistent with public morals, peace or safety."[8]

The ordinances (1) incorporated Florida's anticruelty statute, which provides for criminal punishment of anyone who "unnecessarily or cruelly" kills animals;[9] (2) prohibited the possession of animals for the purpose of ritual slaughter, whether or not the animals were to be eaten as food, with an exemption for slaughtering of food animals carried out by licensed facilities; (3) made it illegal to sacrifice animals (defined as "to unnecessarily kill . . . an animal in a . . . ritual or ceremony not for the primary purpose of food consumption") within city limits, based on a finding that the activity conflicted with "the public health, safety, welfare and morals of the community;"[10] and (4) permitted animal slaughter solely in places zoned for that activity, with an exemption for commercial establishments processing "small numbers of hogs and/or cattle" each week, in accordance with state law.

In addition, the city obtained an opinion from the state attorney general asserting that "ritual sacrifice of animals for purposes other than food consumption" should be defined as "unnecessary" and a violation of the state's anticruelty law.[11] Persons found guilty of violating any of the four ordinances could be imprisoned for up to sixty days and fined up to five hundred dollars.

Pichardo went to federal court to challenge the ordinances as impermissibly interfering with the constitutional right of Santeria believers to practice their religion. Although the trial judge found that the ordinances had the effect of burdening church members' religious conduct, he determined that Hialeah's actions were justified by four compelling governmental interests: (1) protecting the health of city residents, who might be exposed to disease from the decaying bodies of sacrificed animals, as well as the health of participants in the Santeria ceremonies, who could become ill from ingesting uninspected meat; (2) protecting the emotional health of children exposed to animal sacrifice; (3) protecting animals from inhumane killing methods and living conditions; and (4) restricting animal slaughter to areas zoned for that activity. Moreover, the judge determined that a total prohibition of animal sacrifice was constitutionally permissible, because any less-restrictive attempt to regulate the activity to protect the city's interests would be ineffective, due to the private nature of most Santeria ceremonies.[12]

This decision was appealed to the US Court of Appeals for the Eleventh Circuit, which affirmed the decision without discussing it in detail.[13] But then Pichardo petitioned the US Supreme Court to hear the case, and it agreed.

THE SUPREME COURT DECISION

Six years after the church announced its building plans, the Supreme Court issued an opinion striking down Hialeah's ordinances on grounds that they unconstitutionally interfered with the Santeria religion. All nine Supreme Court justices agreed that the ordinances violated the Constitution. Justice Anthony Kennedy wrote the majority opinion. In it, he cited a number of problems with the ordinances, based on the Court's previous decisions construing the First Amendment's ban on any law that prohibits the free exercise of religion.

Three years before deciding the Santeria case, the Supreme Court had issued an important decision interpreting the Constitution's Free Exercise Clause. In *Employment Division v. Smith*,[14] the Court ruled that laws having the effect of restricting religious practices must be both neutral and generally applicable to be valid exercises of state authority. In *Smith*, the Court applied this requirement to uphold Oregon's refusal to exempt from its drug laws the use of peyote in Native American religious ceremonies.

In the Court's view, however, the Hialeah ordinances did not qualify as neutral and generally applicable. First, the Court found that the ordinances' text and their probable practical effect supported the contention that they were enacted to suppress religious conduct, instead of to address legitimate governmental interests. The city's failure to enact laws addressing the animal welfare concerns raised by other practices such as hunting, slaughter of animals for food, pest control, euthanasia of unwanted companion animals, fishing, and other accepted practices "devalues religious reasons for killing by judging them to be of lesser import than nonreligious reasons."[15] Thus, the ordinances constituted an improper singling out of religious activities for punishment, while permitting other activities posing equivalent threats to animals to continue.

Second, the Court found the ordinances impermissibly overbroad, in that they restricted more religious conduct than was necessary to protect legitimate government interests. For example, if the city wanted to address animal welfare issues, it could create and enforce regulations governing how animals are cared for, treated, and killed within city limits, rather than impose a ban on ritual sacrifice. Similarly, it could implement rules on disposal of organic waste to address its purported public-health concerns. In response to Hialeah's claim that the secrecy of the Santeria ceremonies made such regulation impossible, the Court saw no reason why enforcing more narrowly drawn regulations would be any harder than enforcing a ban on animal sacrifice.

Third, the Court found that Hialeah's ordinances were too narrow in scope in their impact on the city's ostensible animal welfare and public-health concerns. Again, if the city had a genuine interest in addressing these concerns, it could enact rules governing many secular activities, such as hunting. In addition, the Court found that records of the city council revealed that the object of the ordinances was to target ritual killing, based on city residents' hostility to the Santeria religion.

For the above reasons, the Court held that the Hialeah ordinances were not neutral and generally applicable. First Amendment doctrine holds that when laws burdening religious conduct fail the test of neutrality and general applicability, they may still be upheld as constitutional if they are necessary to advance a compelling state interest. But again, the Hialeah ordinances failed to meet the constitutional requirements. According to this test, laws needed to protect compelling state interests must be as narrowly drawn as possible to advance the relevant governmental interests. The Hialeah ordinances, however, were both overbroad in their effect on religious conduct and underinclusive in advancing the government's claimed interests, as noted above.

The Court also doubted the city's claim that its ordinances were based on compelling interests in protecting human health and animal welfare. "Where government restricts only conduct protected by the First Amendment and fails to enact feasible measures to restrict other conduct producing substantial harm or alleged harm of the same sort, the interest given in justification of the restriction is not compelling."[16] In sum, before restrictions on ritual sacrifice could be upheld, Hialeah would have to enact comprehensive and consistent laws addressed to all activities, both secular and religious, that threatened its claimed interests in advancing animal welfare and public health.

In a concurring opinion joined by Justice O'Connor, Justice Blackmun expressed his disagreement with the *Smith* rule permitting neutral and generally applicable laws that burden religious practice. He stated his preference for the alternative standard requiring the government to prove that any law burdening religious conduct is justified by a compelling state interest and is the least restrictive means available to advance that interest. Justice Blackmun agreed with Justice Kennedy's conclusions in the majority opinion that Hialeah's ordinances could not meet this standard, because they were "both overinclusive and underinclusive in relation to the state interests they purportedly serve."[17] But he noted that the case would present a more difficult question if members of the Church of the Babalu Aye were seeking to be exempted from the state's general anticruelty law. If government officials had prosecuted members of the church involved in animal sacrifice for violations of this law, and if the government could demonstrate that the anticruelty law "sincerely pursued the goal of protecting animals from cruel treatment,"[18] the Court might have reached a different result than it did in the actual case.

After the *Babalu Aye* opinion was released, news reports portrayed Hialeah's Santeria believers as "jubilant" and "plan[ning] to resume" animal sacrifices.[19] Although the Supreme Court's decision provoked concern among animal protection organizations,[20] lawyers affiliated with these groups emphasized the unusual characteristics of the *Babalu Aye* case, particularly the city's enactment of laws singling out ritual sacrifice for punishment. They echoed Justice Blackmun's assertion that the Court did not resolve the issue of whether religious motivation was sufficient to exempt from punishment those who engage in conduct harmful to animals that is otherwise punishable as a violation of general anticruelty laws. The Court's *Smith* decision, which upheld the constitutionality of applying state antidrug laws to persons using peyote in religious ceremonies, suggests that the justices might be unwilling to exempt from anticruelty laws religiously motivated animal harm.[21]

ANIMAL USE AND THE FIRST AMENDMENT

In today's world, people use animals for a variety of reasons. In the United States, activities such as hunting and fishing; exterminating rats, mice, and other "pest" animals; euthanizing unwanted companion animals; and slaughtering animals for meat, leather, and fur are widely accepted as legitimate, based on the human recreational, sanitary, aesthetic, and related secular preferences these activities satisfy.

In *Babalu Aye,* Santeria members claimed that a particular form of animal use was a crucial part of their religion. If the orishas are denied animal nourishment, they will be unable to help Santeria believers fulfill their individual, God-given destinies. As an analogy, imagine the impact if the government passed laws prohibiting Christians from participating in Holy Communion or baptism, or Jews from fasting on Yom Kippur. For Santeria adherents, the reasons for sacrifice are so vital that they, on balance, decisively justify the infliction of harm on animals.

Yet Hialeah residents opposing the church dismissed the distinctly religious justifications offered for animal sacrifice. At a Hialeah City Council meeting called to consider the church's building plans, speakers referred to Santeria as "'foolishness,' 'an abomination to the Lord,' and the worship of 'demons.'"[22] In the eyes of the majority population, many of whom regarded Santeria as a strange and frightening cult, church members' religious beliefs were illegitimate and insufficient to justify how the animals were treated.

Similar disagreement surrounded the question of whether animal sacrifice qualified as a "necessary" use of animals. According to the attorney general of Florida, religious animal sacrifice performed for reasons unrelated to food consumption was an unnecessary killing within the meaning of this law. On the other hand, the Santeria religion defines animal sacrifice as "absolutely necessary."[23] According to Pichardo, animal sacrifice is "an integral part of our faith. It is like our holy meal."[24]

An explicit values preference is expressed in the First Amendment's refusal to allow laws that interfere with the free exercise of religion. Although subsequent judicial interpretations have permitted some absolute restrictions on religious practices, such as drug use and polygamy, the courts have set strict limits on government attempts to punish or otherwise constrain religious conduct. According to constitutional law, religious freedom is so important that the state may restrict it only when necessary to protect other extremely important values, and even then may apply only the most minimal restrictions on religious conduct necessary to protect the other values.

In light of this values framework, it is easy to see why the Supreme Court struck down the Hialeah ordinances. Hialeah's failure to enact laws interfering with animal harm in other commonly accepted activities revealed the hypocrisy of its claim that the ordinances were designed to protect animal welfare. As the Court noted, the Hialeah City Council's "careful drafting ensured that, although Santeria sacrifice is prohibited, killings that are no more necessary or humane in almost all other circumstances are unpunished."[25] It was clear to the Court that hostility to the Santeria religion, as opposed to the city's claimed interests in animal welfare and public health, motivated Hialeah's actions. In addition to its relatively small number of adherents, Santeria is "mostly a religion of poor people, mostly black Cubans."[26] Because the First Amendment was written to address exactly this situation—a majority's use of its political power to target the religious freedom of an unpopular minority group—*Babalu Aye* turned out to be a simple case for the justices to resolve.[27]

ETHICAL ISSUES

Morally, however, the case is less simple. *Babalu Aye* raises a broad range of questions about how to evaluate the importance of various human interests in killing and otherwise burdening nonhuman animals.

Problems of Conflicting Rights

In essence, Hialeah officials claimed that animal sacrifice was unjustified and unnecessary because Santeria religious beliefs were not as important as many secular reasons for using animals. Hialeah officials may have been thinking that the risks to the community and the harms caused to animals jointly outweighed benefits to members of the Santeria faith. Even if this balancing were accurate, however, it would not decide questions about the *rights* of the members of this faith—or, for that matter questions about the rights of animals. The language of rights has long been used to assert claims that demand recognition, to secure legal protections, and to carve out a zone within which individuals are protected against interventions that benefit the majority but present risks to minorities. (See chapter 1, "Rights Theories.")

The Santeria case is notable for raising questions of both rights of religious freedom and animal rights in circumstances in which a more powerful group seems to deny the importance of those rights: the government appears to deny that the adherents of Santeria have strong rights of religious freedom; the adherents of Santeria seem to deny that animals have significant rights not to be harmed. Moreover, and perhaps paradoxically, Hialeah officials appear to have been appealing to the rights of animals (or at least obligations to animals) as a basis for overriding rights of religious freedom.

Yet neither the Hialeah City Council nor other Florida governmental bodies has erected a significant framework of rights for animals. In Florida, state policy permits and even protects many types of animal use engaged in for secular reasons; but little in the Florida framework of policies protects animals against the forms of treatment involved in Santeria practices. For example, it is a criminal offense in Florida to assist an animal in escaping from a hunter.[28] Children are given the opportunity to learn hunting skills in state-sponsored camps.[29] In his opinion in *Babalu Aye,* Justice Kennedy referred to the determination of a Florida court that using live rabbits to train racing greyhounds was not a violation of the state anticruelty law's prohibition on "unnecessary" killing.[30] In oral argument on the case, Justice O'Connor challenged Hialeah's attorney to explain the city's rationale for banning religious sacrifice while permitting the boiling of live lobsters for consumption in area restaurants.[31] The Supreme Court ruled that the rights framework that underlies the First Amendment did not permit Hialeah officials to deem Santeria religious beliefs a less worthwhile basis for animal use than the preferences underlying practices such as hunting, greyhound training, and eating fresh lobster.

The Standard of Human Benefits

The proper approach to evaluating human rights and obligations to animals becomes more complex when the ethical perspective is broadened. In a brief on the animal sacrifice case filed with the Supreme Court, the Humane Society of the United States and other animal protection organizations asserted, "The 'necessity' of animal killing has generally been determined by reference to tangible human needs such as food, the prevention and treatment of disease, and safety."[32] The brief noted that human survival is the most compelling justification for killing or otherwise harming animals.

But human survival is not at stake in the Santeria case; and even when human survival is at issue, how probable must it be that a certain action toward animals, such as pest extermination or laboratory animal research on disease, will remove the threat to human survival? Does a 10% chance of success justify animal use? Do nonlethal health threats to humans furnish adequate justification for imposing pain, distress, or death on animals? For example, what level of importance should be assigned to the human desire to continue safety-testing new cosmetics on animals to avoid the risk of eye damage? (See chapter 6.) What about interests other than human life and health? What significance ought to be assigned to recreational, pleasure, and aesthetic preferences?

Arguably, given a broad enough understanding of what constitutes a human *good,* almost any human need or desire can be viewed as being of *vital* importance to humans; this standard is already considerably below the standard of survival. Set against such broad understandings of human goods is the view that animals, too, have interests. If one admits that animals have interests, it seems necessary to find a way to balance human interests with the interests of nonhuman animals. This balancing might take a utilitarian or a nonutilitarian form (see chapter 1), but one seems committed to some scheme of balancing.

The Standard of Harm to Animals

In assessing whether animal use is justified or necessary, consideration should also be given to the level of harm imposed on the animal. Animals have interests in avoiding harm and enjoying benefits, interests that may be ranked in terms of importance. According to one commonly accepted ranking, the highest significance should be assigned to avoidance of extreme pain, deprivation, and distress, with interests in receiving species-appropriate living conditions, avoiding premature death, and other interests placed at lower points on the scale. Those who favor a balancing approach to the justification issue argue that a very compelling justification is required for using animals in procedures and activities that pose a deep threat to animal interests.[33] Some who do not favor a balancing approach believe that a threshold or upper limit of pain, suffering, anxiety, fear, and distress should be a stable part of society's network of protections for animals. (See chapter 1, pp. 32–33.)

In its *Babalu Aye* opinion, the Supreme Court relied on the belief that a variety of secular and religious practices subject animals to harm similar to the harm they experience from the Santeria sacrifice procedure. The Court noted that a similar method of killing adopted for Kosher slaughter, for example, is explicitly permitted by state and federal law.[34] It is not clear whether the Court would have responded differently to a religious practice involving an extraordinary level of harm to animals, such as subjecting conscious animals to a lengthy period of extreme pain. Most state and federal laws are unclear on the matter, and very few ethical perspectives on animals (other than those that would prohibit such practices altogether) have presented a clear answer to such questions.

One probable response by the Court is suggested in its remark that, "[i]f the city has a real concern that [Santeria sacrifice] methods are less humane, . . . the subject of the regulation should be the method of slaughter itself, not a religious classification that is said to bear some general relation to it."[35] The Court implicitly acknowledges the legitimacy of official efforts to minimize pain and distress among animals used to advance various human interests, but requires only that such efforts be consistently applied and narrowly targeted when they affect religious activities. The Court does not require that there be a limit or threshold and does not consider the underlying problems of how to handle extraordinary levels of harm to animals and whether human benefits can justify them.

Setting Policies on Animal Use

Traditionally, the rules governing animal care and use have reflected a social consensus regarding which human interests are important enough to justify imposing death and other harms on animals. Over the years, government officials have made some effort to forbid certain kinds of animal use, such as dog and cock fighting, presumably based on the judgment that the enjoyment of the human participants and observers is an insufficient reason to justify the harm such activities cause to animals. Overall, however, regulatory efforts have sought to minimize the pain, distress, and other burdens imposed as part of animal use, rather than to forbid certain forms of animal use or to set thresholds.[36]

As the Supreme Court pointed out in *Babalu Aye,* the current legal consensus seems to be that nearly any human interest can in principle qualify as an acceptable justification for animal use, although there may be legal requirements for humane treatment of the animals used to advance those interests. Whether there is a moral consensus in society to this effect is more doubtful. It also remains to be seen whether animal protection is of sufficient social importance for the citizenry to accept constraints on many now commonly accepted recreational and other pursuits, so that the more consistent policies on animal use demanded by the Supreme Court may be devised.

NOTES

1. Except as otherwise noted, the facts in this case study are taken from the US District Court and US Supreme Court opinions in *Church of the Lukumi Babalu Aye v. City of Hialeah,* 723 F. Supp. 1467 (S.D. Fla. 1989), *rev'd,* 113 S. Ct. 2217 (1993).

2. General descriptions of the Santeria religion and its history can be found in George Brandon, *Santeria from Africa to the New World* (Bloomington: Indiana University Press, 1993); Migene Gonzalez-Wippler, *Santeria: The Religion—A Legacy of Faith, Rites, and Magic* (New York: Harmony, 1989).

3. Gary L. Francione and Anna E. Charlton, "Supreme Court *Did Not* Okay Animal Sacrifice," *Animal People,* July/August 1993, p. 6.

4. Joseph M. Murphy, "Santeria," in *The Encyclopedia of Religion,* ed. Mircea Eliade (New York: Macmillan Publishing Company, 1987), vol. 13 p. 67.

5. Ibid., p. 66.

6. 723 F. Supp. at 1473.

7. Ibid., at 1472.

8. 113 S. Ct. at 2234–35. The text of the Hialeah resolutions and ordinances can be found at 113 S. Ct. 2234–38.

9. Fla. Stat. sec. 828.12 (West Supp. 1994).

10. 113 S. Ct. at 2237.

11. Ibid. at 2223. This opinion and the ordinances' definition of animal sacrifice were intended to exempt from punishment persons performing kosher slaughter, which officials claimed has food consumption as its primary purpose.

12. 723 F. Supp. at 1487 n. 59.

13. 936 F.2d 586 (1991).

14. 494 US 872 (1990).

15. 113 S. Ct. at 2229.

16. Ibid. at 2234.

17. Ibid. at 2251.

18. Ibid.

19. Larry Rohter, "Santeria Faithful Hail Court Ruling," *New York Times,* 13 June 1993, p. A16.

20. Roger A. Kindler, "A Legal Defeat for Animals," *HSUS News,* Fall 1993, pp. 10–11.

21. Francione and Charlton, "Supreme Court *Did Not* Okay Animal Sacrifice," p. 6.

22. 113 S. Ct. at 2231.

23. Douglas Laycock, "Free Exercise and the Religious Freedom Restoration Act," *Fordham Law Review* 62 (February 1994): 890.

24. Linda H. Greenhouse, "Court, Citing Religious Freedom, Voids a Ban on Animal Sacrifice," *New York Times,* 12 June 1993, p. A9.

25. 113 S. Ct. at 2228.

26. Laycock, "Free Exercise," p. 890.

27. Stephen L. Carter, "The Resurrection of Religious Freedom?" *Harvard Law Review* 107 (November 1993): 127–28.

28. Fla. Stat. Ann. sec. 372.705 (West Supp. 1994).

29. Laycock, "Free Exercise," p. 890.

30. 113 S. Ct. at 2229.

31. Henry M. Holzer, "The *Santeria* Case and the Cost of Contradiction," *International Society for Animal Rights Report,* Summer 1993, p. 2.

32. Brief for the Humane Society of the United States et al. at 51, *Church of the Lukumi Babalu Aye v. City of Hialeah,* 113 S. Ct. 2217 (1993) (No. 91–948).

33. Rebecca Dresser, "Standards for Animal Research: Justification and Assessment of Alternatives," *Journal of the American Veterinary Association* 200 (1 March 1992): 668.

34. In enacting the Humane Slaughter Act, Congress permitted as a humane method "slaughtering in accordance with the ritual requirements of the Jewish faith or any other religious faith that prescribes a method of slaughter whereby the animal suffers loss of consciousness caused by the simultaneous and instantaneous severance of the carotid arteries with a sharp instrument." 7 U.S.C. sec. 1902(b) (1988). Florida has a similar statute. Fla. Stat. Ann. sec. 828.22, 828.23(7)(b)(1976).

35. 113 S. Ct. at 2230.

36. Jerrold Tannenbaum, *Veterinary Ethics* (Baltimore: Williams and Wilkins, 1989), pp. 92–94.

Index

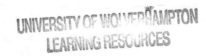